Health, Food and Social Inequality

T0298527

Health, Food and Social Inequality investigates how vast amounts of consumer data is used by the food industry to enable the social ranking of products, food outlets and consumers themselves, and how this influences food consumption patterns.

This book supplies a fresh social scientific perspective on the health consequences of poor diet. Shifting the focus from individual behaviour to the food supply and the way it is developed and marketed, it discusses what is known about the shaping of food behaviours by both social theory and psychology. Exploring how knowledge of social identities and health beliefs and behaviours are used by the food industry, *Health, Food and Social Inequality* outlines, for example, how commercial marketing firms supply food companies with information on where to locate snack and fast foods while also advising governments on where to site health services for those consuming such foods disproportionately. Giving a sociological underpinning to Nudge theory while simultaneously critiquing it in the context of diet and health, this book explores how social class is an often overlooked factor mediating both individual dietary practice and food marketing strategies.

This innovative volume provides a detailed critique of marketing and food industry practices and places class at the centre of diet and health. It is suitable for scholars in the social sciences, public health and marketing.

Carolyn Mahoney Following an extended career in public affairs, as a speechwriter and later as a newsroom journalist and editor, Carolyn Mahoney obtained her doctorate at the University of Sussex, UK. She is based in London and is a Visiting Researcher at the University of Brighton, UK.

Routledge Studies in the Sociology of Health and Illness

Health, Food and Social Inequality

Critical perspectives on the supply and marketing of food

Carolyn Mahoney

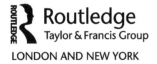

LONDON AND NEW YORK

First published 2015 by Routledge

2 Park Square, Milton Park, Abingdon, Oxfordshire OX14 4RN

52 Vanderbilt Avenue, New York, NY 10017

Routledge is an imprint of the Taylor & Francis Group, an informa business

First issued in paperback 2019

British Library Cataloguing in Publication Data
A catalogue record for this book is available from the British Library

Library of Congress Cataloging-in-Publication Data
Mahoney, Carolyn, author.
Health, food and social inequality : critical perspectives on the supply and marketing of food / written by Carolyn Mahoney.
p. ; cm. – (Routledge studies in the sociology of health and illness)
Includes bibliographical references.
I. Title. II. Series: Routledge studies in the sociology of health and illness.
[DNLM: 1. Food Industry–ethics–Great Britain. 2. Food Preferences–psychology–Great Britain. 3. Marketing–Great Britain. 4. Obesity–etiology–Great Britain. 5. Social Class–Great Britain. QT 235]
RA645.N87
363.8–dc23
2014034587

ISBN: 978-1-138-80129-5 (hbk)
ISBN: 978-0-367-34144-2 (pbk)

Typeset in Sabon
by Cenveo Publisher Services

Contents

Figures

Preface

As this book went to press in the summer of 2014, a new global study of obesity and health was published in *The Lancet* tracing its rise since 1980 (Ng *et al.* 2014). In the intervening period, no country has succeeded in reversing this growth, though the rate of increase has slowed in some developed countries in recent years. But as the authors of the study emphasise, overall rates do not reveal the continued rise of obesity and diet-related illness among some subgroups, including low socio-economic groups. Diet-related illness also affects many who are not obese; nor is a large body-weight a guarantee of ill health.

That is what this book focuses on – the relationship of diet and diet-related health to social status, and the supply side contribution to this relationship. While examining the case of the UK in particular, it encompasses many global aspects of obesity and pulls together evidence from many (mostly developed) countries. As sociological research, it discusses social status in the language of social class, and explores how class, food and health are related. It also examines studies from a broad range of disciplines which substantiate the food–health–class link, including the particular role of bodyweight in health.

Although food, health and class have to be discussed in terms of food *consumption* and dietary types, or what is sometimes called food behaviour, the focus of this book is on the activities and strategies of food *production*: the role the food industry and food marketing play in developing and targeting the food supply at population groups, and how this might reflect and influence social and health inequalities. The new global obesity study itself argued that more effective intervention was needed to tackle the major determinants of obesity, including not only diet and exercise, but also various dimensions of 'a problematic obesogenic environment', including 'the active promotion of food consumption by industry' (Ng *et al.* 2014: 15).

A series of international studies published in *The Lancet* the same week as the global obesity study focused on hypertension. An editorial reviewing the relationship of hypertension to diet and bodyweight concluded that interventions to prevent and treat hypertension in future should be developed in the context of the 'adoption of a healthy food environment'

(*The Lancet*, editorial, May 2014). Furthermore, 'stronger advocacy of this broader approach' was urged among doctors themselves.

This book discusses how and why our food environment has altered and the role it plays in influencing dietary 'choices'. If the food industry is accustomed to researching the power of human psychology in food consumption, and links between social status, neighbourhood and dietary practices, then these food industry understandings need to be studied by social scientists of health, healthcare practitioners, patients and policymakers.

While this is a sociological investigation, it also provides some solid background on the less familiar, supply side of the coin for public health and healthcare practitioners interested in this topic, and perhaps especially those dealing with diet-related illness in patients. Understanding how people are targeted with a particular range of foods in terms of where they live and their socio-economic background can give both practitioners and patients/consumers a deeper understanding of the persistence of dietary patterns and their health effects.

But to challenge an idea as apparently commonsensical as the one which posits that people get fat (and possibly ill) because they've eaten too much purely from greed or at least lack of self-control requires a detailed theoretical analysis. Not everyone will wish to read Chapters 2–4, in which a critical methodology and a range of social theories are investigated, but if they do, they will find that these ideas illuminate empirical reality – and vice versa – throughout. The theoretical investigation discusses the long tradition of the food–class relationship and theorises food production and the role of the food industry in influencing class-differentiated consumption and health. The following empirical chapters then pull theoretical insights through to give greater depth and contextualisation to the topic at hand.

This book also raises questions for public policy. What are the contradictions of the 'nudge' approach to policymaking where food is concerned? What are the implications of voluntary agreements with food producers? How can public health concerns be reconciled with the nature of an ever expanding food supply? What is public policy's role in regulating an increasingly hyperpalatable and omnipresent food supply? Underlying all these questions is the larger issue of diet-related health inequalities.

The food industry, with its roots in an increasingly industrialised, globalised agriculture, and then via the activities of food product development, food science and food marketing, develops the food supply and targets it carefully by population group. The extent and type of consumer research amassed by commercial marketing firms is paralleled by their increasing role in public health research, commissioned by governments. Is there something paradoxical in supplying food companies with information on where to locate foods high in fat, salt or sugar while simultaneously (and quite separately) advising governments on where to site health services for those consuming such foods disproportionately? Could commercial market research be indirectly contributing to a reinforcement of consumption patterns even while it predicts the need for increased healthcare resources to deal with the outcome? At the very least, these parallel activities should be discussed critically by social scientists of health and illness.

Marketing students, academics and practitioners will see frank exchanges regarding marketing education, goals and strategies alongside critiques from within both academic and applied marketing (Chapters 6, 7 and 8). These critiques raise ethical questions about the role and power of marketing, and especially food marketing – a lively and continuing debate in the field. There is also an account of collegial academic and food marketing research co-operation, which might serve as a useful model for future efforts to combine the vast potential of industry data with public health research.

Cumulatively, the texts analysed in this book illuminate the ways in which developments in psychology and consumer research, food chemistry, retail siting decisions, industry logistics and marketing campaigns come together to shape patterns of food consumption. But it is an evolving picture. The food supply is continually expanding into new areas of our daily lives: while writing this book in recent years, I observed new snack and soft drink machines being installed on train station platforms, university buildings and in community sports centres – all in places which did not previously have them. Digitally, too, as we navigate our towns and cities by day and night, we are constantly informed of the nearby location of restaurants or food outlets we have used before, perhaps alongside a discounted offer. These practices and their effects are difficult to trace and quantify but I make a small contribution in this book.

There is much more to the exceptional growth in large bodyweights and chronic illnesses related to diet than simply weak will, emerging some time after 1980. The food supply has changed dramatically, understanding of the psychology of food consumption has advanced, and the capacity of the industry to gather data and target eaters effectively, while normalising large portion sizes and bundling snack products together, has been immeasurably enhanced.

At the time of writing, a New York City ban on ultra-large sodas had just been overturned for a second time, by a second court. Yet the World Health Organisation had recently launched consultations on reductions in sugar intake (WHO 2014), and in the UK, lowered sugar intakes had just been recommended, alongside a suggestion that industry should reduce the sugar content of processed foods (SACN 2014; PHE 2014b). Consultations will take place in the coming months on these proposals. But unless the ever expanding supply and siting of such foods is addressed, alongside the ways in which they are target marketed, it is difficult to see much improvement in terms of overall food consumption patterns – or in the class-differentiated health effects inherent in the way we eat now.

Acknowledgements

I would like to thank the ESRC for funding my doctoral studentship at the University of Sussex, and the University of Brighton School of Applied Social Science for the award of Visiting Researcher to enable me to complete this book. Professor Gillian Bendelow provided continuing guidance and wisdom. Thanks also go to Professor John Abraham, the British Library and the Wellcome Library. Ben Branagan, Maciej Dakowicz, the Wellcome Trust, and the British Heart Foundation graciously supplied images used in this book. Melanie Jervis and Eric Davidson took additional photographs. I am very grateful to them all.

Every effort has been made to contact copyright holders for their permission to preprint selections in this book. The publishers would be grateful to hear from any copyright holder who is not here acknowledged and will undertake to rectify any errors or omissions in future editions of this book.

1 Introduction
The politics of food consumption and health

Setting the scene

While much concern continues to be expressed by healthcare professionals, researchers and governments about high levels of obesity and diet-related ill health in Britain, there is insufficient acknowledgement of the long established social gradient in both these public health issues by policymakers. Lower status people are more likely to experience poor diet, large body-weights, diet-related ill health, and a shorter life expectancy, even though all the way up the social gradient there is evidence of problematic patterns of food consumption.

Much research energy is devoted to asking why people eat the way they do and how they can be encouraged to change their food choices. Less attention has been focused on the role of the food industry – from agriculture to marketing – in shaping the food supply, processing it, developing an array of food products for consumer groups of varying social status, targeting these groups effectively and thereby influencing consumption and health. This book proposes that these forces shape class-differentiated patterns of food consumption and influence diet-related health over the long term, and traces how this process unfolds. Specifically, it examines both public and industry discourses which have constructed and reinforced an understanding of the health effects of food consumption as essentially behavioural issues; it then looks behind what is said publicly to what is acknowledged in texts written by and for industry members, and to a range of academic research which probes the contradictions of both industry practices and public narratives and policies regarding food and health. It asks the following questions:

- What are the discourses which both describe and shape food consumption and its health consequences?
- What health and social phenomena and questions of power and influence do these discourses conceal, whether intentionally or unintentionally? What contradictions do they contain?
- What is the role of both government rhetoric and actual public policy in sustaining these discourses and why might it be in governments' interest to do so?

- What is the food industry's role and interest in sustaining these discourses?
- What is the relationship between government and the food industry in developing approaches to improving dietary quality and health and what are the weaknesses of these approaches?
- How can social theory illuminate our understanding of food-related health trends in recent decades and links between social class and diet-related illness? More broadly, how has the sociological tension between agency and structure been negotiated on the subject of diet and health?
- How does the food industry understand the health effects of diet?
- How do food scientists, food product developers, food retailers and food marketers interact with notions of social class when developing and targeting food products and concepts? What techniques do they use for doing so?
- What can texts by food/marketing industry professionals reveal about industry's role in shaping diet?
- What is the evidence for a diet–class–health link according to epidemiology?
- To what degree does academic research influence the dominant discourses surrounding food consumption, social class and health? In particular, how have the insights of psychology been mobilised in developing and marketing food products?
- What is the larger agricultural, historical, ideological and economic/financial context within which food production and food marketing operate?
- What is the relationship between market research, food retailing, and public health?

My point of entry[1] to the research as a whole is the discourse of healthy eating and the assumption of personal responsibility for healthy diets, as long urged by governments through health policy and health promotion campaigns. For example, the government's obesity announcement of October 2011, calling on individuals to reduce their calorie intake, built on a longstanding yet ineffective strategy. As a press release phrased it, the Coalition government had 'called time on obesity' (Department of Health (DoH) 2011a). In an approach described as novel, people would be urged 'to be more honest with themselves about their eating and drinking habits' (ibid.). Britain was an increasingly overweight nation, and the then secretary of state for health Andrew Lansley concluded that 'reducing the number of calories we consume is essential. It can happen if we continue action to reduce calories in everyday foods and drinks, and if all of us who are overweight take simple steps to reduce our calorie intake' (ibid.). The chief medical officer added that 'as individuals we all need to take responsibility. This means thinking about what we eat and thinking about the number of calories in our diets to maintain a healthy weight' (ibid.).

The previous Labour government had shown an interest in revealing and addressing health inequalities with the Acheson Report in 1998, shortly after being elected to office. Six years later, it was still prepared to acknowledge the role of deprivation in food consumption and high bodyweights, though in veiled terms; the discourse of personal responsibility, perhaps with government-enabled support, is already evident. Its 2004 report, *Choosing Health*, notes that 'it is easier for some people to make healthy choices than others' (DoH 2004: 6). Yet people can be 'enabled to make healthier choices' even if they are coping with 'more immediate priorities' (ibid.: 13). Even so, making healthy choices is a matter of 'motivation, opportunity and support' (ibid.: 12). In a foreword to the report, the then prime minister Tony Blair speaks of 'the responsibility that we each take for our own health'; in that context, the government will 'work to provide more of the opportunities, support and information people want to enable them to choose health' (ibid.: 3).

All this seems quite remote from the realities of class-differentiated growth in bodyweights which are discussed later in this chapter; and somewhat arm's length from the findings and language of the 1998 Acheson Report, commissioned by the new Labour government to research structural, environmental 'determinants' of health inequalities and policies to redress them (Acheson cited in Exworthy *et al.* 2003: v). 'Our report', Acheson noted, 'was based on a socio-economic explanation of health inequalities' (ibid.). The subsequent Marmot Review of health inequalities was set up by the Labour government in 2008, and supported by two health secretaries (Marmot *et al.* 2010: 3, executive summary).

But arguably, neither of these research projects was able to bring about a decisive shift in the discourse away from the notion of personal responsibility for dietary health and bodyweight. If anything, this discourse has intensified since Britain's Coalition government was elected in 2010. Social class and health inequalities are not central to the discussion regarding obesity.

This is also reflected in food industry discourse. In its submission to the 2007 Foresight investigation into obesity, the food industry representative who prepared the document cites factors influencing eating habits: the trend to having children later in life; an ageing society; longer working hours; working mothers; families not eating together as much; less 'perceived' time for fitness and cooking; less physical activity and therefore 'calorie expenditure' (Paterson 2007: 4). Industry-proposed solutions to problematic diets encompass better information and education for consumers alongside product reformulation, with 'nanotechnology, biotechnology and neuroscience' at their core (ibid.: 3). The Foresight report itself recommends addressing health inequalities more broadly in future efforts to tackle obesity (Foresight 2007: 3). In Chapter 6 of this book, industry scientists express concern about the health implications of diets centred on processed foods, the tendency for low income people to eat these types of foods, and acknowledge the powerful role of family background in determining diet.

Where the health effects of food consumption are concerned, there is a tendency for research to focus on 'behaviour' – what people eat, why they eat the way they do, and how they can be influenced to improve their diets. This is natural enough and can yield valuable insights. But there needs to be a greater focus now on the food supply itself, its transformation in the latter half of the twentieth century, and the dietary and health inequalities which are a feature of problems associated with food consumption. In this book I argue that personal responsibility discourse is incapable of explaining embedded, class-related dietary patterns and their health consequences, and that this is due at least in part to a lack of attention to the distorted nature of the food supply and its promotional strategies. The notion of an inadequate degree of individual responsibility for consumption as the underlying cause of the spread of overweight and obesity – and related health risks – cannot explain why bodyweights have increased at the rate they have in recent decades, given that diet is linked to health status and social class as well as the nature and extent of the food supply, and the way in which it affects different sections of the population differently. A decontextualised focus on poor eating habits and campaigns which urge healthy eating do not allow any of these factors to be effectively addressed.

Healthy eating discourse cites the locus of responsibility for food consumption patterns in the individual choices a person makes when selecting and preparing food; this notion underlies both public health and industry pronouncements on dietary health. This book sets out to show what this discourse conceals. But there has long been much valuable, publicly funded research into food consumption and health. At the outset, a review of bodyweight and diet-related health trends in recent decades will help to anchor this exploration in the data.

Diet, health and social class: an empirical introduction

Many studies have demonstrated an association between socio-economic status, diet, and health; this literature is discussed in detail in Chapter 5. But since this introductory chapter begins my investigation of the origins and power of discourse surrounding food consumption and health, it is useful to set out the nature of the problem under investigation. Obesity is one manifestation of the problem, though not the only possible indicator of diet-related illness.

Figure 1.1 illustrates the growth of obesity since 1993, for women and for men. There has been a notable increase in obesity throughout the period, though the rate of increase looks less steep in latter years. However, the trend of extremely high bodyweights ('severe obesity') continued to increase throughout most of that period, rising more dramatically among women before dipping after 2010, while continuing to rise for men, as Figure 1.2 shows.

Obesity statistics also show a social class gradient, revealing a much more nuanced picture than for the adult population overall. Prevalence rates are

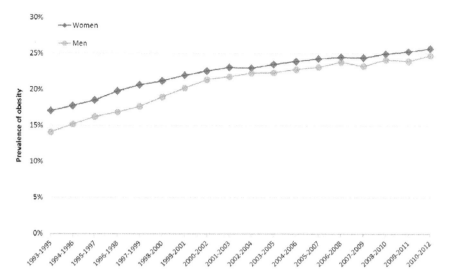

Figure 1.1 Trend in obesity prevalence among adults (Health Survey for England 1993–2012; three-year average). Data source: Health and Social Care Information Centre. Chart by Public Health England.

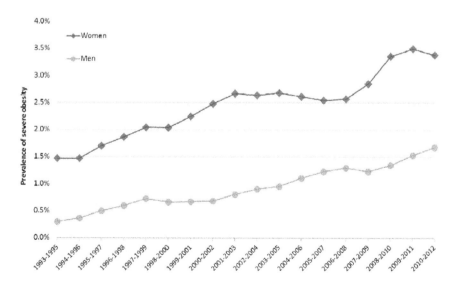

Figure 1.2 Trend in severe obesity prevalence among adults (Health Survey for England 1993–2012; three-year average). Data source: Health and Social Care Information Centre. Chart by Public Health England.

Men   **Women**

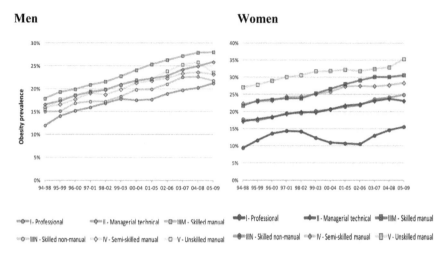

Figure 1.3 Trend in adult obesity prevalence by social class (Health Survey for England 1994–2009; five-year moving average). Data source: Health and Social Care Information Centre. Chart by Public Health England.

Note: This chart has not been updated because the social class of respondents was not noted in subsequent HSE 2010 data (Public Health England 2014a).

markedly higher among lower social classes, particularly for women, and have been steadily increasing. Among men, the gradient is somewhat less consistent (see Figure 1.3). One study speculates that male and female obesity patterns across occupational social class measures may not be comparable, since women often earn less than men; they may therefore experience much greater disadvantage (El-Sayed *et al.* 2012).

Statistics for obesity among children also tell a more nuanced, class-differentiated story, with those who are most deprived twice as likely to be obese as those who are least deprived (see Figure 1.4).

These graphic representations of patterns of obesity make the discourse of individual responsibility (or the lack thereof) appear one-dimensional as an explanation of food consumption and bodyweight patterns, particularly where children are concerned. Overall obesity statistics do not reveal the underlying disproportionate distribution of obesity by social class or differences in prevalence rates between different categories of obesity.

Studies have long shown that those on lower incomes spend a larger proportion of their incomes on food. The Food Standards Agency's Low Income Diet and Nutrition Survey (LIDNS), last done in 2007, and the government's Family Food Survey, carried out annually, also observe social gradients in the nutritional quality of diets (FSA 2007a; Defra 2012). The LIDNS survey found that low income earners tend to eat less wholemeal bread and vegetables and more fats and oils, meat dishes and processed meats, non-diet soft drinks, pizza, whole milk and table sugar (FSA 2007a: 17).

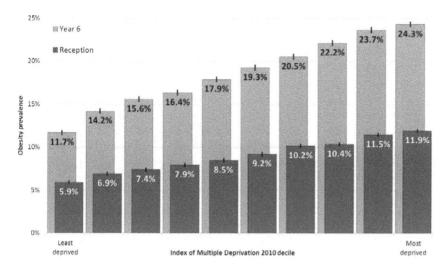

Figure 1.4 Obesity prevalence in children by deprivation decile (National Child Measurement Programme 2012/13). Data source: Health and Social Care Information Centre. Chart by Public Health England.

Note: Data for 2012/13 showed that overall child obesity rates were lower than the previous year for the first time; 'further years' data will be required to see if this is the start of a decline' (NCMP 2013: 11). The strong relationship between obesity and deprivation remained for both age groups measured (ibid.: 10). Overall obesity rates in year 6 were double those in reception year (18.9 per cent and 9.3 per cent respectively; the rates for combined overweight/obesity were 33.3 per cent in year 6 and 22.2 per cent in reception year) (ibid.: 9).

Food inequalities have intensified in the years since the economic crisis began in 2008. Overall, British households are spending more on food since 2007 while purchasing smaller amounts. For 4.2 per cent less food in 2011 (the latest year for which data is available), spending was 12 per cent higher than it was in 2007 (Defra 2012: 54), the year that food prices began to rise in real terms after a period of stability since 2001 (ibid.: 67). But, as with obesity statistics, a more nuanced picture emerges by tracing the patterns of different income groups. Those in the lowest income decile spent 17 per cent more on food between 2007 and 2011 (ibid.). They also purchased 29 per cent less fruit and 20 per cent fewer vegetables than in 2007 (ibid.: 51), a greater decline in fruit and vegetable purchases than for the population overall (4.4 per cent), following a peak in fruit and vegetable consumption in 2005 in the UK (ibid.: 56).

No income group eats sufficiently healthily according to the recommended 'eatwell' plate, but fruit and vegetable consumption showed the most marked difference by income (ibid.: 59). Defra's subsequent report found that all income groups exceeded recommended intakes of non-milk extrinsic sugars but that the lowest income group had by far the highest consumption; the highest two income groups had the lowest consumption (Defra 2013: 43). Once again fruit and vegetable purchases increased with income (ibid.: 44–5) and an income gradient was observed for fibre consumption (ibid.: 46; but no group consumed enough according to the recommended average). A 2014 study of the cost of living in the UK found that the cost of food had increased by 26 per cent since 2008, faster than prices overall, or indeed incomes or benefits payments (Davis *et al.* 2014).

Throughout this book, the role of social class will be central to the discussion, since it reveals much about how people experience financial pressures, health and food itself. The inequalities reflected in food consumption are not cited by governments when individual responsibility for diet and health is urged. Yet the class-differentiated nature of society is central to understanding both 'lifestyle' behaviours and the way the food industry designs and markets its products, as will be discussed in Chapters 6, 7 and 8.

A note on the data

In the Family Food Survey published in 2012, the authors acknowledged the limitations of the data. Food intake reporting is notoriously unreliable, and those who responded to the survey (54 per cent) sometimes supplied incomplete data (Defra 2012: 73). One solution, they propose, would be 'to obtain data from the KANTAR household panel which records household food purchases' (ibid.). Despite the views of some academics that commercial data is inappropriate for social or health research (see Chapter 7), market research data is being increasingly used by governments. It has the potential to provide more data, from more participants, faster, and with a higher degree of technology use by participants. For example, in one market research example, 30,000 panel participants are given handheld scanners so all in-home purchasing can be recorded; they are supervised and motivated to continue by research staff; and they are incentivised. Participants are categorised by marketing category (marketing's version of socio-economic status) and all products purchased are analysed by market research staff for their nutritional breakdown, including amounts of saturated and unsaturated fat (Interviewee B 2012). The sociologists Burrows, Savage and others have urged academics to try to get access to market research data (see Chapter 7); now Defra's public sector food consumption research seems to be reaching the same conclusion. In Chapters 7 and 8, there are examples of market research analysis of class-differentiated food consumption and health, and the use to which this data is put.

Inequality, diet, and health

Poorer diets and higher rates of obesity among those of lower social class are accompanied by disease/risk gradients which have arguably been somewhat obscured by the focus on the rapid growth in obesity itself.

In March 2013 in the UK, 'almost two-thirds of the burden of cardiovascular diseases [could] be attributed to the combination of all dietary components and physical inactivity', quite apart from body mass index, which is an additional factor (Murray *et al.* 2013: 21). People are living longer, but this can mean more years spent living with disability, which was the focus of the study. Dietary factors contributing to health risk included low consumption of fruit, vegetables, nuts, whole grains, seeds, fibre, seafood, omega 3 fatty acids and polyunsaturated fatty acids, diets high in sodium (an associated condition, high blood pressure, is one of the major risk factors identified for the UK), and high total cholesterol (ibid.: 19). This study did not investigate social class dimensions of these experiences, though it acknowledges the role of resulting health inequalities. However, the nutrition surveys cited in this section, and epidemiological studies discussed in Chapter 5, note the poorer quality diets characteristic of lower social groups. This is also acknowledged by food industry scientists in the texts cited in Chapter 6, and by some marketers and marketing researchers in subsequent chapters.

Levels of cardiovascular disease risk factors are differentiated according to socio-economic position. Diet, a key risk factor, is 'dependent on macrosocial forces'; in turn, one's socio-economic position is also affected by these macro forces (Harper *et al.* 2011: 40). Mortality rates from circulatory disease have fallen in the last 50 years, thanks to better prevention of stroke and heart attack, as well as more effective treatments and a decline in smoking (Weissberg 2011: 4). But as life expectancy has increased, the numbers of those suffering from circulatory illness has increased; and social class disparities in incidence have continued (Marmot *et al.* 2010: 153, full report). There has been no narrowing of the gap between the most deprived and least deprived groups (Scarborough *et al.* 2010: 16). In 2010, 1.5 million people had a heart attack in the UK; another 2 million had diagnoses of angina or heart failure (Weissberg 2011: 4). Between 1994 and 2006, cardiovascular disease increased from 7.1 per cent to 8.1 per cent for men and from 5.2 per cent to 5.6 per cent for women (Scarborough *et al.* 2010: 44).

Yet, in addition to existing social class and area (deprivation) differences in prevalence, the impact of obesity, with its class-differentiated patterning among children and young people, has not been fully expressed in disease statistics; this will take more time to emerge, as these younger cohorts age (Weissberg 2011: 4). Circulatory problems increase with age, and poor diet and/or overconsumption would need to be experienced over the long term before a circulatory condition became apparent.

Diabetes is another health problem associated with food consumption and bodyweight. By 2013, 3 million cases of diabetes had been diagnosed in the UK (Diabetes UK 2013), up from 800,000 in 1980 and 1.4 million in 1996 (Diabetes UK 2004). By 2025 an estimated 5 million people will have diabetes in the UK. The Health Survey for England first assessed diabetes prevalence in 1994. Since then, prevalence has increased from 2.9 per cent to 7 per cent of men and from 1.9 per cent to 4.9 per cent among women (HSE 2011: 11).

Diabetes, too, exhibits a class gradient. Those in the lowest socio-economic groups are 2.5 times more likely to develop Type 2 diabetes, and 3.5 times more likely to develop associated complications (such as heart disease, stroke and kidney disease) (Diabetes UK 2006: 5; the former figure is still cited in Diabetes UK 2012, with complications rates not cited). Diet-related factors contributing to the risk of diabetes for those from lower socio-economic groups include poor diet, higher cholesterol levels and higher salt consumption (Diabetes UK 2006: 8).

Health and the contribution of diet to health is a nuanced, class-differentiated picture, then. Establishing this at the outset strengthens the case for analysing the role of structural forces in shaping diet and health, and sets the scene for the focus of this book, which is to investigate a key structural force – the food industry – as it designs the food supply and engages with social class and health issues in marketing it.

This brief introduction to the literature on health inequalities precedes a fuller discussion of the evidence for a link between diet, health and social class in Chapter 5. The literature is primarily epidemiological in nature, but also spans some international political analysis linking higher obesity rates with more neoliberal regimes. The patterning that is observable in studies of social class, food intake and diet-related health can be traced to deeper political and economic trends and ideas. It is these larger forces which anchor and reinforce the personal responsibility discourse, in spite of the evidence which challenges it, revealing underlying social and health inequalities and the activities of the food industry (see Chapters 6–8). But how is this discourse associated with neoliberalism?

A neoliberal discourse

> Neoliberalism has ... become hegemonic as a mode of discourse and has pervasive effects on ways of thought and political-economic practices to the point where it has become incorporated into the commonsense way we interpret, live in, and understand the world. (Harvey 2007: 23)

In the neoliberal era described by Harvey, which began in the 1970s, there was an effort by major Western economies, and particularly the UK and the US, to 'liberate' the market, reducing government interventions aimed at altering the course and functioning of markets. In addition to the economic and regulatory policies carried out to achieve this, 'neoliberal philosophy has also generated ideas of self governance and citizenship that further help the neoliberal political-economic project' (Guthman 2011: 18). This perspective emerges in the work of Guthman, a geographer, and others who analyse food systems, beginning with agriculture, and builds on the ideas of

Harvey, whose writings have theorised neoliberal practices. These ideas link the liberalisation of markets with an accompanying strategy emphasising 'the liberty of consumer choice, not only with respect to particular products but also with respect to lifestyles, modes of expression, and a wide range of cultural practices' (Harvey 2005: 42). Neoliberalism, in social Darwinist tradition, values 'individual achievement, entrepreneurial prowess, and competitive spirit'; and as it applied to 'the care of the self, bodily practices that seem to indicate self-efficacy and self-control were readily associated with personal qualities that lead to both individual and collective success' (Guthman 2011: 53). Under neoliberalism, people are encouraged 'to make few demands on the state but rather to act through the market ... by exercising consumer choice ... and striving for self-actualization and fulfilment' (Rose 1999 cited in Guthman 2011: 18).

With these messages communicated, state intervention could recede as the individual became responsible for self-improvement, and answerable for his or her choices, including any risks taken (Dean 1999 cited in Guthman 2011: 54). Nevertheless, neoliberal discourse is somewhat paradoxical. Alongside the notion of self-reliance, neoliberalism also fosters a role for the state and, increasingly, multilateral institutions to intervene and set standards, creating markets and favourable market conditions even while the accompanying discourse champions the market as 'the most natural (and optimal) way to regulate social life' (Guthman 2009: 1115; McMichael 2000: 23). The state must also, of course, ensure that healthcare is provided.

Seen from this perspective, healthy eating/personal responsibility discourse, invoked by governments, the food industry, or even well meaning healthcare providers, health researchers and health promoters, is part and parcel of policy measures and economic strategies which have redesigned economies along neoliberal lines in recent decades. Thus an increasingly free market is portrayed as being populated by freely choosing individuals, who are then, logically, responsible for those choices. When things started to go wrong in population health terms, as bodyweights and the risk of chronic diseases increased alongside the accelerated production of foods high in fat, salt and sugar, the logical (neoliberal) solution was to point to individual choices and urge behaviour change.

But the discourse of individual dietary 'choice' – and therefore responsibility – is seriously challenged by the epidemiological picture which emerges linking diet, class and health; by social theory and psychology as they separately track how food behaviours are formed and become habit; by developments in agriculture, processing and logistics technologies that have transformed the food supply; by food industry scientists and product developers as they concede the role of early and lifelong habit formation in food consumption, and admit to concerns about health implications of diets based on snack and convenience foods; and by market research and marketing techniques which both track and target consumers according to their social rank and existing consumption patterns.

Healthy policy elites and healthy eating discourse

The emphasis in healthy eating discourse on the responsibility of individuals for choosing a healthy diet in a foodscape[2] which is both omnipresent and obesogenic has long been reflected in government policy (see DoH 2007 and 2004, both featuring 'choice' in their titles, along with talk of voluntary partnerships with industry, which the present government has continued to emphasise).

Even the work of the respected health research charity the King's Fund reflects the wider, taken-for-granted discourse and focus on 'unhealthy behaviours'. A King's Fund study speaks of 'helping people to kick bad habits', and its solution – 'the use of commercial marketing techniques to promote socially desirable outcomes' (Boyce *et al.* 2008: vii) – seems destined to merely shadow much more pervasive and well resourced commercial marketing campaigns to promote hyperpalatable foods and efforts to site them ever more conveniently for their targeted eaters. This key element underlying food consumption is explored in this book.

The King's Fund report acknowledges that poor diet and obesity are associated with social class and the latter also with gender (Boyce *et al.* 2008: 3). As far as the activities of the food industry are concerned, the report backs the plea made by government to the food industry and advertisers in a 2004 policy document 'to make healthy lifestyles an easier option for people' (DoH 2004 cited in Boyce *et al.* 2008: xi). The focus in the 2004 government document is on the role of the NHS in changing health behaviours, alongside an emphasis on the 'responsibilities of individuals in maintaining their own health' (ibid.). Yet the King's Fund report admits that 'a strong evidence base is lacking' on the effectiveness of such interventions; of those evaluations that had been done, few looked beyond the short term, and some were not considered robust (Boyce *et al.* 2008: 20). A subsequent King's Fund study reported that multiple unhealthy behaviours including poor diet were more prevalent (and increasing) among those on low incomes and with the least education. The study acknowledged the ineffectiveness of health promotion efforts which did not consider the role of social class in such behaviours (Buck and Frosini 2012).

Two years later, NICE guidelines acknowledged structural barriers to healthy diets and bodyweights: 'The environment in which people live may influence their ability to maintain a healthy weight ... Tailoring advice to address potential barriers (such as cost, personal tastes, availability, time, views of family and community members) is particularly important for people from black and minority ethnic groups, people in vulnerable groups (such as those on low incomes)' and others at risk of weight gain (NICE 2014: points 1.1.3 and 1.1.2). The guidance also highlighted a role for local food suppliers to promote healthy foods and drinks (NICE 2014: point 1.1.3.7).

Nevertheless, healthy eating/personal responsibility discourse has performed the co-ordinating function typical of discourse 'by providing the frame within which policies can be elaborated and justified by the key policy elites involved in the construction of the policy programme' (Schmidt 2000: 286). These elites then influence the 'fleshing out [of] the policy programme ... even ... promoting a particular discourse and policy programme' (ibid.). So the focus is on supporting people to change their behaviour (possibly helpful in individual cases, but not in itself thus far able to change population health trends), and calls to food producers to consider how the food supply might become healthier (the effectiveness of this approach remains to be seen).

The NHS medical advisory group the Future Forum focused on lifestyles in a 2012 report, advising medical professionals to 'make every contact count' to emphasise healthy choices, 'whatever their specialty or the purpose of the contact' (NHS 2012: 17). Thus pharmacists might raise 'lifestyle' matters (diet, fitness, smoking, alcohol) even with customers picking up prescriptions for unrelated conditions. The *Guardian*'s health correspondent accompanies the news report on this policy with a commentary on 'the brutal truth that more people are harming and killing themselves with their lifestyles' (*Guardian* 30/12/11), as though there were a conscious death wish at work. The Patients' Association acknowledged the need for health advice but questioned the appropriateness of all contacts being diverted to discussions of lifestyles; they called on government to examine underlying factors including poverty (ibid.).

A 2004 House of Commons Health Committee report did take account of the influence of structural factors in rising obesity, citing the obesogenic environment; 'the promotional efforts of the food industry' which drowned out health promotion messages; inadequate food labelling; and pricing strategies which made unhealthy foods so attractive (Health Committee 2004: 3). They also located some of the problems in agricultural policy, which they recommend should be shaped around public health needs (ibid.: 4). The committee was sceptical of food industry responses to criticism of their products, particularly the frequent statement that

> 'there are no such things as unhealthy foods, only unhealthy diets', a phrase we have also, perhaps surprisingly, heard from sports officials and Government ministers. But it is patently apparent that certain foods are hugely calorific in relation to their weight and/or their nutritional value compared to others. (Health Committee 2004: 25)

It is also true that unhealthy foods[3] are often marketed in combination, for example as meal deals, or in discounted offers, and consumed disproportionately by some groups.

The Health Committee's analysis, specifically mentioning industry influence on obesity, is unusual (and its influence on public policy seems limited), though more characteristic of committees of both houses of parliament. By contrast, Miller and colleagues trace the greater, if mostly invisible power and influence of corporate actors via lobbying and public relations, including that of think tanks, trade associations and front groups which may appear independent, but are not (Miller and Harkins 2010: 568; Miller and Mooney 2010: 468). Another factor is that corporations seeking 'policy capture' may one day offer board memberships for those leaving public service, a path many public servants, elected and unelected, have followed (ibid.).

Supply side: the role of the food industry in shaping diet

The food industry and food marketers have been continually refining techniques for tracking consumption patterns and matters of taste, social background and neighbourhood, often in interactive ways, in order to develop and target their food products efficiently at segments of consumers who will grasp, intuitively, that a given range of food products is for people like them. Examples of this are given in Chapters 6–8. Healthy eating discourse has never fully taken account of this powerfully structuring influence on our food intake, though many social scientists point to marketing and advertising as key factors to consider when trying to understand dietary patterns and increasing bodyweights (for example, Nestle 2002; Lang and Rayner 2005; Hawkes 2006, 2007). Several academic marketing scholars and some food scientists have analysed the contribution of low nutrient foods to obesity, and the role marketing might play in this phenomenon. Their insights are discussed in Chapter 6.

Some consumer groups, social scientists and health bodies have urged stronger regulation of the food industry and food marketing. A 2014 report by Consumers International and the World Obesity Federation made a range of recommendations, including improving public awareness and support for good eating habits, but also calling for controls on food advertising and promotion, improvements in the nutritional quality of foods, and nutritional standards for schools and other public sector institutions (CI 2014). The report also urged the use of retail licensing measures and other economic tools such as taxes, levies and subsidies in support of healthy food consumption (ibid.: 18).

What about the role of the vast amount of academic and other public sector research into diet-related health? The previous secretary of state for health, Andrew Lansley, said he was influenced by academic research, referring to 'nudge' theory and the work of Christakis on obesity and social networks (see Chapter 5). The evidence-based social science and epidemiological studies linking diet, health and class and even the health effects of free market policies (also discussed in Chapter 5), have not been popularised as has the social network research, yet it reveals a more nuanced picture.

The food industry's defence in the face of criticism regarding its production of unhealthy foods rests on its patent inability to *force* people to buy their products and consume them to the exclusion of more healthy foods. In any case, as Kraft's vice-president, marketing put it, 'There is no such thing as unhealthy foods, just unhealthy diets' (*Marketing Magazine* 10/08/11), recalling the Health Committee's citing of this industry argument several years earlier. It is true that no one food producer or retailer is responsible for the overall pattern of someone's diet or the quantities of specific types of food consumed. However, food consumption is closely monitored by the food industry and the expertise developed by market research is very clear on the social patterning of diets. Insights gleaned from this research inform industry decisions on where to site food outlets or products, who to market it to, and how (including the language and style of promotions). People who consume a certain type of food will probably consume a range of similar foods. Marketing firms openly discuss this type of dietary profiling on publicly accessible websites, including frank discussions of 'unhealthy diets' and their social and neighbourhood characteristics. One outcome of industry understanding of the social patterning of diets is bundling – the widespread practice of offering several food products together in 'meal deals', such as sandwiches, fizzy drinks and crisps.

But governments in the two decades since obesity has become a growing public health concern have largely backed the individual choice/responsibility discourse. 'The healthy choices are the easy ones,' as a Heartbeat Wales health promotion campaign once phrased it (cited by Bury 1997). We are all responsible for our diets and, by implication, the health effects that can be linked to our diets.

In a further example, the then minister for public health stressed in a 2010 speech the importance of individual responsibility for healthy choices. Regarding salt consumption, she said, 'Government can only reach so far. We can't step into people's homes and stop them reaching for the cruet' (Milton 2010). In fact, most salt consumed is in processed foods, not added in the home (SACN 2003: ii).

In any case, the discussion of food industry strategies in Chapters 6–8 shows that target consumers are already embedded in foodscapes based on where they live and work, and what they have come to expect people like themselves will eat. This involves an intuitive, not entirely conscious approach to food consumption based on both their social background and the way in which they are marketed *to*; both of which limit and shape their 'choices'. This book substantiates this argument in detail.

A public–private partnership to promote health

We need to be honest with ourselves and recognise that we need to make some changes to control our weight ... Each of us is ultimately responsible for our health. (DoH 2011b: 3–4)

After the election of the Coalition government in 2010, it was not long before examples of individual responsibility discourse began to emerge in the context of diet and health, as in the report on obesity, quoted above. There was also a decision to build on the previous government's approach and look to the food industry to take over some degree of responsibility for offering and promoting healthy diets, indeed seeing it as a 'force for good': 'The food industry has unparalleled ability to influence our diet through the food it offers and the way it promotes and markets it. Yet up to now we have not made enough use of its reach as a force for good in nutrition' (DoH 2011b: 41).

In the Public Health Responsibility Deal (DoH 2011b), the government asked various organisations including food businesses to sign pledges addressing some of the public health issues associated with processed food; this was interpreted by critics as an offer which, if complied with, might pre-empt future regulation. It was just the latest illustration of a shift in the balance of governance responsibilities from the public to private sector: 'The advent of "partnership" governance, where public policy is not simply "influenced" but is actually co-created and delivered by the private sector, indicates the increasingly shaky grip of concepts of governance developed before neoliberalism' (Miller and Harkins 2010: 582).

The arrangement was also regarded with some scepticism by public health representatives in subsequent oral and written evidence to the House of Commons Health Committee because it set no measurable expectations or time limits for the food industry; nor did it say what it would do if the industry did not take sufficient action or how this might be judged (Health Committee 2011: 41). While aiming to avoid 'regulation or top-down lectures', the report noted that the government reserved the right to ascend the 'intervention ladder' if voluntary agreements failed to work (DoH 2011 cited in ibid.: 95). Commenting on the public–private sector co-operation inherent in the Responsibility Deal, the committee report concluded:

> Partnership with commercial organisations has a place in health improve-
> ment. However, those with a financial interest must not be allowed to
> set the agenda for health improvement. The Government cannot avoid
> its responsibility for constantly reassessing the effectiveness of its policy
> in delivering its public health objectives. (Health Committee 2011: 87)

A House of Lords Science and Technology committee report similarly found that 'obesity is a significant and urgent societal problem and the current Public Health Responsibility Deal pledge on obesity is not a proportionate response to the scale of the problem' and that the government 'should consider the ways in which businesses themselves influence the behaviour of the population in unhealthy ways' (House of Lords 2011: 57). This statement is one of few by political representatives (albeit unelected ones) suggesting that the influence food businesses have on consumers needs greater consideration. The mechanics of this influence are investigated in Chapters 6–8.

The contradiction in 'nudge' thinking

In a key shift in policy orientation, the new government came to power enamoured of 'nudge' theory, a fusion of behavioural economics and psychology which relies on tweaking behavioural cues in various decision-making processes and environments, and popularised by academics Thaler and Sunstein in their book *Nudge: Improving Decisions About Health, Wealth and Happiness* (2008). A 2008 newspaper editorial authored by the current chancellor promoted 'nudge' thinking (Osborne 2008), as did another co-authored with Thaler shortly before the Coalition government came to power (Osborne and Thaler 2010). David Cameron apparently suggested that his entire shadow cabinet read *Nudge* in the summer of 2009 (BBC 2011c). A behavioural insights team was set up within Cabinet Office soon after the election; apparently the only one in the world (BBC 2011b). A seemingly new approach to public policy was under way.

This unit is looking at a range of policy issues in which changing behaviour is thought to be key, including health/lifestyle behaviours such as food consumption and physical activity. The former head of Cabinet Office and the civil service, Gus O'Donnell, was enthusiastic about the potential for 'nudge' thinking in public policy, calling it simply 'applied common sense' (BBC 2011b). Thaler himself hints at a more ideological foundation for 'nudge' thinking, describing it as 'libertarian paternalism' (ibid.). In fact it occupies a curious middle ground, challenging the neoliberal parallel between market freedoms and individual responsibility via nudge's acceptance of problems of consciousness in some behaviours including problematic food consumption. In such cases, individuals cannot be fully responsible, and there is therefore a role for the state in seeking to influence individual behaviour in a subtle, even undetectable manner. This shadows existing industry expertise in 'nudging' consumers to purchase items targeted at them, and does not seek to force industry to alter the food supply in ways that might address public health problems more directly.

The unit's 2010 discussion paper cites healthy eating 'nudges' such as shopping trolleys with a designated area for fruit and vegetables, perhaps featuring photographs or 'social norm' messages, or other visual prompts such as placement of healthy products on shelves where people are most likely to see them (Cabinet Office 2010: 24). There is also a partnership with an Icelandic TV programme called *Lazy Town*, which rewards children for eating healthily and being active (ibid.: 25). This seems well in line with Thaler and Sunstein's conviction that choice should not be forbidden. Thus 'putting the fruit at eye level counts as a nudge. Banning junk food does not' (Thaler and Sunstein 2009: 6). Choice should be designed so that the desirable option (from a public policy point of view – in this case, public health) is the most obvious. People may remain unaware of how 'choice architecture', as it is termed, has been rearranged for this purpose; 'in these circumstances, nudges can be understood to have influenced the non-deliberative aspect of a person's choices or actions' (House of Lords 2011: 12).

An investigation of the appropriateness of 'nudge' theory for guiding government policy was undertaken by the House of Lords Science and Technology Committee in 2011. While the minister for public health told the committee that 'nudge' initiatives *can* encompass regulation (House of Lords 2011: 12), the government's chief social scientist at the Department for the Environment, Food and Rural Affairs (Defra), reported that 'in her experience within central government, "behaviour change is very much used as a shorthand for alternatives to regulation and fiscal measures"' (ibid.: 11). This is in line with the government's goal of minimising intrusiveness (ibid.: 13).

'Nudge' theory is distinct from previous health promotion approaches and, indeed, previous assumptions of economics: it acknowledges that human beings are not fully rational beings making rational choices, but instead are creatures of habit, not fully conscious in all areas of decision-making; indeed, sometimes – in health behaviours – quite automatic and unthinking. There is an ideological character to the 'nudge' approach to public health, one which admits to human frailty and develops imaginative techniques to tap into our unthinking behaviour, but does not acknowledge the influence of structural and structuring factors emerging from the activities of consumer industries, socio-economic status or social capital. At the same time, the 'nudge' framework resists interference in market freedoms – indeed, it warns against doing so. It is a highly ideological policy framework.

The House of Lords report raises doubts about the ethics of 'nudging' as public policy, given its lack of transparency (House of Lords 2011: 13). As leading food policy academics Rayner and Lang wrote in defence of more traditional policy frameworks, 'at least nannies are overt' (Rayner and Lang 2011: 2). For nannies, read regulation (ibid.).

But outside the public policy context, 'nudging' is not new. It is, more or less, the basis on which the consumer economy and the 'consciousness industries' of marketing and advertising have long operated. Discussing the potential for 'nudging', which derives from behavioural economics (BE), as a marketing strategy, one marketer said, 'This label provides an academic underpinning for techniques and approaches that have been used for years' (*Marketing Magazine* 14/09/11a). BE or 'nudge' techniques are not transparent in the consumer world, either: 'retailers do not, for example, tell consumers that they have designed their stores in a way that is intended to encourage purchasing of specific types of product' (House of Lords 2011: 14). The food industry's expertise and success in marketing and siting snack and convenience foods in an ever expanding concept of public space may be a major obstacle to the success of public policy 'nudging'. Minimally resourced health-promoting 'nudges' are no match for lavishly resourced, highly technical, continually updated consumer research and marketing techniques.

As 'nudging' gathered pace in public policy, *Marketing Magazine* discussed how BE can be used by marketers. For example, digital marketing can best adopt BE 'because it applies to user experience and design' (*Marketing Magazine* 18/05/11a). A pizza chain was using BE to overhaul its marketing with a planning tool to help it understand how consumers decide what to purchase (*Marketing Magazine* 04/05/11). Another marketer describes using BE as 'going with the flow of human judgement ... people are poor witnesses to their own deeper motivations and are simply unaware of some of the factors that influence their decisions' (*Marketing Magazine* 27/07/11). One agency has adapted BE 'to create roadmaps for brands that enable them to identify a desired customer behaviour or attitude and plan a realistic way to bring this about' (*Marketing Magazine* 14/09/11a).

This expertise and the sheer weight and reach of commercial food marketing and advertising, the profusion of cheap agricultural commodities and the food products developed from them, and the pervasive and ever expanding nature of the processed foodscape in which we live will be a formidable challenge for healthy eating 'nudges' to counteract. Simply put by the House of Lords report, 'the ready availability of cheap and unhealthy food ... makes it more likely that people will consume it' (House of Lords 2011: 17).

Furthermore, the report notes the gap in evidence for the success of 'nudge' thinking in public policy; doubtless future evaluations of such initiatives will aim to measure their effect. Thaler cites growing evidence that 'nudging' works in areas of 'prompted choice', for example in organ donation questions on driver registration forms, and joining pension schemes (BBC 2011c). However, there are no countervailing structural forces here – merely individual unwillingness to consider these matters – which battle against decisions regarding organ donation or joining company pension schemes (though there may also be financial considerations in the latter case). With food consumption, the countervailing, structuring forces of targeted marketing, advertising and the blanket siting of foods are powerful cues – as is the class-differentiated, non-deliberative nature of food consumption, food-health awareness, and questions of purchasing power. All these matters are explored in this book.

'Nudge' theory operates on the basis that a lack of consciousness – a lack of common-sense thinking – can explain why 'undesirable' behaviours persist, even at some cost to the individuals concerned. Thus the two prongs of the government's healthy lifestyles thinking display incompatible notions of what makes people behave the way they do. Lansley, for example, accepted that 'psychosocial' influences and particularly 'low self-esteem' influenced health behaviours. While these factors cannot be dismissed (and there are countless studies on the psychology of problematic food consumption), they are only one area on which to focus investigation and intervention. Obesity cannot be attributed to a relatively sudden emergence of weak will in a growing number of people when obesity has only increased so dramatically amid the food oversupply and hyperpalatability so characteristic of recent decades; nor can we have had a sudden epidemic of low self-esteem and food overconsumption that is unrelated to these food production trends. Gard (2009) makes similar observations in Chapter 5.

But government rhetoric about individual responsibility for health behaviours does not register the important admission inherent in its adoption of 'nudge' thinking: namely that food choice is not fully conscious or rational. Instead, as an emerging consensus understands it, it is shaped by strong forces, both social and psychological, and has a highly automatic character.

All in all, the contradiction manifested in exhortations simply to eat more healthily, alongside 'nudge' thinking's acceptance that eating behaviours are often automatic, culturally and socially embedded and unthinking, demands exploration. In particular, neither 'nudge' theory nor healthy eating/lifestyles discourse acknowledges the role of social class in the formation of habits and behaviours where food is concerned. This book will redress that neglect, and show the weakness of approaches such as 'nudging' in the face of marketing strategies and distinct consumption patterns which the industry itself, alongside epidemiologists, has traced among different social groups. Government approaches to obesity do not acknowledge the blanketing of our digital and physical worlds with food marketing, nor the highly sophisticated techniques by which food manufacturers develop products that build on our unconscious tendencies to overconsume unhealthy but palatable products and to do so by, broadly speaking, social class; nor the way in which the food industry targets different consumer groups with food products of variable quality. The government may not always acknowledge the role of food budgeting in food consumption, but the food industry is acutely aware of its importance for people on low incomes. Much, though not all, food developed for and marketed at such groups is of low nutritional value. The overall result is a widely varying dietary quality among different social groups.

Response to the Coalition government's healthy eating initiatives

There has been some controversy over the Coalition government's approach to healthy eating. Many public health specialists, researchers and commentators feel that the food industry is incapable of addressing the grave risks posed by diets increasingly high in fat, salt and sugar (HFSS), though some progress in lowering these substances in some foods has already been made, and potential for further reformulations surely remains. This varies from country to country: there is evidence that even some established global brands contain widely differing amounts of salt in different countries (World Action on Salt and Health 2009). Kellogg's accounts for the difference in its salt levels in breakfast cereals by citing variations in tastes (*Guardian* 23/07/09). In any case it is clearly possible to adjust formulations of processed foods.

In Britain, it has taken ten years to get salt consumption down from 10g per day on average to 9g a day; 6g is the current goal, yet 2–3g per day are sufficient (and NICE 2011 recommends reducing the daily maximum salt intake to 3g by 2025). Diets that remain heavily reliant on processed foods will not be dramatically improved by marginally or selectively lowering fat, salt or sugar content, though the government did ask the food industry to remove 5 billion calories daily from British food products and 'to extend and intensify their efforts to help people make healthier choices' (DoH 2011b). While many snack and convenience foods will be reformulated, some will not be. As one marketer put it, 'If there's a market for the healthy stuff, brands will make it, but if people want unhealthy stuff, they will make that, too' (*Marketing Magazine* 26/10/11).

In addition, it is difficult to see how the removal of calories from an ever shifting food supply can be measured, given the constant changes and expansion of such products. There is also the matter of size; in announcing a maximum of 250 calories per chocolate product, it was unclear whether this would be achieved through product reformulation, smaller product sizes, or both (*Marketing Magazine* 15/02/12a).

The food industry publishes information regarding the growth in sales of its snack and other processed food products, a success achieved at least in part by ever more pervasive product siting. These processes are tracked in this book. The government does not acknowledge this dimension of a constantly expanding food supply, nor the difficulty of tracking food consumption outside the home.

It would not be in the industry's overall interest to encourage people to reduce their consumption of processed meals and snack foods or to eat whole foods themselves; food industry profit lies mostly in the processing of foods and the adding of value through pre-cooking, packaging, bundling and branding. Even attempts to lower fat have not been without problems; paradoxically, there is evidence that substitution of low fat foods (often high in sugar) has increased consumption, with resulting risks for weight gain. This is explored in Chapter 6.

Furthermore, while the Coalition government has suggested the food industry reduce calories, they do not address (and may not be aware of) other health concerns about processed food, such as those by food industry scientists regarding emulsifiers. Drawing on the work of Millstone (2009 and 2010), these are discussed in Chapter 6.

The government and its policies of imperceptible 'nudges' and voluntary action by firms do not address the relative power of the industry, its ability to influence us according to our social rank, or the growing pervasiveness of the foodscape. This latter point is evident from observations of shops and public spaces: snack foods and drinks machines have been installed in community fitness centres, a range of previously non-food shops, local train station waiting halls, train station platforms, and commuter station concourses and tunnels. It is a process that is difficult to quantify, either in terms of the growth in product availability or the ultimate effects on consumption and health, but it must surely be a factor to consider when government points to industry efforts to make the food supply healthier.

In this context, it is difficult to see how 'nudge' policies could succeed in changing population trends to consume large quantities of processed food, leading to weight gain and health risk – a pattern more prevalent in some social groups than others.

Summary: aims of this book

> Good access to the use to which market research puts the word life-style is not readily available to academics, and systematic scrutiny of the obtainable reports and journals to establish a well-substantiated analysis has, as far as is known, yet to be undertaken. (Murcott 2000: 122)

In a field that has seemingly been studied from every conceivable vantage point, there was one path of study that remained relatively unexplored: a sociological analysis of the language and techniques of food market research and food marketing, and the understanding by food product developers and food marketers of social ranking and segmentation (the industry does not speak of class). This is the central task of this book, and is in line with what Murcott, the British sociologist who led the first major ESRC research programme into food choice (Murcott 1998), argued for in the article cited above and again in 2011 (Murcott 2000, 2011). In the intervening period, research agendas in the sociology of food have tended to focus on consumption rather than production, of which marketing and market research is one (two-sided) important dimension. The focus on recent food trends, including healthy alternatives and food behaviours, has been in evidence at the BSA's Food Study Group conferences since they began in 2008. Murcott wonders whether this might be because sociologists researching food tend to have the concerns of 'thoughtful, well informed members of the public' regarding health and provenance. Their research interests emerged 'in the kitchen, the university common room, being ill now and then, as parents, of a left-leaning political persuasion' (Murcott 2011: point 3.5).

Thus there has been much sociological interest in farmers' markets, organic food, healthy eating and growing food at home, but 'noticeable by its absence is attention to the supply side' (Murcott 2011: point 3.6). This is also symptomatic of a longstanding and continuing split between the sociology of food and the sociology of agriculture (Murcott 2011: point 4.1). The former has traditionally focused on eating and culture, while the latter has been guided by agrarian political economy (Carolan 2012: 305). While it is beyond the scope of this book to fully unite these two bodies of research (Carolan himself does so in his 2012 book), I bring food production and consumption together and show how they interact and influence each other. Clearly both sociologies stand to benefit from extending their focus on agriculture/production or food/consumption, to take in its opposite.

Developing the sociology of food choice

Sociological explorations of food 'choice' have primarily focused on how food is consumed, often in small-scale, qualitative studies (as noted by Murcott). Some of these studies from recent years, linking food and social class, are referenced in Chapter 4, in the discussion of Bourdieu. But as long ago as 1986, sociologists Charles and Kerr traced the link between low social class, low income and dietary restrictions in a study of 200 families in the north of England (Charles and Kerr 1986).

An ESRC research programme in the 1990s resulted in the book *The Nation's Diet: The Social Science of Food Choice* (1998), edited by Murcott. Seven of the 18 chapters involved sociologists; ten projects studied food choices in the context of health/risk, the home, family and/or culture. Several of the *Nation's Diet* studies observed social class differences in consumption, and addressed the relationship between diet and health. There was also some interest in the food industry's role in constraining food choice. An economic geographer, Wrigley, researched how British retailers have shaped food choice; a researcher in consumer behaviour, Gofton, examined British market research data on food in studying food choice; Flynn *et al.* looked at the structuring role of food retailers in shaping food choices; and Fine *et al.*'s combined expertise in economics and food policy examined the propensity of different socio-economic groups to purchase given food types and investigated food processing and retailing (all in Murcott 1998). I cite more recent such research in Chapters 6–8, but note its early appearance in the ESRC collection (Murcott 1998).

Sociological contributions to *The Nation's Diet* and in the years since have variously researched how ethnicity, class, gender, age, peer group, family, marital status, schools, income, media influence and the (in) adequacy of benefit levels/low income have affected food choice. What this book adds is a clear description of the role of food production in its various permutations, from agriculture to food marketing, in shaping food 'choice', and along social class lines.

It is tempting to use quotation marks around the term 'choice', since the degree to which *conscious* choice is taking place is unclear where food consumption is concerned. There are structural limitations to choice imposed by the siting of the food supply itself, and by habitus, with the resulting poorer quality diet, particularly among those of lower social class. I investigate sociological theories and empirical research into food, but I emulate *The Nation's Diet* in seeking out the complementary perspectives of other social sciences. I also broaden the sociological critique of social class/low income and diet by examining the ways in which food is designed for and targeted at consumers by the food industry, based on their social status, and investigating the outcome for public health. Arguably no social science analysis of food consumption can be complete without recognising the activities and the power of the food industry.

While many social scientists acknowledge the role of food marketing in influencing diets, this is the first sociological research, as far as I am aware, to examine and critique in detail how marketers research and interact with society to understand and shape consumption, how they understand the consumption patterns of different social groups, and how the industry constructs new products and markets them to fit those distinctions – thereby contributing to social class differentiation in dietary and health terms.

In order to make this argument, it was essential to unpack the role of social class in food consumption, since this aspect so often escapes health promotion policy and discourse and because it is not overt in food industry discourse. I begin this task in Chapters 3 and 4 with a theory-testing analysis. Though few theorists address food consumption specifically, I trace the rise, fall and rise of social class in sociology and social theory, and examine several theorists for their insights into the nature of food production and consumption as it began to change dramatically during the late twentieth century.

Chapter 5 reviews the obesity critique and the health effects of food consumption, and discusses epidemiological understandings of associations between class, diet and health. Although my main research interest was in the influence of food marketing on diet, it was apparent that marketers work closely with food product developers, and food product developers must in turn engage with agricultural production and trends. All these forces are fed by global investment flows and technological advances in logistics and consumer research.

I argue that marketing is a crucial factor in extending the appeal and consumption of processed foods. The primary texts analysed for this book are concerned with market research and food marketing, but my analysis is set within this larger context, tracing the food industry's influence on the food supply from its origin in agriculture through to its health effects. This is the work of Chapters 6, 7 and 8. In these chapters I cite discussions of food products and dietary health by product developers and food scientists, plus strategies and approaches used by commercial marketers, in texts written by and for those working in the food industry – as well as research articles from academic marketing journals and books, which evaluate the nature, practice and effects of commercial marketing. The writings of industry practitioners and business/marketing academics are relevant and revealing sources for a critical analysis of the role and influence of marketing on patterns of food consumption. Critiques by academic marketers reveal a layer of commercial and ideological reality – and industry power – underneath the activities and discourse which characterise commercial marketing. Since these critiques come from within the discipline of marketing, albeit situated within the academy, they merit particular scrutiny, as they challenge the commercial marketing discourse of an altruistic focus on serving and involving the consumer in improving products and services. This 'insider' critique could also be mobilised to bolster 'outsider' monitoring and analysis of food industry activities.

A summary of research conclusions and ideas for future directions for research constitute Chapter 9. In the following chapter, I discuss the analytical framework which guided my research.

Notes

1 Fairclough writes of objects of research allowing for various 'points of entry' for social researchers; discourses can be useful points of entry (Fairclough 2010: 5).
2 The term 'foodscape' is used by Winson, a Canadian sociologist of agriculture and food. He defines this term as 'the multiplicity of sites where food is displayed for purchase and where it may also be consumed' (Winson 2004: 301). The notion of the ever spreading foodscape will be useful in analysing the activities of the food industry. It is discussed in detail in Chapter 4, 'Foodscape and lifeworld'.
3 As the food industry comment cited by the Health Committee shows, these are contested terms. A UK study by an expert group representing scientists, nutritionists, the food industry, consumer groups and policymakers, cited on the government's food.gov.uk website, consulted a range of terms in developing a nutrient profiling model and lists of healthy and unhealthy foods (Rayner *et al.* 2004 for the British Heart Foundation Health Promotion Research Group, Department of Public Health, University of Oxford). They wrote: 'Throughout this report the terminology of the brief for this project i.e. "foods high in fat, salt or sugar" and "healthier food choices" has been used. These terms are cumbersome and in future it might be simpler to use "healthy" and "unhealthy" foods or "healthier" and "less healthy" foods' (ibid.: 36). In this book I use both 'foods high in fat, salt or sugar' and 'unhealthy foods'. As future chapters clarify, it is such foods consumed regularly, in combination and disproportionately to healthy foods, that pose risks to health; and it is among lower status groups that this pattern and the attendant health risks are disproportionately observed.

2 Analytical framework and methodology
Critical realism and critical discourse analysis in food and health research

Introduction

Since I am arguing against a simplistic reliance on individual dietary choice to explain population trends in obesity and diet-related ill health, I was committed from the outset to a critical investigation of underlying explanations for the social gradients in both bodyweights and health and differing patterns of food consumption. The surface level explanation of obesity and/or poor health resulting from poor dietary choices ignores a complex relational context structuring both the production *and* consumption of food. So a critical sociology, and in particular critical realism, with insights from critical discourse analysis, all shape my analytical and methodological framework.

A critical sociology finds theoretical grounding in critical theory, broadly conceived, and critical realism in particular. For critical theorists it is essential to examine the knowledge 'which structures our perceptions of the world', and analyse the social process of knowledge 'to reveal underlying practices, their historical specificity and structural manifestations' (Harvey 1990: 3–4). Critical social scientists note the potential for scientific knowledge to be skewed by unacknowledged social, political and economic factors, and they therefore enquire 'how ideology or history conceals the processes which oppress and control people' (ibid.: 6). A critical approach has 'distance to (sic) the data … [while] embedding the data in the social' and aims to 'root out a particular kind of delusion' (Wodak 2007: 209). The notion of 'hidden forces' and the need to unmask them is central to critical theory (Delanty and Strydom 2003: 215) and it has particular relevance for the enquiries made by this book.

Critique, critical realism and positivism

Critical theory emerged as a response to positivist thinking focused on agency rather than structure, and aimed to examine concepts such as the 'systemic integration of modern societies in such mechanisms as the market' (Bohman 2003: 93). The very identification and formulation of problems to examine would result in different choices for critical social scientists and positivists, even though both are committed to discovering the truth about our world.

Of the dozens of research studies reviewed for this book from the fields of epidemiology, psychology and nutrition, most are empirical and might well be considered positivist. There is a clear dedication among these researchers to understanding the reasons for overeating or unhealthy eating, and to tracing the possible origins of dietary quality in the eventual emergence of cancers and metabolic and circulatory illness. Some of this research links disease levels and dietary types to social/structural factors such as social class in ways that critical researchers would find equally 'critical'.

However, there is, understandably enough, a tendency for much research into diet and health to focus on overeating as a behavioural matter, assessing phenomena and patterns of behaviour among individuals, or even groups or networks of actors, which can be observed and measured. As discussed in the previous chapter, a major strand of this research has been absorbed by 'nudge' theory, and the growing acceptance by economists, psychologists and policymakers of a high degree of habit and unconsciousness where diet is concerned. This converges with a long tradition of sociological, especially Bourdieuan, investigation of how habit shapes diet. But arguably this pan-disciplinary shift has *not* challenged the personal responsibility discourse where 'overeating' is concerned; paradoxically, government policy and rhetoric now backs both the personal responsibility and unconsciousness/'nudge' explanations for overweight and obesity. Yet the progress made in understanding problems of consciousness in food choice could and should lead to a critical investigation of structural factors which interact with actors' states of mind.

Hammersley has questioned what he found to be an increasingly meaningless use of the term 'critical'; in particular, the tendency among those who claim to be 'critical' social researchers to find that empirical research conceals ideological underpinnings which may render findings invalid (Hammersley 1995: 22). I do not find such underpinnings where epidemiological and other studies are concerned; though, as I have already discussed in Chapter 1, such ideological underpinnings arguably do underlie the notion that we are individually responsible even for the dramatic increase in the public health problem of large bodyweights and diet-related illness in recent decades.

It is only relatively recently that we have begun to see firm evidence of hitherto opaque but powerful corporate forces which influence public policy. The Leveson inquiry on relations between the press and political parties and governments has been instructive on this point. Recent years have also revealed the little understood power of Britain's financial sector to influence regulatory policy, contributing to the economic crisis beginning in 2008. Pollock (2005) has documented corporate influence on healthcare policy in the UK, with its interconnected policymaking and healthcare company elites. And since Hammersley wrote his views cited above, social and health inequalities have widened and deepened, as major transformations in diet have taken root around the world. There is much more evidence that social and dietary inequalities influence health and longevity; yet this is not the most salient dimension of public policy approaches to obesity and poor diet. Food policy seems either hesitant to challenge the food industry or ideologically aligned with it in a neoliberal conviction that less regulation is better. So there *is* a need for research which is critical; which seeks to reveal hidden realities; which looks beyond behaviour and queries the nature of the food supply itself, the multi-faceted industrial activities which produce it, and the way it is marketed – alongside public policy responses to date.

But how can a critical realist framework assist this sort of inquiry, and how is the research distinct from positivist research, then? Crossley describes one useful way of thinking about the difference in approaches to causation. While, broadly, for positivists, 'a' causes 'b', critical realists search for a mechanism or mechanisms linking 'a' and 'b' to explain more fully why 'a' brings about 'b' (Crossley 2005: 246). These mechanisms may be 'out of phase' with 'the course of actual events' (Bhaskar and Lawson 1998: 5). So, for example, overconsumption of food can bring about obesity, and potentially illness, over the long term, but this apparently closed sequence of events needs to be understood in the context of social and economic structures and processes, operating at rhythms or in cycles that may be 'out of phase' with the growth in bodyweights and the emergence of diet-related health problems. A critical realist framework can guide this kind of exploration.

Scambler, a medical sociologist, finds limitations in the paradigms which have long underpinned health investigations and influenced medical sociology, particularly positivism and its persistence as 'neo-positivisms', and postmodernism (Scambler 2002: 3). He also critiques the mid-level theorising of much medical sociology as inadequate for understanding health in its wider social, economic and political context (ibid.: 1–2). In sociology more widely he finds a persistent underestimation of structure (ibid.: 156) and calls for a critical sociology to examine the problems of late modern capitalism in a neoliberal era – including health problems, and in particular health inequalities. Williams (2003: 45–6) similarly finds the neo-positivist paradigm both dominant and restrictive in health research, with a decontextualised focus on the empirical world, relational explorations lost and accounts of power submerged in survey data.

One other problem is that in looking beyond conventional, surface-level explanations, researchers may focus on psychosocial pathways to ill health, as Wilkinson did in his research on health inequalities, and for which he has been critiqued (Scambler 2002: 97; Scambler also cites critiques of Wilkinson by Coburn 2000 and Scambler and Higgs 2001). The former secretary of state for health, Andrew Lansley, interpreted this notion to mean that people's self-esteem must be bolstered so that they are encouraged to make better choices for themselves (DoH 2011b). It is not clear how this could actually be done or what the role of the state would be in this endeavour. The psychological experience of low status and consumption may well have links to ill health, but research needs to go beyond this, drawing out the structural forces influencing health inequalities (Scambler 2002: 96–7).

Critical realists acknowledge that some dimensions of reality, including structural forces, might not be experienced knowingly; they might remain unperceived or even unperceivable. Furthermore, the capacity for perception may be more limited for some actors than others (Bhaskar 1997: 24). So health research which privileges lay narratives may miss 'the world beyond what people think and/or say about it' – Williams cites the lack of awareness of health inequalities even by those who experience them (ibid.: 47). Equally, Blaxter noted the pointlessness of asking health research partici-pants 'to place themselves in a class structure, especially when asking about an embodied life ... asked for general accounts of health, they are hardly likely to invoke the class structure' (Blaxter 2003: 79).

For Bourdieu it is similarly unreasonable to ask research participants to explain how their actions are structured, 'precisely because much of this is accomplished, via habitus and the logic of practice, unthinkingly and unknowingly' (Bourdieu cited in Williams 2003: 56). Scambler concludes that 'sociology cannot take people's own narratives at face value' (2007: 312) when seeking the effects of social structures on people's lives. Yet differing levels of 'health capital' among social groups can account for rates and experiences of depletion of such resources (ibid.: 80).

Just as individuals are unlikely to relate their health or diet to their social class, well intentioned healthy eating discourse does not usually discuss class, often focusing instead on the avoidability of many 'lifestyle'-related illnesses. For example, the National Diabetes Audit found that there were as many as 24,000 'avoidable' deaths among people with diabetes each year; avoidable, that is, had people made healthier lifestyle choices (NHS NDA 2011). While the terms 'avoidable' and 'lifestyle' reflect personal responsi-bility and choice discourses, this study did acknowledge that there were twice as many deaths among those from 'deprived backgrounds' as those from the 'least deprived backgrounds' (ibid.). Supposed lifestyle 'choices' have a strong correlation with social class, and serious questions about free-dom of choice can be raised, as they are in this book. Of the tendency to mask or dismiss class issues, Bourdieu makes the point that 'misrecognition of the reality of class relations is an integral part of those relations' (Bourdieu 1990: 136). Denial or unconsciousness of class is part of what allows it to be reproduced; in this way it is not sufficiently investigated for it to be effec-tively addressed. Chapters 3–5 examine sociological and epidemiological understandings of class and Chapter 8 analyses the language used by consumer marketing to denote and target people by social rank.

Levels of reality

Critical realism makes a useful distinction between the empirical, the actual and the real (Bhaskar 1989: 208; 1997: 41). The empirical is derived from observable experience, the actual from events and experiences which are not necessarily observed, and the real consists of 'generative mechanisms', which exist whether we are aware of them or not, along with events and experiences (Bhaskar 1997: 41). Generative mechanisms are inherent in structures, but may not be recognised in social life: 'some things do go on behind our backs and the effects of many that go on before our faces do not require us to face up to them ... not all is revealed to consciousness and sometimes that is because it is shaped outside our conscious awareness (Archer 1998: 199).

To illustrate this point in the context of food production and consumption, a person buys food and eats it (observable experience); those purchases and eating habits are shaped by social status and past experience, consumer research, product development and promotional activity by producers and retailers (real but not necessarily observable by consumers); the range of food options are laid out by the food industry based on changing transnational agricultural, processing, distribution, consumption and health trends (again, real, and potentially observable, but many people remain unaware of such phenomena – and the combination of their effects is observable only in overall consumption and health patterns or tendencies). These three domains of reality 'are not naturally or normally in phase. It is the social activity of science which makes them so' (ibid.: 42).

As Bhaskar, founder of critical realism, points out, studies of natural phenomena are often characterised by complexity. The empirical does not 'exhaust the real ... [and] positivists are wrong to expect the social sciences to find constant conjunctions in the human world, for they are scarce enough in the natural' (Bhaskar 1998: xv). Illustrating this point, a study by Cancer Research UK in December 2011 outlined evidence that multiple, overlapping lifestyle factors contribute to cancer (Parkin 2011a). While the relative contribution of each risk factor to the overall number of cancers in the UK could be quantified, it is of course more difficult to say in which proportion or at what rate these factors might combine to cause cancer in an individual patient (ibid.). Predicting the effect of proposed interventions is also an uncertain matter (ibid.). The conjunction of poor diet with ill health is not instantaneous; there is usually a substantial time lag between a given pattern of problematic eating and subsequent illness. In cases of diet contributing to cancer, Cancer UK estimates this to be about ten years (Parkin 2011b: S4).

When studying the effect of diet on health, although the weight of an individual, dietary type, the rate of weight gain, and metabolic tests can be assessed in attempts to trace the presence of illness related to diet, both the pathology and timing of any resulting disease is often uncertain. So is its relationship to changes in different dimensions of food production, including the nature and development of agricultural production and food processing. The very act of measuring weight and asking people to record their food intake can alter their consumption (and possibly weight) and in a societal context, an array of economic, agricultural/technological and cultural forces structure the food supply and influence consumption. Calculating the effect of food consumption on health is not an exact science in individual cases, but looking at populations, useful measurements can be made, and tendencies or probabilities established. The rise of obesity is measured by increases in population bodyweights, but we need to look beyond the consumption of food to explain this rise. Hence, in this book, the role of social class, the nature of choice and habitual behaviours, and industrial influences on human bodies via the food supply are all explored. Critical realism allows us to reclaim such 'vital lost dimensions and domains of reality' (Williams 2003: 51) and to analyse and assess their influence.

This can also be done in the context of marketing. For example, marketers are taught that when shoppers are interviewed by market researchers, they give only 'a partial, post-event rationalization for their actions ... we as shoppers are consciously aware of only a fraction of our actions' (Scammell-Katz 2012: 26, 29). Scammell-Katz advises marketers to observe what shoppers actually *do*, and when they are interviewed, to read between the lines to understand unspoken, unconscious motivations. The phenomenon of not perceiving 'reality' is key to nudge thinking and to food marketing, which relies on subtle cues to activate consumer behaviour. Research into these techniques and approaches should note the missing level of conscious perception of at least some dimensions of 'reality' – something openly acknowledged by food industry and marketing literature.

Tendencies and demi-regularities

Whereas political, food industry and even well intended public health approaches to diet and health emphasise the potential for individuals to improve their diets and associated health by making better choices, critical realism would observe that underlying structures with a role in causation are not being addressed. Yet these structures are a dimension of reality influencing human life, food consumption and health; 'social structures may be just as "coercive" as natural laws' (Bhaskar 1979: 446). So 'causal structures' (Bhaskar 1997: 41) must be investigated and an explanatory critique developed to illuminate a given social problem or phenomenon (Delanty and Strydom 2003: 377). Bhaskar derives his theorisation of causes and events from a transcendental analysis of science which understands causal laws as the expression of 'the tendencies of things, not conjunctions of events' (Bhaskar 1979: 444). One must search for 'the distinct structures that mesh together in the field of social life' (ibid.: 446).

In seeking to understand the patterning of phenomena in social life, and to build a critical realist framework for understanding the role of tendencies, Lawson has theorised the concept of partial or demi-regularities. A demi-regularity, or demi-reg, to use his shorthand, is 'a partial event regularity which prima facie indicates the occasional, but less than universal, actualization of a mechanism or tendency, over a definite region of time-space ... Where demi-regs are observed there is evidence of relatively enduring and identifiable tendencies in play' (Lawson 1997: 149). These partial regularities are highly significant in the context of a perpetually changing social world in which experimental closure is not possible, and are central to understandings of population diet and health. They can also claim to be scientific: both natural and social science must accept the concepts of tendencies, probabilities and uncertainties which, while not delivering full predictability, are nevertheless useful in advancing knowledge.

Partial regularities are observed in the largely epidemiological research discussed in Chapter 5 of this book. Much of this research, as with health research in general, might be considered positivist: after all, the cause of some ill health *is* associated with overconsumption of unhealthy foods and/or inadequate intake of nutritional foods. But some epidemiologists take this further and link the overall *quality* of food consumption with health outcomes, and further link the quality of *diets* with social class (typically referred to as socio-economic status in epidemiological studies).

In this kind of health research, we can only ever have tendencies (or probabilities). Obesity has increased dramatically with the production and increasing availability of snack and convenience foods, but many people are still of 'normal' weight. People of lower social classes are more likely than those of higher social classes to have an unhealthy diet, and larger bodyweights, but not in all cases; a significant proportion of people even in the highest social classes are overweight or obese; and while obesity is associated with a range of health problems, some people are healthy and fit even with large bodyweights (see Chapter 5).

Nevertheless, in what Lawson would term a contrastive social demi-reg, there is a *tendency* for people of higher social classes to eat a higher quality diet and have better health and lower levels of obesity than those of lower social classes. This is a persistent and enduring phenomenon. Scambler notes the consistent reporting of demi-regs like this in the socio-epidemiological research tradition, but he then urges a sociological interpretation 'on retroductive grounds for asserting the *reality* (in Bhaskar's sense) of relations of class and command' (2007: 309; author's emphasis). Otherwise, neoliberal rhetoric will simply emphasise the role of individual responsibility (Scambler 2007: 311), as indeed happens in the case of diet and health.

Thus, a critical realist approach to food consumption and health can look to the underlying structures of social class, how these are understood or ignored by governments, and how they are engaged with by the food industry – to the general ignorance of consumers themselves. We are often warned of the risks of overeating. But the growing spread of non-nutritious foods into a variety of social spaces, and the targeting of intensively tracked, class-differentiated consumer groups, neighbourhood by neighbourhood, goes largely unremarked in public policy and public health discourse on increasing bodyweights and associated health risks. Even further upstream in terms of causation, and equally unremarked, are the activities of a transnational agri-food industry in shaping our diets. An interdisciplinary group of social scientists has been challenging this omission in a global health context, noting that although agri-food systems are closely implicated in dietary shifts which have increased health risks, the 'agriculture and health sectors are largely disconnected in their priorities, policy and analysis, with neither side considering the complex inter-relation between agri-trade, patterns of food consumption, health and development' (Lock *et al.* 2010: 1699; also Hawkes 2008, 2009; Hawkes *et al.* 2010).

Retroduction in critical research

Retroduction is a critical realist concept in which a researcher moves from a concept in one category or dimension to another concept of a different order: for example, from health inequalities to class relations, which give a partial explanation for the initial phenomenon (Scambler 2007: 307). In critical sociology, a 'retroductive mode of inference' moves from 'a knowledge of events to a knowledge of mechanisms' (Scambler 2002: 10).

Both qualitative and quantitative research techniques are useful in studying food consumption and health, yet even a combination of these approaches seems incomplete without additional elements of both investigation and interpretation which are retroductive – neither exclusively qualitative nor quantitative, at least not as these approaches are traditionally understood. However, if the former can encompass 'qualitative investigations of the agencies and structures that produce [a given] behaviour' (Downward and Mearman 2007: 94) then much of my research and analysis has been qualitative. It is also true that many quantitative studies discussed in this book embraced imaginative interpretive linkages which might be thought of as more typical of qualitative (and indeed critical) research: for example, those studies investigating relationships between socio-economic status and diet; income inequality and obesity; agricultural policy, saturated fat intake and cardiovascular disease; and obesity prevalence and the degree of market freedom in different countries. Retroduction unites these variations on qualitative-quantitative research in pursuit of 'a nexus of mutually supportive explained propositions' (Downward and Mearman 2007: 92).

Thus the critique of obesity discourse by a group of sociologists is assessed by testing their claims through reviewing large-scale epidemiological studies. This includes epidemiological and social science research linking food and health, health and class, and food and class, to find patterns and connections which make the demi-regularities of Lawson's concept apparent. Then, in examining how food industry professionals approach questions of food, class and health, industry texts describe the processes of food product development, marketing, consumption, health and illness, revealing what various industry actors say about what they think and what they do, through their own literature and discourses. These texts sometimes contradict more public portrayals and perceptions of industry activities. I also discuss some insightful marketing research into the influence of processed food on obesity. Working through healthy eating and obesity discourses, investigations by epidemiology, food sociology, medical sociology, psychology, geography, food chemistry, economics, class theory and academic marketing, as well as market research techniques, product development, technological change, capital flows, and agriculture itself – it became possible to make multiple linkages in a retroductive manner, as suggested by critical realism.

Critical discourse analysis and food consumption

There is an important role for spotting and analysing discourse in the process of retroduction. Using the language and paradigm of critical realism, Fairclough, who pioneered critical discourse analysis (CDA), recommends a critical, relational analysis of discourse in the context of neoliberal economics, since 'the character of the economic system affects all aspects of social life' (Fairclough 2010: 1).

Fairclough finds critical realism a particularly fruitful philosophy of social science for the exercise of critical discourse analysis (Fairclough 2010: 361). Critical realism has provided the methodological basis for dozens of social science studies of health-related subjects in recent years, but the combination of critical realism and critical discourse analysis is unusual in health research. In this book I undertake a version of critical discourse analysis, identifying key discourses, phrases and terminologies and analysing their role in either indicating or obscuring some of the deeper generative mechanisms and ideologies which structure food consumption and its health effects.

CDA was developed by Fairclough partly as a response to Habermas's warnings that communication is easily distorted, and thus public debate can be harmed because clear information is not freely available. Both Habermas and Fairclough concern themselves (rather unusually for social theorists) with the capacity for advertising, marketing and promotional discourses to 'colonise' many domains of contemporary social life (Fairclough 1993: 139); this was a guiding insight for this book, one that is analysed in Chapter 4, with examples of this 'colonising' effect given in Chapters 6–8.

The problem, as Fairclough poses it, is this: 'Given that much of our discursive environment is characterized by more or less overt promotional intent, how can we be sure what's authentic?' (Fairclough 1993: 142). This creates challenges for consumers targeted by food industry promotions of a wide array of 'healthy foods', as outlined in Chapter 6, which may in fact be problematic for health, and which may obscure genuine public health advice on healthy eating.

There are limits to an analytical focus on language alone in social research; the relations of social life in a neoliberal era include both discursive and non-discursive elements (Fairclough 2010: 12). As Williams has observed, medical sociology has often focused too narrowly on more Foucauldian traditions of discourse analysis, leaving structures unexplored (Williams 2003: 50). By contrast, adopting a critical focus similar to that of critical realism, Fairclough has concepts of power and structure clearly in his sights.

He also urges researchers to work in a transdisciplinary manner, moving from discourse to other social processes and back again in a manner which recalls retroduction. This can lead us to delve into exactly the 'deeper ontological levels of enquiry' urged by Williams, who notes much discourse analysis which does *not* engage in such layered investigations (Williams 2003: 50). So, in terms of the topic at hand, it is clear that food marketing activities have a strong discursive element, but also that they emerge from a food production process embedded in developments in agriculture, international trade and investment, processing technologies, transport logistics and insights from transactional data, and additionally the need to make profits, which are all different orders of reality from discourse per se. Yet it is changes in all these domains which have shaped the activities of food product developers and food marketers as they design and promote new foods. In turn, all these important dimensions of *reality* are obscured by healthy eating/individual responsibility discourse.

For Fairclough, discourse is not so much defined as 'arrived at' through analysing sets of relations between discursive and non-discursive elements 'including objects in the physical world, persons, power relations and institutions, which are interconnected elements in social activity' (Fairclough 2010: 3). This recalls Bhaskar's observation that sociologists should focus not only on the behaviour of large groups but also on the relations between, for example, individuals/groups/structures/nature, and even the relations which emerge as the result of various other relations. We must aim to give social – relational – explanations of human behaviour (Bhaskar 1989: 209). Arguably it is only by considering the 'relational' dimensions of food consumption that the patterns which emerge can be fully understood. On this point, critical realism and critical discourse analysis are united.

Thus in this book a wide set of relations – between science, medicine, governments, media, the agri-food industry, individuals as consumers, shoppers, cooks, eaters and members of social classes, and the rhetorical forms which describe and pervade the relationship between food and bodies – are analysed. All are interconnected elements in the processes of food production and food consumption, and together they explain the problems which can emerge in the chain of events beginning with agriculture and ending with eating (and its health consequences).

Foucault: discourse and health

While CDA is the main approach to discourse adopted in this book, Foucault's influence on the role of discourse in social research and its importance (and limitations) for medical sociology cannot be ignored. Most relevantly for the topic at hand, Foucault developed the concept of biopower, in which the state has an interest in monitoring and controlling the movement and activities of human bodies – and a growing capacity to do so (Foucault 1972–77: 64). While this framework illuminated Foucault's writings on the history and discourses surrounding sexuality and mental illness, the failure of the promotion of healthy lifestyles arguably challenges his analysis. Foucault provides a model for what government has *tried* to do with health-promoting discourses, which have doubtless reached some social groups who *have* absorbed messages regarding risk and diet. But if the rise in obesity and diet-related ill health is anything to go by, bodies have *not* overall been rendered 'docile' (Foucault 1975) by health-promoting discourses.

On this point, Crossley (2004) queries sociology's preoccupation with body control. The individualised sense of discipline which is encouraged by state discourses (Foucault 1975: 182) has evidently *not* increased 'the forces of the body' in a healthy direction, at least in terms of bodyweight trends in recent decades. In this case, discourses of healthy eating and fitness have *not* been powerful in terms of reforming overeating and lack of exercise: 'the obesity trend suggests a rather different picture … [and] provides an excellent case study for thinking about the interaction of biological and social processes' (Crossley 2004: 222).

Rose and Miller refer to the '"will to govern" fuelled by the constant registration of "failure", the discrepancy between ambition and outcome, and the constant injunction to do better next time' (Rose and Miller [1992]2010: 288). It is difficult to think of a more apposite summary of government dietary health/bodyweight policies and the discourse surrounding them in recent decades.

Nevertheless, government approaches to obesity have arguably reinforced understandings of it as a matter of behaviour and individual choice, considerably restricting the terms of the discussion and blocking a comprehensive search for both causes and effective policy solutions. In this sense, Foucault's ideas hold some relevance for diet-health discourse, which closes off debate even as it fails to solve the problems associated with food consumption.

Ideology and discourse

This closing-off is achieved with the help of what Fairclough describes as 'ideological-discursive formations' – discourses containing 'ideological norms' (Fairclough 2010: 30). The subjects described or instructed by the discourse and even those who articulate it may not be aware of its ideological underpinnings. Ideology as it becomes embodied in discourse, then, is powerful. This is how ideologies are normalised, so that they seem to be not ideologies at all, but simply common sense. An example of this is the comment by the then head of the Cabinet Office and the civil service, Gus O'Donnell, that 'nudge' thinking as a framework for government policy was simply 'applied common sense' (see Chapter 1), when it is actually more complex and ideological than that. 'Nudge' strategies have been criticised for lacking an evidence base and resisting acknowledgement of structural inequalities or industry practices. They also contradict the government's accompanying discourse of individual responsibility, which assumes a level of consciousness and awareness which 'nudge' thinking denies we have. In focusing on individual behaviour and not structural factors, 'nudge'-inspired policies are ideological in nature, *not* merely common sense.

The suggestion that the problems of obesity and dietary health can be addressed by individual behaviour change diverts attention from underlying, perhaps more opaque but vital explanatory factors; this limits both the terms of the debate and the effectiveness of 'solutions' adopted either by individuals on diets or by governments funding health promotion activities. It may be that what this discourse really conceals is a conclusion by politicians and governments that the problems of food consumption and related ill health are simply unsolvable, at least by governments disinclined to intervene substantively in industry practices. If diet-related illness is an insurmountable problem, then politicians, by articulating the individual responsibility discourse, can at least 'dim the critical insights' that could turn this problem into a stronger challenge to government itself (paraphrasing Scambler 2002: 158).

Values and objectivity in critical research

Fairclough has warned that the loss of authenticity in our discursive environment and 'the colonisation of discourse by promotion may also have major pathological effects upon subjects, and major ethical implications' (2010: 100). The question of values should thus enter considerations of how to research promotional activity such as marketing.

Critical sociology, critical realism and critical discourse analysis are not value-free stances; each hypothesizes that something is wrong in the situation being studied and takes issue with it. The explanatory critique that results cannot then be value-neutral; but it can still be objective as it pursues its search for the deepest layer of explanation. The research process itself can reveal values held by the object of the critique; values which were not known by the researcher at the outset (Bhaskar and Collier 1998: 387). For example, while some social research has acknowledged the role of marketing in consumption-related health behaviours, there is also a lively debate among both applied and academic marketers regarding marketing ethics.

Critical research places a value on fair and reasoned public depictions of problems and debates about them. This is not possible when the problems are described by some actors in rhetorical terms which conceal (however unintentionally) underlying causes and prohibit deeper understandings. Terms such as 'lifestyle' and 'lifestyle choices' (and the need to make better ones) and even 'health behaviours' appear routinely not only in government pronouncements but also in mainstream, highly empirical, non-ideological health research. These terms imply free choice, mask what can be a limited set of options for people in given social groups and neighbourhoods, and may (unintentionally) divert attention from the growing evidence of the forces of social background and habit in food consumption. A critical sociology is able to observe in a non-partisan way that there is something wrong with a lack of acknowledgement of these factors. The values which are intrinsic to critique here are to do with a commitment to 'the public use of reason' (Scambler 2002: 154).

One of the problems for critical theory in general is that an 'illusion of objectivism' can conceal 'the connection of knowledge and interest' (Habermas [1965]2003: 239). In seeking where power and responsibility lie in the health effects of food consumption, it is important to examine how knowledge claims regarding the problem are communicated, the language that is used, the interests of different actors in framing issues in certain ways, and the ideology in which those interests are embedded, even if some actors are not aware of this. This is critical discourse analysis in practice.

Critique must aim to reveal how ideologies represent the world and the potential they have to distort understandings of it. For Fairclough the concept of normative critique is central to critical research: a critique 'grounded in values ... [assessing] what exists, what might exist and what should exist on the basis of a coherent set of values' (Fairclough 2010: 7). Such values might well be contested, and critical social research must be able to explain and justify the values which guide it.

Conclusion

In discourse analysis, the objective is not to outline all possible perspectives on a problem, but 'to examine how particular attitudes are shaped, reproduced and legitimized', to seek to expose contradictions within discourses, and to query 'taken-for-granted meanings' (Tonkiss 1998: 253, 259).

The contradictions of healthy eating discourse were the point of entry for this research, especially the notion that 'individual responsibility' (and the lack thereof) was either the problem underlying or the solution for population health concerns, emerging as they did alongside an industrially transformed and marketed food supply in recent decades. Chapter 5 challenges an emerging obesity critique among social scientists and presents a wide range of evidence linking diet with obesity, ill health, social class, regulatory regimes and even ideology. This evidence poses a strong challenge to the notion (and discourse) that a little more self-control is all that is needed to address problems arising from food consumption.

If discourse is also notable for what it conceals, then the systematic, highly technologised and pervasive market research activities which continually track and rank consumption habits, food products and consumers themselves, and the scope for marketing to shape and reinforce those habits, have remained largely absent from both individual and public policy understandings of dietary health. Chapters 6–8 analyse these activities, including marketing discourse regarding consumer choice and healthy eating, with its range of rhetorical proxies for social class. Both positive and negative views of marketing and assessments of its influence, intentions and its inner logic are presented. Many instructive market research studies into food consumption are cited, along with thoughtful marketing commentaries on these matters.

While critiquing the structuring effects of food industry activities and especially marketing, it was clear that the food supply is the logical result of constant advances in an array of technologies, alongside the need for the industry to grow and profit, and that the context of these activities is very much a global one, even when examining primarily British consumption patterns and health outcomes. The globalised food industry is itself a generative mechanism for food product development and food marketing, for patterns of food consumption and ultimately for diet-related health, so in Chapter 6 I also set out this larger agricultural/industrial context.

But in Chapters 3 and 4, which follow, I test a range of social theories on class, habitual behaviour, reflexivity, consciousness, consumerism, the economy and systems of governance for their insights into food production, consumption and health.

3 Applying social theory to food production, food consumption and social class

Introduction

Behavioural economics and its operationalisation as 'nudge' theory have made a strong case for force of habit and a lapse into routine, unthinking behaviour in many different contexts, including food consumption. Yet the discourse of personal responsibility for dietary choice persists and is mobilised as the way forward in dealing with diet-related health problems. It constitutes the rationale for both food industry and government resistance to more structural reform of the food supply. Moreover, much academic study is devoted to the study of eating behaviours, and while much of this research is insightful, this can reinforce the personal responsibility/individual choice discourse, however unintentionally, and leave structural factors insufficiently explored.

In seeking to dislodge the dominant and misleading individual responsibility discourse, which has driven policy (or the lack of it) since obesity rates began their accelerated increase in the late 1980s, I turn in this and the following chapter to social theory. Amid some internal debates and disagreements, sociology has produced a rich vein of argument and ideas which can strengthen the core of behavioural economics by giving it a social context – a social structure in which the forces of class and habit are observable as intertwined. This addresses a lacuna in 'nudge' approaches where food consumption is concerned.

But while social class has seen a rebirth in sociological analysis, other disciplines, along with political commentary and public debate, do not often acknowledge class as a formative, structuring force, nor query how class is perpetuated. Even within sociology, there continues to be much focus on how culture – excluding both class and economic forces – shapes social life. This risks giving an incomplete picture of what happens when changing consumption patterns begin to yield troubling population health consequences, as in the case of diet. If the food industry engages with social structure, social rank and psychology in developing and marketing food products, then social scientists need to explore these activities. As a critical realist framework suggests, structural forces, whether social (class) or agro-industrial (the nature of the food supply) or psychological (the emotional resonance and routine nature of foods embedded through family background, habit and marketing), are not observed or experienced consciously.

In Chapters 3 and 4, therefore, social theories are applied to the empirical worlds of food production, food marketing, food choice and health promotion, testing each theory for its capacity to illuminate how food is produced, consumed and how it influences health. In challenging healthy eating/ personal choice discourse, the theoretical arguments mobilised here reveal the weakness of assumptions that lifestyles, including diets, are consciously chosen or easily changed. In subsequent chapters, the disciplines of epidemiology, psychology and marketing will also call these assumptions and the resulting dominant discourse into question.

Developments in the sociology of class are debated by Scambler, Savage, Crompton, Skeggs and others. The central role of the 'cultural turn' in deflecting attention from class is key, along with its interaction with the sociology of consumption, drawing particularly on Crompton and Edwards. A persistent analysis of health in the context of capitalism remained in medical sociology, and this will be traced.

Since much use will be made of official national statistics in Chapter 5's discussion of studies of diet, health and class, and because they are incorporated into consumer marketing classifications, this book would not be complete without a discussion of how official national statistics classify social groups, and in particular, how the Registrar General's classification has been reformed in response to sociological critique (Crompton 2008b). Graham's analysis of health inequalities also discusses these innovations (Graham 2007).

In addition to the wealth of late twentieth century social theory, explored here and in Chapter 4 for its application to matters of food consumption and health, it is also illuminating to turn to the nineteenth century for an examination of Marx, not least because we will see his insights reproduced or contradicted by our modern theorists and even by the contemporary and highly empirical world of food itself. Marx's thought provides a clear view of the interlocking relationships between the forces of history, family, culture and economic change in structuring social life, including eating. It is a line of thinking which will be traced throughout this book, later illustrating how alert food marketers mobilise this understanding even today.

Marx, class and food

> Life involves before everything else eating and drinking. (Marx [1845]1997: 100)

Marx's theorising of social class was very much of its time, and notoriously incomplete; a section on classes in *Capital* is only two pages long and he never theorises the nature of social classes (Pierson 1997: 15). But his analysis of capitalism and history is grounded in a very empirical concept of human action and societal development which is still fruitful. For Marx, the development of human life and indeed history itself is not a matter of advancing, disembodied consciousness but 'a quite material empirically verifiable act, an act the proof of which every individual furnishes as he comes and goes, eats, drinks and clothes himself' ([1845]1997: 108). This wording strikingly reflects contemporary market research techniques which are now, in the digital age, able to track consumers in highly 'empirically verifiable' ways as they carry out exactly these kinds of actions in their residential and working neighbourhoods and 'foodscapes'.

It is natural that Marx's highly materialist view of history and human life would include references to food and health. He was conscious of the central role of food in human history, referring, for example, to the lack of key commodities contributing to the Napoleonic wars in the nineteenth century ([1845]1997: 107), and of the significance for human societies of the shift away from small-scale food production to industrial production and industrial work.

Marx was also acutely aware of the poor living conditions of industrial workers, their stunted bodies and shortened lives ([1867]1997: 235) in which inadequate diets had a major role to play (Burnett 1989; Steel 2009). 'Capital', he avowed, 'is reckless of the health or length of life of the labourer, unless under compulsion from society' (Marx [1867]1997: 235). His concern for the health of workers was not universally shared at the time; a common view of the poor health and circumstances of some sections of society was that these resulted from a failure of initiative and resolve. Popular ideas of human character in Marx's time included 'two sorts of people, one the diligent, intelligent, and above all frugal elite; the other, lazy rascals, spending their substance, and more, in riotous living' (ibid.: 236). The notion that the poor were responsible for their low status and any problems accompanying poverty, such as ill health, was evident in both the nineteenth and twentieth centuries (Burnett 1989; Pember Reeves 1913; Steinbach 2004) and arguably its residues can be traced in the discourse of individual responsibility regarding diet and health. Giddens refers to a middle class tendency to deny the importance of social class in people's lives, and to believe instead that individual initiative accounts for personal achievement (or lack thereof). This is a powerful discourse in British society and politics, one which some of Giddens's work would subsequently reinforce (Giddens 1982: 162, 166; 2007).

It has been pointedly displayed in some British television programmes on the subject of weight, in which lower status overweight people are taken to task for their nutrition-poor diets by higher status experts; Gillian McKeith's *You Are What You Eat* (Channel 4, 2004–07) was one early example. The Duchess of York appeared in a 2008 series (*The Duchess in Hull*, ITV) in a more sympathetic, less judgemental role, advising a low income family with multiple diet-related health problems how to make better food choices.

These are modern versions of the practice of higher social classes providing a supervisory role regarding the diet of the poor, as depicted in the nineteenth century illustration in Figure 3.1. It is a social practice with a long history in the UK. One historian cites the early nineteenth century example of the politician and journalist William Cobbett, who wrote a series of 'cottage economies and penny cookbooks aimed at stopping the working classes from squandering money in the pie shop' (Hughes 2014).

Even when it was well intentioned, such cross-class intervention could not resolve food inequalities in the nineteenth century, and cannot do so now. Televised interventions have, perhaps unintentionally, reinforced an image of ignorance, incompetence and fecklessness among those of lower social class who have a poor diet. This in turn bolsters the discourse of personal responsibility for dietary practices: if these people cannot

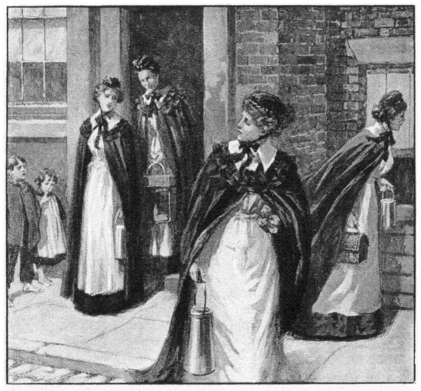

VOLUNTARY LADY ASSISTANTS TAKING OUT FOOD TO THE SICK POOR

Figure 3.1 An image of food and class in the nineteenth century. © Wellcome Images.

improve their diet even when coached by their 'betters', then they must surely bear the responsibility for their food consumption and diet-related illness.

Marx portrayed industrial workers as 'determined and regulated on all sides by the movement of the machinery, not the other way round' ([1857]1997: 199). In recent decades, a radically altered concept of health and safety at work and a much higher overall standard of living and health have transformed the picture – not least because of the ways in which capitalism *has* come under compulsion from society via health and safety standards. Yet there are parallels: workers in offices now find themselves at the opposite extreme of physicality – sedentariness – which carries its own health risks and alienation from the body. Their working days are shaped by the nature of the technology they use. The link between obesity, sedentary lives, including working lives, and health problems including musculoskeletal disorders is now widely acknowledged.

Food, drink and the nature of choice

On the question of the power of the individual to act, Marx famously insisted that 'Men make their own history, but they do not make it just as they please; they do not make it under circumstances chosen by themselves, but under circumstances directly encountered, given and transmitted from the past' (Marx [1852]1997: 156). In terms of the grand scale of historical change, he describes the inherited nature of the productive forces:

> In each stage [of history] there is found a material result: a sum of productive forces, an historically created relation of individuals to nature and to one another, which is handed down to each generation from its predecessor ... which ... is modified by the new generation but also prescribes for it its conditions of life and gives it a definite development, a special character. (Marx [1845]1997: 108)

So the freedom of the individual is circumscribed by these inherited 'circumstances', which can only be modified but not discarded altogether. Giddens, Bourdieu and Habermas all accept varying degrees of limitations placed on individual action, though ultimately Giddens emphasises the conscious reflexivity inherent in human life and choices. Marx describes a historical *process* which has a degree of reflexivity to it (though he did not use this term) as systems of various kinds (financial, agricultural, familial/cultural, technological) interact with one another. This process brings about change, but interacting systems over time do not offer to everyone the same opportunity to interact with what is new in each system or domain, and therefore to make fully free and informed choices. There are limitations on individual agency, since 'man is not free to choose his productive forces ... for every productive force is an acquired force, the product of previous activity'

(Marx [1846]1997: 121). The productive forces shaping agricultural development – the forces of science, technology, labour and capital, including agricultural subsidies – generate the basic commodities that constitute our diet, including, in recent decades, the crops (such as corn and soya) on which many snack and convenience foods high in fat, salt and sugar (HFSS) are based.

Marx's writings are primarily associated with production as the determining force of economic and social life, but he also acknowledged the role of agriculture in the development of capitalism: 'Agriculture comes to be more and more merely a branch of industry and is completely dominated by capital' (Marx [1857]1997: 190). The separation of human beings from their role as producers of their own food was an 'epoch-making' development; Marx describes 'the expropriation of the agricultural producer, of the peasant, from the soil, [as] the basis of the whole process' of class formation in capitalism and the history of capital itself (Marx [1867]1997: 239–40). It was certainly to alter the character of people's diets.

The need to eat and drink for survival is the basis of the first productive activities. Satisfaction of these very material, physical needs then 'leads to new needs' (Marx [1845]1997: 100). There is a way in which 'new needs' are engineered so as to increase consumption (and profits). Marx is explicit about this, talking about 'the production of new consumption ... [by] quantitative expansion of existing consumption ... creation of new needs by propagating existing ones in a wide circle ... [and] production of new needs and discovery and creation of new use-values' (Marx 1973 cited in Pietrykowski 2009: 89). This is a prescient description of a key strategy of consumer industries and their marketing arms.

Examining these 'new needs' in the context of food and drink – once basic needs have been met – we might consider the array of foods and techniques of food production and preparation throughout history, or, within the context and timespan of an individual human life, the gradual expansion of the types of foods consumed from infancy, throughout childhood and into adulthood. Both these processes take place in geographic, agricultural, technological and social contexts: no individual begins the process of food consumption anew and independently. A system is in place to grow, process, distribute and prepare food, and a constantly extended range of foods is presented to us. As Marx outlined above, something very different from a merely 'quantitative increase in consumption of extant goods' is taking place (Pietrykowski 2009: 89).

As infants, our 'consciousness is ... merely consciousness concerning the immediate sensuous environment and consciousness of the limited connection with other persons and things outside the individual who is growing self-conscious' (Marx [1845]1997: 101). Consciousness in the context of eating is thus shaped by the foods produced, sold, and then prepared and fed to us, usually by family members. Bourdieu's work and much empirical research has provided evidence for this model of dietary development,

along with psychology research which builds on both cultural and evolutionary influences in food consumption patterns; food marketing and food
science research concurs (see Chapters 6–8).

But Marx made it clear that consumption helped to 'differentiate
consumer/workers through the diversification of consumption patterns'
(Pietrykowski 2009: 89). This is as true of food consumption as of any
other consumer good, as Bourdieu would emphasise a century after Marx.
Such differentiation is described as segmentation in consumer marketing
(see Chapter 8).

Marx could not have envisaged the technological developments that
would enable the expansion of consumption in the twentieth and twenty-
first centuries. Food processing, the tracking of food consumption and
marketing of new products would all play a powerful role in reinforcing
consumer identities and the instinctive notion that 'this is food for people
like me'. But Marx knew that technology was a key structural force bolstering both production and consumption. Capital would always remove any
obstacles to 'the development of productive forces, the expansion of needs'
(Marx [1857]1997: 95) – wording which acknowledges the symbiosis of
production and consumption (Edwards 2000: 16). Yet Marx's analysis of
the relationship between production and consumption is 'underdeveloped
and open to interpretation' (Edwards 2000: 16, 176).

Some late twentieth century social theorists, turning to culture rather
than class to analyse societal change, would conclude that this 'expansion
of needs', generating an endless array of consumer goods, would eliminate
structured social classes as people constructed their own identities via
consumption. But not all consumers are equal; our consumer status and
profile are connected to our social class, even if this term is not used by
consumer/retail industries.

Consumption and the division of labour

The division of labour which develops in capitalism leads to a varying
distribution 'both quantitative and qualitative, of labour and its products'
(Marx [1845]1997: 102), a process which will be reflected in the distribution of foods among different segments of society. Foods are purchased and
consumed in ways which flow from an individual's education, family background, labour and wages, indicating gradations in consumption in terms
of both quality and quantity of food. Official statistics still assess food
consumption and health in terms of a socio-economic structure largely
based on employment, with its implications for income. Marketers also
consider consumers in terms of their occupations (among other
categorisations).

Marx writes that the division of labour 'fixes' each individual into a
specific 'exclusive sphere of activity which is forced on him and from which
he cannot escape' (Marx [1845]1997: 104). Such language may overstate

restrictions on occupational mobility nowadays, but it is useful for analysing food consumption patterns by category of employment. The inescapability of labour-related 'spheres of activity' can animate the concept of the individual's foodscape in the areas where he or she lives and works. Technology makes it possible to trace – and, arguably, 'fix' (embed) – individual consumption patterns along geographic/spatial lines, and to inform food suppliers of the tastes and purchases of consumers in a given area, for which they then cater, in a process that seems self-reinforcing (see Chapter 7).

In this process, dietary alternatives are geared to different classes of workers/residents/consumers according to their known tastes. As illustrated previously, our consciousness of the kinds of food we *can* eat and *want* to eat is shaped from earliest infancy, throughout our school years, and into adulthood, by food providers throughout the food chain – from agriculture, to industry, food retailing and through the influence of the family and social networks. By adulthood, the foodscape through which we move responds to and reinforces the tastes and practices we have developed through this process.

Marx acknowledges those who subjectively raise themselves socially, but insists the individual cannot really transcend the social relations 'whose creature he socially remains' ([1867]1997: 205). Bourdieu also articulates this notion: 'the dominated have only two options: loyalty to self and the group ... or the individual effort to assimilate the dominant ideal which is the antithesis of the very ambition of collectively regaining control over social identity' (Bourdieu [1984]2010: 385). At the very least, then, there can be a kind of alienation when the individual makes this sort of attempt; even if she/he succeeds in assimilating the dominant ideal (or transcending the social relations of the habitus), some aspects of it may be retained. In explaining change and continuity in food consumption patterns, it is possible that even where there is some degree of social mobility, perhaps via occupation/income, dietary patterns may not change significantly for the better. In seeking to understand levels of obesity among men, who do not exhibit as clear a social gradient in bodyweight as women do, this insight may have some purchase.

Marx and 'lifestyles'

The term 'lifestyle choices' where food and drink are concerned would not withstand close scrutiny under a Marxist framework, given his focus on the restrictions of human life and the circumstances we find ourselves in, rather than actively create. But lifestyles and lifestyle choices are commonly cited by food companies, doctors, government ministers, researchers and health promoters when they discuss diet-related health. It is a concept picked up by Giddens, with some qualifications, but much critiqued by other sociologists.

That the individual is primarily responsible for his or her food consumption and consequent diet-related health is a 'ruling idea', to use a Marxian term ([1845]1997: 109), articulated independently by the groups listed in the preceding paragraph. Given their widely varying skills, occupations, educational background, salaries, influence and lack of cohesion, these dominant groups are not a Marxian 'ruling class', although arguably all have a role in governance. But where food and health are concerned, they collectively constitute an example of Marx's material and intellectual forces generating a ruling idea, shaping the prevailing public understanding of diet and health. The benefits of a healthy diet are clear, but the accompanying notion – that we are responsible for achieving a healthy diet, regardless of our circumstances, the limitations to consciousness in food choice, and the structuring of our diets by the agri-food industry – is more suspect. But the lines between the two are blurred in the discourse surrounding this ruling idea.

Marx was concerned to reveal the connections between ruling classes and ruling (or dominant) ideas, as the latter do not arise unbidden out of nowhere ([1845]1997: 110). Who produced the ideas? In whose interests are they? Marx writes of the tendency of the dominant class 'to represent its interest as the common interest of all the members of society … It has to give its ideas the form of universality, and represent them as the only rational, universally valid ones' (ibid.: 111). For Marx, 'the class which has the means of material production at its disposal, has control at the same time over the means of mental production, so that … the ideas of those who lack the means of mental production are subject to it' (ibid.: 109).

Marx's concept was developed by Gramsci in the early twentieth century, who described the 'hegemony' of ruling ideas by dominant forces, which, despite their power, do not merely impose their ideas – they seek the 'active consent' of those who are subordinate (Crompton 2008b: 43). Hegemonic power is a kind of continually renegotiated dominance 'across the economic, political, cultural and ideological domains of a society' by one class over others (Fairclough 2010: 61). The dominant group builds alliances, making concessions as necessary. Applying this concept to an analysis of food consumption, we can observe the adoption of healthy eating discourse, and some at least apparently healthy products, as part of 'corporate social responsibility' efforts on the part of food manufacturers and retailers to convince government that tighter regulation of the food industry is unnecessary. Hegemony is achieved on the consumption end of the spectrum when those who have unhealthy diets can be seen (in the context of healthy eating discourse) as 'consenting' to or integrating the idea that individuals are responsible for their food choices, and consequently, their health. Ideology, then, becomes 'naturalised, automatised' – simply '"common sense" in Gramscian terms' (ibid.: 67).

But a focus on the genesis of these ultimately hegemonic ruling ideas among influential elites could reveal 'enduring continuities in the way that powerful groups organize society in their own interests' (Savage and Williams 2008: 4). Scambler has identified a 'striking empirical neglect of the rich and powerful' (Scambler 2002: 156) in terms of research tracing their political influence. Much energy is wasted arguing for a stronger role for government policy in alleviating inequalities if we do not understand how politicians and senior civil servants are connected with the commercial world out of which they often emerge – and to which they often return (Scambler 2002: 100–5). Elites lobbying for deregulation or resisting regulation should also be tracked for their influence on policy while ensuring larger returns on 'entrepreneurial activities' (Scambler and Higgs 2001: 4).

Pollock has documented the career path of elite individuals from private healthcare management consulting companies into the NHS and back again, noting the effect on health policy (Pollock 2005). Lee and Goodman (2002) traced a similar phenomenon internationally, among global health policy experts. Buse cites evidence of transnational companies influencing health and regulatory policy regarding 'sugars, pesticide use and residues, transfatty acids, additives and dietary guidelines' at global level (Buse 2005: 191). Abraham and colleagues trace the phenomenon of regulatory capture in medicines regulation (for example, Abraham 1997; Abraham and Lewis 1999; Abraham and Davis 2005, 2006). Miller and Harkins (2010) monitor efforts to influence policy by the food and drink industries.

But there is more to do, given the power of ruling ideas in a neoliberal era. At such a time, and despite the insights of both Marx and Gramsci, 'the possibility ... that the ruling ideas might be those of some ruling class is not even considered, even though there is overwhelming evidence for massive interventions on the part of business elites and financial interests in the production of ideas and ideologies' (Harvey 2005: 115).

In the present context, the food industry finds it needs to do more than simply produce food: a set of ideas must also be constructed to support consumption. This was particularly true once agricultural shortages became surpluses in the second half of the twentieth century. Thus advertising messages tell targeted groups that they deserve snacks and convenience foods; they are busy people; they can eat while working or in the cinema or watching television (i.e. without really thinking about it or being fully conscious of what they are doing). Furthermore, these foods will be available everywhere they go, as the potential for siting foods continually expands.

Since the early 1990s, food technology has been taught in schools. Students learn about industrial processes, design, packaging and marketing food in a shift in educational practice which has been little analysed by social scientists. While many teachers continue teaching cookery within the rubric of food technology, the shift from one to the other at least in name seems to have been intended to prepare future consumers (and possibly food industry workers) for an uncritical familiarity with food industry activities and products (BBC 2012).

The food industry is a powerful productive force – productive of both food products and the ideas we need to absorb in order to consume them.

If one of these ideas – that we are all individually responsible for our food choices – is accepted as true, there is little need for the state to intervene in matters of food consumption, except perhaps to promote healthy eating and fitness as a lifestyle.

Consciousness and diet

But how conscious are we of what we eat? If it is our social being that determines our consciousness and not the other away around, as Marx argued ([1859]1997: 119), then our consumption of food will be shaped by our social life and experience. Food consumption is a matter of routine, in which conscious choice is often not required, particularly when we are moving through habitual foodscapes. Research into food consumption by psychologists indicates a high degree of unconsciousness in eating patterns (see Chapter 7).

Some contemporary theorists feel we must break with the classical Marxist concept of the power of one group to exploit another 'in favour of the recognition that the capitalist system as a whole exerts particular systemic powers over all its members' (Postone 1993 cited in Savage 2000: 12). An analysis of food marketing by social group will provide some backing for this argument – we are all targeted in different ways by the food industry and most of us are now overweight or obese. But in examining states of diet-related health, it is undeniable that lower status groups tend to consume less nutritious food and more processed foods of poor dietary quality. They also have worse health throughout the lifecourse, which is itself shorter for lower social groups. The system's power has more serious consequences for some than others.

Sociology of class and food

> How and why have sociologists, in general, found it less useful to use the concept of class at the very same time that economic polarization has reached unparalleled depths?' (Savage 2000: 70)

In his book *Class Analysis and Social Transformation*, Michael Savage tries to answer this vexed question, first tracing the linked history of social class and the social sciences, and sociology in particular, in Britain. Tracking and measuring social class after 1945 gave sociology both intellectual credibility and legitimacy, and supported social policy's emphasis on 'political arithmetic' (Savage 2000: 5, 6).

Marx's influence had extended beyond the collapse of communist regimes around 1990, but the tradition of Marxist class analysis, rooted in the exploitation inherent in industrial production, as well as class consciousness and the anticipated culmination of class conflict in revolution, had weakened by the late twentieth century (ibid.: 9, 43, 58). Class distinctions became less easy to observe; 'class relations as generative mechanisms simply do not straightforwardly express themselves in social worlds which are complex, dynamic and open systems,' Savage writes, though arguably this can be overstated. Food consumption patterns based on distinct products aimed at different social groups are one example of a 'straightforward' expression of class relations. For Scambler and Higgs, class relations are no less real even if they are sometimes less visible than they once were (2001: 3).

Bourdieu saw in the retreat from class analysis 'the expression of the class interests of a group of relatively powerfully placed professional intelligentsia' (Bourdieu 1988 cited in Skeggs 2004: 54). He rejected criticisms of a more 'rigorous' sociology which some had described as 'doomed to appear deterministic and pessimistic because it takes account of structures and their effects' (Bourdieu 2003: 36). Bourdieu felt that sociology needed to resist the 'de-politicisation' of the study of economic and social policy, staying alert to the state's relaxation of attempts to control economic forces and retreat from regulatory responsibilities (ibid.: 38). Savage also critiqued an increasing abstraction within sociology, and the view that social change is 'beyond anyone's direct purview or control' (Savage 2000: 151). This, he argues, simply releases academics from the moral dimensions of their research (ibid.: ix).

While medical sociology and some social scientists of food continue to address connections between class, capital and health, the discourse of individual responsibility for dietary intake and health remains dominant. This is in spite of a critique of industrialised food dating back decades: 'over-processed foods treated with chemicals' were critiqued by McKee in 1988, as were advertising and marketing of unhealthy foods by a range of authors between 1978 and 1990 (cited by Lupton 2003: 10). As these analyses see it, 'capitalism produces health needs which are treated in such a way as to obscure their origins' (Lupton 2003: 10), so in this way, class differentiation in the context of health can be missed.

By 2008, Crompton reported a resurgence of class analysis in sociology generally, although she regretted the resulting 'fragmentation' of class studies. Studies of cultural aspects of class formation have usefully redressed an economistic focus (Crompton 2008b: 93). But an interest in culture has been for some an alternative to class analysis.

Savage acknowledged the problems inherent in contemporary efforts to trace the salience of class, but felt that broadening class analysis from the long-established occupational connection might reinvigorate it (Savage 2000: 8). He has analysed the structuring categories of 'property, organisation and culture' and the processes by which they relate to class formation' (ibid.: 20). More recently, he and colleagues reconstructed Bourdieu's research on class and culture in Britain (Bennett *et al.* 2009). Four years later they presented a new class schema based on a BBC survey of social class among self-selected participants and a supplemental survey commissioned to ensure representativeness (Savage *et al.* 2013; see next section below).

Most centrally for this book, Savage and other sociologists considered 'place' in the context of geodemographic and social sorting by neighbourhood (see Chapter 7).

While theories of individualism, social mobility and reflexivity attempted to displace class analysis, class itself is 'simultaneously being institutionalized and reproduced' (Skeggs 2004: 53). Even the process of individualisation involves both 'differentiation from others and differential access to resources' (ibid.: 53). But rather than concentrate sociological energies on mapping class structures, Savage urges us to 'see class cultures as contingently embodying forms of individualised identities which operate relationally' (Savage 2000: 150). This individualising process has led to the paradox that 'the structural importance of class to people's lives appears not to be recognised by people themselves' but it has not, he insists, obliterated the salience of class itself (ibid.: xii).

Alongside research interest in the rise of consumption and culture, other concepts such as 'disorganised capitalism, post-Fordism and post-industrialism' all assumed the waning of social class (Savage 2000: 6). State benefits and returns on capital investment (mostly via pension schemes) are now widely received, though many pension schemes have weakened and will no longer provide the guaranteed level of income they once did. There have also been capital increases for homeowners resulting from increases in house prices (Savage 2000: 44). Self-employment has increased markedly since the 1980s (ibid.: 48), weakening the labour–capital–exploitation dynamic. All these factors have influenced perceptions of social class and the way society is segmented into classes for analytical purposes. Nevertheless, most people earn their income via their labour, and if shareholding has expanded, it has also increased economic inequality (ibid.: 51). But inequality is apparent in gradations rather than between distinct social groups with uniform interests, so where would one draw class boundaries (ibid.: 44)?

How official statistics draw class lines

Researchers grappled with this question in redrawing the categorisations of official national statistics, following long-held reservations among social scientists about the previous Registrar General's system of five hierarchical/occupational rankings (professional, intermediate, skilled manual and non-manual, partly skilled, and unskilled) (Crompton 2008b: 53). This ranking left out the long-term unemployed, retired, disabled, and those not working for other reasons – who, collectively, constitute most of the population (Graham 2007: 53). The underlying criticism was that the RG scheme was poorly conceived, even atheoretical. The new system, the Official of National Statistics Socio-Economic Classification (NS-SEC) addressed these concerns and viewed occupation in the context of employment relations (whether one is supervisor, supervised or self-employed, for example) and size of employment organisation (Crompton 2008b: 64). This system attempts to be non-hierarchical, with three different sets of classes (eight, five or three), though the latter (managerial/professional, intermediate, routine/manual) does not escape this characterisation (Graham 2007: 55). For Rose and Pevalin, who wrote the 2003 *Researcher's Guide to the National Statistics Socio-Economic Classification*, occupation combined with employment status is a 'reasonable indicator of overall social position ... because the life chances of individuals and families depend mainly on their position in the social division of labour and on the material and symbolic advantages they derive from it' (cited in Graham 2007: 52).

There are criticisms that the new scheme still gives an incomplete portrayal of societal inequalities and makes unexplained assumptions about culture and norms, and its class divisions are somewhat arbitrary (Crompton 2008b: 68). For all social groups, 'socio-economic indicators serve as markers for a concept which they partially, but never wholly, represent', focusing as they do on associations between measures (Graham 2007: 62). Whichever indicators are chosen, they may only reveal symptoms of an underlying factor which may 'not only be unmeasured but [also] as yet, unknown' (ibid.: 62). It is just such a low-lying factor – the understanding of our social worlds by the food industry and its marketing arm, and its role in influencing food consumption by social group – that is highlighted in this book.

Despite the drawbacks of the NS-SEC, it has been useful in both measuring and predicting health outcomes and in operationalising class inequality (Crompton 2008b: 67; 2008a: 1221). However, it does not distinguish 'substantial holders of wealth or capital', or the link between wealth and occupation (Crompton 2008b: 68, 70), reducing the potential for insight into the lives of elite members and classes. But Savage and Williams (2008) acknowledged potential in the new classification system for exploring small groupings, including elites. For example, the highest occupational class can be subdivided into '"employers in large organisations", "higher managerial occupations" and "higher professional occupations"' (ibid.: 6).

Ultimately, a 2013 study by Savage and colleagues, based on the BBC and supporting survey, proposed a new series of groupings taking into account socio-economic changes in the UK since the economic crisis beginning in 2008, and combining Bourdieuan ideas about social, cultural and economic capital. They delineated seven social classes: elite, established middle class, technical middle class, new affluent workers, traditional working class, emergent service workers, and the 'precariat' (those with no or insecure employment, reflecting zero-hours contracts and other types of irregular employment seen in recent years; this group constitutes 15 per cent of the UK population) (Savage *et al.* 2013). The authors acknowledge that their schema differs from the NS-SEC and does not seek to compete with it, but rather to present a more fine-grained interpretation of class boundaries – and one which responds to recent developments. While not exploring matters of diet and health, the surveys did enquire into types of food consumed, reflecting the class–diet patterns which have long been revealed (and which are discussed in Chapter 5). But their schema suggests considerable potential for further exploration of class-differentiated food consumption which takes into account recent developments and emerging trends.

In this book, official statistics are cited in assessments of food consumption patterns and health outcomes. As Graham concludes, when researching social influences on health, we must work with 'a range of imperfect measures, trying to remain alert to their limitations while seeking to exploit their strengths' (Graham 2007: 61); no classification system will ever meet every need.

But we can deepen our understanding of the power of social class in shaping social life by examining theories of human action; this takes us beyond the quantitative portrayal of class as supplied by statistical studies.

Inequality, class and capitalism

Habermas saw no paradox in the receding of class identities and analysis in late modern capitalism. It is a process with a long history, as primitive societies characterised by age and sex roles and a system based on kinship became traditional ones, characterised by a system based on class domination. Ultimately, a liberal-capitalist society emerged, characterised by the relationship between wage labour and capital (Habermas [1973]1996: 241–3). In liberal capitalism, the growth of commerce leads ultimately to 'civil society', with its 'depoliticization of the class relationship, and ... anonymization of class domination' (ibid.). In these circumstances, 'the theory of class consciousness loses its empirical reference' (Habermas [1981]1996: 292).

The economic polarisation Savage decries has taken place in the latter stages of liberal-capitalism, with the development of the welfare state, and is, for Habermas, the logical outcome of liberal-capitalist society (Habermas [1973]1996: 243). The welfare state addressed the most egregious sufferings experienced by the lowest social classes, with sufficient redistribution of resources to see off any serious social upheaval (though this has not been true of some countries experiencing severe austerity in recent years). The benefits of some measures, including free education and healthcare, extended far beyond the lowest social classes. Collective bargaining arguably further pacified class conflict (Habermas [1981]1996: 287). Yet underlying structural inequalities have never been effectively addressed (Habermas [1981]1996: 287). Previously existing class conflicts have become institutionalised in the mass democracy of the welfare state, and class differentiation has developed along the lines of 'functional position, income and way of life' (Outhwaite 1996: 270).

The UK has seen the fastest growth in income inequality of any OECD country since 1975 (OECD 2011: 1). But despite some protests from time to time, including the early twenty-first century, with the introduction of austerity measures, the welfare state has been a relatively stable container for discontent. This might be Habermas's answer to Savage's paradox. Habermas's theory of human action and communication, and his notion of the colonisation of the lifeworld, has much to offer our understanding of patterns of food consumption, and their consequences for health. His ideas are analysed in detail in the following chapter.

Gender and ethnicity versus social class

Savage speculates that the disconnect between economic inequality and social class is also linked to the growth of interest in other dimensions of inequality, such as gender and ethnicity. The path of class analysis in the academy and the competing concepts that arose to challenge it are worth tracing here.

Scambler (2002) takes issue with the notion of gender and ethnicity studies as competitors with social class analysis, particularly in the context of health. Gender and ethnicity, once the objects of some very bad science (Oakley 2000: 96; Bhopal 1997: 168), then almost a replacement for class in academic research, are clearly powerful influences on health. But while these are factors which must be addressed in tackling health and healthcare inequalities, 'socio-economic differences should be considered as an explanation of differences in health between ethnic groups' (Bhopal 1997: 177). Epidemiologists Marmot and Mustard found that levels of economic development over time of 'cultural groups' in the societies to which they had migrated was *the* decisive factor in their health, certainly in terms of mortality (1994: 208). They detect 'a dynamic and evolving relationship with class status' even for individual risk factors. The 1998 Acheson Report into health inequalities concluded that 'within minority groups, there is a clear association between material advantage and poor health' (cited in Scambler 2002: 107). For Scambler, class is the 'core' property of 'disorganised capitalism of relevance to health'; since the genesis of capitalism in the sixteenth century, 'its class relations have always been gendered (just as they have always been racialised)' (Scambler 2002: 117).

One illustration of this arises in the relationship between gender, age group, obesity and health, in which a social gradient is apparent for women, children and adolescents, but the pattern is less clear for men, though men share the relationship between rising obesity prevalence and lower educational attainment (HSE 2006-11 cited in PHE 2014c). Occupation-based measures also links with obesity among men (NOO 2012a), as does low income, though the association between low income and obesity is stronger for women (HSE 2012b: 2). Lower status men who are obese have worse health and shorter lives than higher status men who are obese. Moderate obesity is not associated with worse health for men unless they are in lower status groups (see Chapter 5). This seems to sharpen the case for examining gender differences in the context of class–obesity–ill health. And if current bodyweight trends among boys do not change, a clearer social gradient among men may be observable in future.

Skeggs notes that the return to class research since the 1990s has been most marked in feminist and queer theories, along with geography, media studies, history and to some degree sociology (Skeggs 2004: 47). These different approaches are thus not mutually exclusive; integrating class with other research interests can bear fruit.

Perhaps a more damaging divide has taken place between empirical and theoretical researchers within sociology, described as a 'huge gulf', with the former finding continuity in the 'class character of culture' while the latter, by and large, do not (Milner 1999 cited in Skeggs 2004: 53). The cultural turn prompted a major shift in approaches to class analysis.

The cultural turn

In the 1990s, Warde challenged sociological research which rejected materialist/political economy critiques and embraced the notion of culture in studying consumption. For such researchers, 'signs, discourses and mental constructs' (Warde 1997: 1) were the path to understanding social action in this domain; the role of prices and incomes became almost ignored after the materialist trend in sociology in the 1960s and 1970s (ibid.: 97).

Culture encompasses 'both the meanings and the values which arise amongst distinctive social groups and classes, as well as the lived traditions and practices which these meanings are expressed and in which they are embodied' (Hall 1981 cited in Crompton 2008b: 44). This resonates with Bourdieu's observation that class and status are connected via 'the role that different class-based principles of taste play in organizing the cultural values and practices through which classes organize, symbolize and enact their differences from one another' (cited in Bennett 2010: xx). Such a concept of culture can coexist alongside observations of structural influences on cultural meanings, values, traditions and practices.

But this was not the only approach to interpreting the role of culture in social life. The cultural turn in social science saw cultural factors as more appropriate for analysing society than economic ones (Crompton 2008b: 13). Cultural consumption generating 'symbols, discourse and difference' was viewed as a defining force of postmodern society (Pahl 1989, Beck 1992, Clark *et al.* 1993, Pakulski and Waters 1996, all cited in Savage 2000: viii).

Consumption, together with increasingly available credit, was thought to have made social status a matter of fluidity, as the constraints of hierarchy and tradition receded (Pakulski and Waters 1996 cited in Webster 2007: 85). The ways in which consumer goods were themselves stratified and marketed by social group – categories in which social status has always been a dominant factor – seem not to have been noted; nor was the substitution of credit for a rise in wages in real terms. Yet consumer marketing was, by the 1990s, building ever more refined techniques for segmenting society into distinct, status-based consumption groups.

Crompton disagreed that culture and consumption constituted an epochal social shift, finding neoliberalism and an intensified capitalism sufficient to explain social change (Crompton 2008b: 83). But with the postmodern cultural turn, consumption was split off from its socio-economic and political context, and its role in identity formation became central (Edwards 2000: 27). Early theorists of consumption (Veblen, Simmel and the Frankfurt School) had questioned its consequences; Marxist analysis focused on the alienation resulting from consumption as both exploitative and a mere 'palliative' for hard work (ibid.: 27, 17). By contrast, postmodern interest in 'the symbolic aspects of consumption ... diverts attention from issues of the material resources required for survival' (Warde 1997: 175) and from the connections between consumption and social class (Edwards 2000: 129). Yet consumption is connected to 'economic systems of provision and production and is central to the shaping and reproduction of social practices and social divisions' which are not merely stylistic, but rather structural in nature (ibid.: 29–30).

A related cost of the cultural turn is the resistance among theorists of social class to studying consumption. Edwards finds that 'class and consumption act precisely in conjunction with one another to maintain individual and group identities' (Edwards 2000: 130). Consumer marketers track and understand this very well; the interaction between class, consumption and marketing is a key observation of this book.

Tomlinson's study of data from the 1985 and 1992 health and lifestyles survey found that 'contrary to many current theories of consumption and lifestyle ... traditional notions such as social class and gender are still highly relevant to a discussion of lifestyle and consumer behaviour and may even be better determinants' (Tomlinson 2003: 97). He noted a tendency for people to imitate health behaviours witnessed in their environment in ways which show a clustering along social class lines (ibid.: 97, 109).

Moreover, the cultural factors relevant to food consumption are not distinct from the purchasing power of different social groups. A kind of 'reflexive' relationship exists between them, in that industry is increasingly adept at studying and then using an understanding of socio-cultural trends to promote and target new forms of consumption. Innovations in agricultural, financing, transport, processing, packaging, retailing, advertising and marketing technologies and styles also interact with socio-cultural factors and trends. In the context of marketing, culture has become a 'plundered' resource (Skeggs 2004: 153).

The social mobility debate

Skeggs highlights the role of academics in retreating from class studies and setting research agendas which excluded it. In search of alternatives to class analysis, 'academics *who could* looked for something else as the site of social change, usually themselves, via theories that could explain *their* mobility and *their* social networks' (Skeggs 2004: 47, author's emphasis). In doing so, they described what happened to 'a privileged few' and then applied this more widely (ibid.).

For Skeggs, it is not mobility which counts, it is control: who has the power to move or remain fixed, to connect with others, or even to withdraw (Skeggs 2004: 50)? In order to exert such control, one needs access 'to resources and resourcefulness' (ibid.: 51). One way of observing the degree of control individuals have is to look at where they live. Thus 'a geography of placement becomes a way of speaking class indirectly' (ibid.: 50). Chapter 7, describing the power of geodemographics for both retail and healthcare planning, provides evidence for Skeggs's concern. She references the fixed locations of the working class, who are thus rendered both 'identifiable and governable' (ibid.). In fact, all social groups are targeted as consumers of geographically placed goods and services via a range of market research techniques, though with varying degrees of information and type and quality of product or service.

Conclusion

This chapter has provided some historical-sociological context to the debate over social class – its trajectory in the academy, the ways it is measured, and how it is influenced by questions of culture, ethnicity, consumption and social mobility – in preparation for situating the notion of class in the field of diet and health. Savage urged researchers to find 'more effective ways of drawing out the implications of different kinds of empirical research for class analysis' while fully theorising developments (2000: ix); thus the linkage of theoretical and empirical contexts in this chapter. It is a call broadly echoed by Crompton, though she valued existing methodologies in pursuing such research (Crompton 2008b: 149–50). Both Crompton (2008b) and Edwards (2000) see a role for linking analyses of consumption and social class; this is done in a highly empirical manner in Chapter 5, which discusses both social and health epidemiology in the context of food consumption.

But the following chapter pursues the theoretical questions raised in the present one. I have mentioned the work of Giddens, Bourdieu and Habermas in passing; their ideas are now discussed in detail, as the insights of these key theorists are applied to social class, food production and food consumption.

4 Reflexivity, habitus and lifeworld

Applying the theories of Giddens, Bourdieu and Habermas

Introduction

This chapter focuses on three key theorists whose ideas, applied to food production and consumption, can help to reveal some of the contradictions inherent in the way we eat, why we eat what we do, and the way we are differently affected by what we eat.

Giddens's writings on reflexivity are deserving of detailed discussion here because of their prominence within the academy, their influence on both discourse and policy, and arguably a degree of inconsistency where questions of diet and choice are concerned. His references to diet are casual observations – no more than personal views – but, along with his notion of lifestyle and individual responsibility, and the influence these ideas and Giddens himself had on public policy under New Labour, they also merit close examination. But Bourdieu's concept of habitus and Habermas's analysis of the colonisation of the lifeworld by external forces take us further in theorising why and how we eat the way we do; their work will also be analysed in depth in this chapter.

Although Giddens's thinking on reflexivity is ultimately problematic in the context of diet, health and class, he devoted himself to an investigation over many years of what drives human action and how to explain social change. His work is useful for understanding food consumption and health 'behaviours', but his notion of reflexivity is challenged here.

How reflective is reflexivity? A critique of Giddens

Anthony Giddens was a leading figure not only in British sociology but also, by the 1990s, government policy circles, influencing New Labour rhetoric and policies with his 'Third Way' programme, and eventually taking his seat in the House of Lords (Reyes 2005: 237–45). In this section his ideas are applied to developments in healthy eating discourse, with its notions of individual responsibility for diet and health, based on conscious, 'reflexive' choice.

While Giddens gave much early attention to class analysis in ways which are still instructive, class was already in retreat in the 1980s as a sociological subject of enquiry. Initially, he was interested in returning class to its central role in sociology, but his focus gradually shifted to the philosophy of human action and to what he believed was the reflexive nature of such action. Yet he continued periodically to refer to the collective behaviours of social groups in a class context; Savage sees class appearing in Giddens's work in 'hidden and indirect ways' (Savage 2000: 8). Arguably his writings indicate contradictions regarding freedom of action for individuals from different social groups which he never fully resolved.

In an early essay, Giddens acknowledged the 'conceptual confusion' inherent in the term 'class' (Giddens 1982: 157) and identified a 'blank spot' in the transition from 'economic classes' to 'social classes' (ibid.). But this did not alter the continuing appropriateness of the term 'class'. Capitalism had generated a 'class society' more emphatically than any previous era or system, given the central role of labour as a commodity, and therefore the labour contract, the inherently exploitative nature of the production process in capitalism, and the connection between production and consumption in the context of labour and capital (Giddens 1982: 169–70). All these processes influence and shape the real lives of individuals.

Still, he cautioned against using the term in the context of market-generated interests or divisions: 'while there may be an indefinite multiplicity of cross-cutting interests created by differential market capacities, there are only, in any given society, a limited number of classes' (Giddens 1982: 158). There is a parallel here with Marx's admission of the difficulty of demarcating classes: 'middle and intermediate strata' proliferate around the three main social groups he identified: labourers, owners of capital and landlords (Marx [1867]1997: 247). And what of the 'infinite fragmentation of interest and rank into which the division of social labour splits labourers as well as capitalists and landlords' (ibid.: 248)?

Decades after the Giddens work cited above, the dozens of consumer group profiles produced by market research firms arguably constitute just such a distillation of Giddens's 'indefinite multiplicity' or Marx's 'infinite fragmentation' of social groupings – and they are *not*, admittedly, 'classes'. These groupings instead make a very utilitarian accommodation with the difficulties of stratification and, for their commercial or public sector clients, usefully construct some order out of a society apparently in flux.

For Giddens, income and occupation are important elements in identifying and measuring social groups in national statistics, but one cannot demarcate 'classes' per se in this quantitatively tidy way. Giddens instead finds mechanisms such as the potential for social mobility, which link market dynamics with the shaping of class relationships (Giddens 1982: 159). The more rigid the limitations upon mobility, the more likely it is that identifiable classes are formed in a process which reproduces itself over time (ibid.). Thus individuals in succeeding generations will tend to get similar types of work which yield similar material outcomes (ibid.). This would traditionally stem from differing market capacities in terms of ownership of means of production, educational qualifications or manual labour skills, in what might be termed 'mobility closure' (ibid.).

But such definitive closure never truly exists in capitalism, and Giddens finds the potential for mobility in society as it develops. Yet more recent empirical research shows that those born to unskilled parents are most likely to enter unskilled work themselves, the corollary being true for children of professional parents (Breen and Rottman 1995, Breen 2004, both cited in Graham 2007: 123; BBC 2010). Social elites have been reproducing themselves with surprisingly little change, given the narrative of class mobility in recent decades (Cabinet Office 2009). This report concluded that powerful, embedded – indeed, structural – constraints are in fact limiting social mobility. The experience of social class is also reflected in the British Social Attitudes Survey of 2011, in which both class status and subsequent advantages of private education are 'robust and substantial' (National Centre for Social Research 2011: 41–2). The May 2012 report by the government's independent reviewer on occupational mobility found that significant barriers remained: 'There is no one profession that can say it has cracked the fair access problem. Indeed, almost no profession has a clear plan for doing so' (Milburn 2012: 7).

Giddens on class and consumption

Alongside the structuring of classes within the domain of production, Giddens believed that consumption patterns also influenced what he called class structuration (1982: 159). Structuration theory aimed to bring together the poles of agency and structure, emphasising the interaction between the two. Structure is reproduced and gradually modified by individual actions taken in the context of a given structure, which constrains, and yet changes over time by the collective actions of individuals. So for Giddens, structures are flexible, providing resources upon which actors draw (Shilling 2003: 174).

But for critical realists, agents find themselves in a pre-existing structure, which they '*re*create, *re*produce and/or *transform*' (Bhaskar 1987 cited in Scambler and Scambler 2013: 84). According to this formulation, the interaction of agent and structure will often entail reproduction of pre-existing circumstances, with transformation of reality a potentiality, but no more than that. In the context of food consumption, the potential for transforming one's diet for the better is limited when resources are few and/or exposure to and identification with the discourse of healthy eating – and reflexive interaction with it – is limited. New technology in agriculture, production, distribution and packaging may present consumers with new food items, but these tend to be developed and marketed according to existing tastes and patterns of consumption, as described in Chapters 6–8.

Distinguishable status groups can emerge on the basis of socially differentiated consumption, an insight fundamental to consumer marketing. The most notable groupings that emerge in the sphere of consumption are based on 'community or neighbourhood segregation' (Giddens 1982: 161); here he anticipates geodemographic tracking of exactly this phenomenon (see Chapter 7). His observation also recalls Skeggs's concerns with the geography of class: fixed in space, hence more governable.

However, he also noted the impact on lifestyles of the spatial disconnectedness of modern life, as people move through their day in different locations (home, school, work, leisure, errands, and the spaces which connect them). These locations will have an underlying unity for a particular class or group, and will shape lifestyle options (Giddens 1991: 83); there will certainly be implications for the character of the food supply.

Groups of people inhabiting the social realities of their neighbourhood are likely to have distinct styles of life, behaviours and attitudes (Giddens 1982: 162). This is a phenomenon which consumer firms harness as they target consumers spatially, reinforcing the identification with place and social class. It is difficult to see how individual actions or choices can be seen as free of class influences in such an analysis.

Giddens, diet and lifestyle

Although not concerned with questions of diet and health in any detail, Giddens discusses them periodically. He writes, for example, that 'the question "How shall I live?" has to be answered in day-to-day decisions about how to behave ... and what to eat' (Giddens 1991: 14). Yet studies of the psychology of eating (see Chapter 7) show that the process of deciding what to eat can be deeply unconscious, with any 'choice' emerging from what Bourdieu describes as our habitus. This is what behavioural economics and psychology have come to accept, and what has led to 'nudge' theory.

Giddens did not acknowledge an unconscious quality in what he considered reflexive 'lifestyle' choices; instead he cites Freud's diagnosis of the 'compulsiveness of modernity', with compulsion substituting for tradition and remaining distinct from the unconscious (Giddens 1994: 68). Habermas speaks of the colonisation of the lifeworld by such externally introduced compulsions. This is illustrated by the extremes of food consumption in an obesogenic foodscape: compulsive eating can lead to obesity or bulimia, disorders which have emerged as food-related pathologies in late modernity. For Giddens, these are both social and psychological phenomena illustrating the disintegration of tradition in society (Giddens 1994: 71), a conclusion with Habermasian overtones.

The term 'lifestyle' is associated with, among other things, dietary choice, alongside connotations of individual responsibility for such choices. For Giddens, as society becomes de-traditionalised with the advance of modernity, the notion of lifestyle becomes predominant (Giddens 1991: 5). Lifestyle choices then take the place of constraints imposed by class in formulating action (Atkinson 2007: 536, analysing Giddens). But how can lifestyle choices be made without emerging from within an already existing lifestyle (Atkinson 2007: 542)? If, as Bourdieu found, 'lifestyle choices' are shaped by one's habitus, then such choices are not as free as Giddens implies in his 'tokenistic attempts to pull lifestyle into the definition of class and stratification' (Atkinson 2007: 542).

The language of 'lifestyle' can slip into discussions about diet and health all too easily; it is a central plank in the individual responsibility/choice discourse where health is concerned. Warde warned that the displacement of class by lifestyle as a determinant of social identity is misleading (Warde 1997: 7). He challenged the notion that consumption had become individualised, that lifestyle is a matter of choice, and that personal taste and an aesthetics of everyday life have overtaken the role for class or social rank in social science.

Giddens acknowledges that the term 'lifestyle' is problematic because of its association with affluence (Giddens 1991: 5). In late modernity, 'access to means of self-actualisation becomes itself one of the dominant focuses of class division and the distribution of inequalities more generally' (ibid.: 228). But he does not concede the role of this limited access in blocking self-actualisation. Instead, he finds a link between life chances and lifestyle via work and the varying material opportunities it provides (ibid.: 82). The only way to ensure access to this world of opportunity – and a better lifestyle – is 'emancipation from situations of oppression [as] the necessary means of expanding the scope of some sorts of lifestyle option' (ibid.: 86). Emancipation would enable an individual to make free, independent and responsible choices (ibid.: 213). But how is this emancipation to come about? The very restrictions of some 'lifestyles' must often preclude the possibility of self-emancipation. Skeggs finds his concept of the self 'detached from structure ... Giddens relies completely on everybody having equal access to the resources by which the self can be known, assessed and narrated' (Skeggs 2004: 53).

Giddens grants that access to health and lifestyles expertise may be limited: only those who have 'the time, resources and talent to grasp' expert advice can absorb it (Giddens 1994: 85). Leaving aside the linking of 'talent' with those who have time and resources, there must be a class/social background/status element here: some social groups are more likely to be targeted effectively by messages regarding health and diet and better able to implement the advice and benefit from it. A study substantiating this showed that while higher status groups were, over time, demonstrating fewer unhealthy behaviours, lower status groups were demonstrating more of them (Buck and Frosini 2012).

This differential of access, receptiveness and benefit was not acknowledged in the 'social exclusion' discourse which arose during New Labour, replacing the terminology of underclass or 'culture of poverty' (Skeggs 2004: 47). Indeed, it became a mechanism for avoidance of acknowledging class itself (ibid.: 54).

But Giddens thought that those living in poverty might be *more* susceptible to the disintegration of traditional practices than others, making lifestyle choices more fundamental to such individuals. They become 'virtually obliged to explore novel modes of activity' (Giddens 1991: 86). Even so, he admits that all choices 'refract upon pre-existing power relations' (Giddens 1994: 76).

Giddens's understanding of lifestyle is connected to the idea of habit, which is shaped 'within relatively set channels' (Giddens 1991: 80). Choice is circumscribed by the force of habit and the limitations of individual lives. Nevertheless, he concludes that the lifestyle we end up having is an 'integrated set of practices' chosen by individuals (ibid.: 81).

Just such a concept of an 'integrated set of practices' typifying social groups, derived from detailed market research, is the basis for consumer marketing; but are these practices really freely chosen? The discourses of free choice and individualism are indissolubly linked, and constitute the basis of consumerism itself (Cronin 2000 cited in Skeggs 2004: 56). Marketing profiles describe, for example, the types of work, housing, educational background, family structure, entertainment, health and diet that characterise various groups, in an attempt to understand consumer behaviour and predict purchasing patterns.

For Giddens, lifestyles are a feature of modernity. In contrast, traditional cultures are handed down and received more or less unquestioningly, precluding any real role for choice. Yet lifestyles, too, can become routinised, including our eating habits (Giddens 1991: 81). But Giddens veers away from the unconscious dimensions of routine and habit: 'the routines followed are reflexively open to change in the light of the mobile nature of self-identity. Each of the small decisions a person makes every day ... [including] what to eat ... contributes to such routines' (ibid.).

The order resulting from routines gives us a sense of ontological security, for which we have a psychological need (Giddens 1994: 101). So strong is this need that we are powerfully drawn to creating and sustaining routines; thus there is something deterministic, *not* free, and *not* reflexive, about our near-compulsion to institute routines, as Giddens describes it (Atkinson 2007: 544). Our habits cannot be 'wholly optional'; they are 'effectively beyond question' and circumscribed by power relations (Giddens 1994: 75–6). Yet they are also 'reflexively open to change in the light of the mobile nature of self-identity' – a self-identity we consciously construct as we make our daily choices (Giddens 1991: 81). How can both be true? Perhaps conscious reflexivity in the context of diet becomes possible (or even compulsive) for *some* individuals, as part of their habitus, social rank and lifeworld, but not for others; or such reflexivity may take place in different areas of their lives and consciousness.

Giddens acknowledges that different types of lifestyles do not merely *emerge* from social stratification, they *reinforce* it (Giddens 1991: 82). Individuals form habits, and this gradually becomes a collective process; habits are shaped by forces of commodification in a case of institutional reflexivity (Giddens 1994: 101). To apply this to consumption, trendsetting individuals might start to buy something in a habitual manner and locale; similar individuals are then targeted with a similar product in similar locales; the habit extends and the product is anchored in the lives of a certain type or group; and their lives are in turn anchored by the repeated purchase and use of the product.

Lifestyles are also formed by socio-economic circumstances (Giddens 1991: 82). Yet Giddens assumes that those who have unhealthy diets have decided to ignore research indicating the health risks of diets featuring insufficient fruit and vegetables, for example; instead, they choose to eat an excess of fatty, sugary foods, as previous generations of their families might have done (ibid.). For Giddens, this still constitutes a lifestyle (ibid.: 83). They might only be convinced or forced to change their choices when faced with changes in manufacturing or design, which are non-negotiable (Giddens 1994: 101).

The appearance of new products, marketed according to an understanding of existing tastes or budgets, for example, leads many people to absorb these products into their diets. Some groups are alert to nutritional information and products geared to healthy eating – but not everyone. Differing degrees of reflexivity and receptivity are at work. Yet Giddens is not able to explain 'behavioural (and thus lifestyle) variations between individuals and groups in a way that would be consonant with his comments on social differentiation' (Atkinson 2007: 544).

The reflexive body

For Giddens, reflexivity is practised in a bodily sense: we consciously observe the body's processes, and the influences upon it within the environment. We even become 'responsible for the design of our own bodies' via the adoption of body regimes (Giddens 1991: 102). There is ever refreshed guidance on health matters, as we engage in 'reflexive appropriation of bodily processes' (ibid.: 218). Giddens views this bodily reflexivity as emancipating, despite the pathological preoccupation with body shape among those with eating disorders. He also describes the body as being 'invaded' by the 'abstract systems' of a post-traditional world (ibid.) in language which resembles Habermas's colonisation of the lifeworld.

Human bodies are both 'the medium and outcome of human (reproductive) labour' for Giddens (Shilling 2003: 174). But in the context of structuration theory, it remains unclear 'how we go about ascertaining the conditions under which bodies constrain and enable action' (ibid.: 174–5). Giddens seems to alternate between voluntaristic and deterministic versions of the body (ibid.: 175), reflecting his dichotomous views of human action in general.

A disembedding modernity

Giddens admits that 'disembedding mechanisms' intrude into our experience of life. For example, there are 'foodstuffs purchased with artificial ingredients [which] may have toxic characteristics absent from more traditional foods' (Giddens 1991: 20). Even dietary advice from experts can be 'disembedding' in that it is 'non-local' and 'impersonal' (Giddens 1994: 84–5); this may be why some people reject it. Authentic expert advice can also be overwhelmed by marketing campaigns promoting certain foods as healthy, when this is not necessarily the case (Herrick 2009). Nevertheless, for Giddens, these kinds of challenges simply prompt a continual revision in our understanding of our lives and identities (Giddens 1991: 20).

Giddens's prescription

So how are we to emancipate ourselves and acquire the freedom to choose wisely? Giddens finds some value in both Rawls's theory of justice, in which justice is the 'organising ambition' of emancipation but human behaviour is left unaddressed, and Habermas's theory of communicative action (Giddens 1991: 213; 1995: 256), in which society aspires to operate on the basis of clear, open communication among individuals and between system and lifeworld. Ultimately Giddens finds this inadequate for explaining how society actually reproduces itself. Instead, he looks to autonomy – freedom balanced by responsibility to the collective – as the 'mobilising principle of behaviour' (1991: 213).

But by 2007, in a book for non-academic audiences, Giddens was urging quite radical measures. Beyond improved food labelling, which he supported, he also suggested that restrictions on advertising, along with health warnings on some food products, should address the 'severe health implications' of current dietary habits (Giddens 2007: 100). Even 'quite draconian action' against calorie-dense foods would be justifiable (ibid.: 128). Yet he also recommends behavioural 'remedies' in addition to economic ones, including measures to address 'the failure to take exercise' (ibid.: 114, 128). There should be an acceptance of 'greater responsibility for one's own health [as] a fundamental part of active citizenship' (ibid.: 132); there was no acknowledgement of the obstacles to achieving such goals for many people. Lifestyle change should become the core objective of the welfare state, using both incentives and sanctions (ibid.: 131). In an approach described as 'positive welfare', 'personal autonomy and self-esteem' should be encouraged. This would enable people to 'adapt to change and to make the most of their opportunities' (ibid.: 122–3).

But Giddens acknowledged that a lack of capability can prevent some people from improving their circumstances (Giddens 2007: 123) and spoke of the need to 'invest in people's capabilities', citing low self-esteem as a block to capability (ibid.: 127, 131).

A concluding reference to class notes that the growing use of complementary healthcare was an encouraging sign that more people are taking personal responsibility for their health. But this phenomenon 'is heavily class-based, with poorer people making much less use of such treatments – at the same time as they follow less healthy lifestyles' (Giddens 2007: 132). The term 'follow' seems to indicate an elective character. His earlier acknowledgement of the limits of reflexivity, and the shaping of choice by structural forces including power relations, personal circumstance and locale, recede in these closing remarks on class. Emancipation is only available through fresh lifestyle choices (Atkinson 2007: 540).

Giddens has been criticised for imposing observations of middle class experience on other social groups in ways that powerfully situated his ideas in neoliberal politics (Atkinson 2007: 536). For Skeggs, reflexivity itself is a mode of living characteristic of middle classes, precisely because of the resources and privileges available to them (Skeggs 2004 cited in Atkinson 2007: 536, 545). She describes 'the middle class imperative to produce oneself as a choosing, self-managing individual' (Skeggs 2004: 57). Giddens had once acknowledged this himself, when he critiqued consumption theorists who saw class distinctions disappearing; new flows of information, he insisted, would be differently interpreted by different groups and this would reinforce 'patterns of social differentiation' (Giddens 1981 cited in Atkinson 2007: 543). As Atkinson advises, only empirical research can really confirm this. Such data is available as evidence for the relationship between diet, health and class and is evaluated in the following chapter. Food marketing research also discerns subgroups which practise what Giddens might term reflexive eating habits driven by health concerns.

Whimster criticises Giddens for taking action theory and mixing it with ethnomethodology, with the result that 'Brit (sic) sociology ended up with the inward-looking idea of reflexivity. That version of action theory is unable to depict sociological determination and de-mystify the exercise of power' (Whimster 2011: 38). But other theorists *are* able to address these tasks more satisfactorily, none more so than Bourdieu.

The relevance of Bourdieu

> Bourdieu's metaphors enable us to understand who *can* move and who *cannot*. (Skeggs 2004: 48, author's emphasis)

Pierre Bourdieu offers solutions to the contradictions inherent in Giddens's thought; Atkinson concludes that Giddens himself hinted at this (Atkinson 2007: 542, 544–5). In this section I argue that Bourdieu's depiction of habitus takes us further than Giddens can in understanding human action in the domain of diet.

Earlier I discussed the 'cultural turn' in sociology and its role in deflecting attention from social class analysis, instead viewing consumption as the defining principle of late twentieth century society. Yet consumption was arguably simply a new way for social stratification to be manipulated and embedded (Crompton 2008b; Edwards 2000).

Edwards locates what modernists and postmodernists share on the subject of consumption: both would agree that it is an important dimension of social life, and even postmodernists, focused on consumption as culture, would not necessarily deny that consumption has socially divisive and exploitative aspects. Where they *would* differ is in the degree to which these aspects 'centre on matters of class or underlying economic mechanisms' (Edwards 2000: 50). Bourdieu resolves these tensions, seeing consumption as 'a cultural site of social stratification through which the wider economic and political tensions of contemporary capitalism are played out', and recognising consumption's role in forming both individual and group identities in terms of both culture and status (ibid.: 36). Bourdieu also links production and consumption: recalling Marx's statement that 'the division of labour brands the manufacturing worker as the property of capital', Bourdieu locates the 'branding' to which Marx refers in lifestyle itself, which is expressed through consumption (Bourdieu [1984]2010: 174).

Bourdieu's empirical research published in *Distinction* (Bourdieu [1984]2010)[1] portrayed French society of the 1960s, and included diet as a cultural practice. Even at the time, food consumption in France and Britain would have differed widely; several decades later, there are aspects of Bourdieu's class ethnographies which have no parallel with British practices and stratifications. Bourdieu predicted such variation, but insisted that the basic analytical principles should apply over time and space – especially, that education, occupational structure and status shape tastes according to class cultures.

Bourdieu based his class groupings on 'the fundamental determinants of the material conditions of existence and the conditionings they impose' – hence a focus on occupation (Bourdieu [1984]2010: 100). We automatically associate a series of secondary characteristics when a single criterion such as occupation is used as the basis for social segmentation (ibid.).

Before outlining Bourdieu's thinking about food and class, and the embodiment of class via diet, it is necessary to place Bourdieu's most fundamental concept, that of the habitus, in the context of food consumption.

Habitus

As Habermas was to develop the previously existing concept of lifeworld, so Bourdieu did with habitus, which is also to be found in Weber, Mauss,

Husserl, Schutz, Merleau-Ponty, Elias, and possibly even Aristotle (Bennett 2010: xix; Scambler 2002: 74; Crossley 2005: 104). Bourdieu's focus on habitus reflects his concern with challenging a voluntaristic concept of agency and demonstrating the underlying 'pre-reflective' nature of habitus (Crossley 2005: 108–9). He includes diet in his empirical research and shows how it is shaped by the habitus of different social groups.

Lupton describes habitus in the context of food consumption as a set of 'unconscious preferences, classificatory schemes and taken-for-granted choices' as subcultures pass on 'food practices and beliefs' (Lupton 2003: 44). People are not necessarily making free choices (ibid.: 44); the context is given and practice begins in the absence of conscious thought. This recalls Marx's depiction of man finding himself in a set of circumstances which he has not chosen, but with which he must interact.

An element of routine is generated by the habitus. For Giddens, routine was an ontological necessity which sustained frail psyches in a challenging world. For Bourdieu, routine is not something we *need* so much as something we naturally *do*; a practical matter, arising unquestioningly out of our habitus and our relationship to the world (Atkinson 2007: 545). It is not that choices in routine contexts such as eating are *entirely* automatic – but that those choices, and the capacity for reflection itself, are shaped by the habitus (Crossley 2005: 110). Whatever degree of choice exists, the 'prerequisites of choice cannot be chosen' (ibid.).

Much of the meaning of Bourdieu's use of the term 'habitus' is captured in its definition as 'acquired disposition' (Crossley 2005: 104). This encompasses the notion of behaviour as emerging from the set of circumstances into which we are born and raised; but it also alludes to the tension between structure and agency. Structure shapes the circumstances we 'acquire' through birth, and within those limitations, we are 'disposed' to act in a given way. However, we might acquire resources of one kind or another during our lives which will allow for degrees of departure from inherited habitus.

But such acquired dispositions are not necessarily expansive in a positive way. In the context of food consumption, as agricultural production and food processing technology advanced, particularly since the nineteenth century and accelerating throughout the late twentieth century, snack and meal products emerged which had little or no connection to previous modes of eating. Some have little recognisable connection to original agricultural constituents. As the epidemiology will show in Chapter 5, and food industry scientists and marketers will acknowledge in subsequent chapters, people from the lowest socio-economic groups consume more highly processed snack and fast foods and are more likely to experience the health effects of a nutrient-poor diet. Even some of those in higher socio-economic groups may be consuming a high degree of processed snack foods and too many calories overall for optimum health. This is where Bourdieu's idea of the habitus has its limits. Habermas's notion of lifeworld colonisation, discussed later in this chapter, helps to bridge this gap when we seek to understand dietary practices which have altered dramatically in recent decades. At the very least we need to see food industry influences (both products themselves and the marketing/advertising of them) as phenomena which can be absorbed into the habitus; as this happens, dietary practices shift to absorb the products the industry is targeting at us.

But an altered, increasingly industrialised and highly palatable food supply does not discount early, familial influences on food tastes and practices. Describing the shaping of human action by the circumstances into which he is born (and in a way which recalls Marx), Bourdieu concluded that

> it is probably in tastes in food that one would find the strongest and most indelible mark of infant learning, the lessons which longest withstand the distancing or collapse of the native world and most durably maintain nostalgia for it. The native world is, above all, the maternal world, the world of primordial tastes and basic foods. (Bourdieu [1984]2010: 71)

Bourdieu, like Freud, believed in the power of the 'oldest and deepest experiences' and noted that tastes in food are 'deeply rooted in the body and in primitive bodily experiences' (ibid.: 73). Food industry scientists and marketers reach similar conclusions (see Chapters 6–7). Thus a taste for sweet, fatty foods established in childhood can remain decisive throughout adult life, even as products containing these elements constantly evolve in the marketplace. Lustig, an endocrinologist who treats obese infants, describes a can of infant formula which contains over 43 per cent corn syrup solids and an additional 10.3 per cent sucrose, and asks if this could be why some six month olds are already obese (Lustig 2009).

Barker's epidemiological research backdates the role of habitus in diet even further, through his investigation of 'foetal programming', and in particular, the connection between maternal ill health, foetal undernutrition and ill health in adulthood (Barker 1998 cited in Graham 2007: 153). Other studies show a relationship between early cognitive development and later socio-economic position, alongside the role of family background in shaping 'cognitively strong' children (Esping Andersen 2004 and Machin and Vignoles 2004, both cited in Graham 2007: 154). So how does the 'inherited capital' that flows from such early experiences interact with or allow for 'acquired capital'?

A certain standard of education is generally what equips one to move from 'merely knowing' to valuing 'ways of using knowledge' (Bourdieu [1984]2010: 73). This is a useful way of conceptualising what happens for some social groups: their diet evolves as they take into consideration and put into practice information about nutrition. This move from 'knowing' to 'using knowledge' about food doesn't necessarily produce a uniform result: one group of people might become (possibly overly) concerned about dietary health risks, amid ever shifting warnings absorbed by those alert to them; another might more proactively adopt a Mediterranean-type diet rich in fruit, vegetables, fish and olive oil – possibly for health reasons, but also for taste reasons. Such practices presume, for Bourdieu, a certain standard of education. This could be what trumps the restricted diet of a British childhood (even in a middle class family) from the 1960s, say, in which Mediterranean food was little known. The educational aspect of the habitus can be the mechanism for enlarging it beyond its earliest or most 'primitive' inputs.

But the habitus can also go 'backwards' in nutritional terms. This seems to be happening with the ever increasing consumption of highly palatable snack and meal combinations, and the use of prepared foods at mealtimes which may not represent a healthy diet. This consumption is cued by the production, marketing and display of new non-nutritious foods, which are more likely to be consumed in large quantities among those of lower socio-economic status.

A crucial aspect of the habitus is that it is internalised. However, even if it is not consciously experienced by individuals, habitus will be observable in 'categories of perception and appreciation' (Bourdieu [1984]2010: 95). A habitus imposes societal norms and restraints which may conflict with strong impulses (Crossley 2005: 105). This process may be at work in the clash between the dominant societal norm regarding slimness and the fact that increasing numbers of people do not attain it. Overconsumption of calories, lowered sensation of fullness or satiety, a primitive urge us to eat as much as we can, while we can, even amid a plentiful food supply – these factors might have trumped the widespread desire in the late twentieth/ early twenty-first centuries to be thin. Only when this is mediated by vigilant and, to some degree, class-associated ideas of healthy eating and slimness is overconsumption of unhealthy foods avoided.

For Bourdieu, culture and class were interconnected in a dynamic relationship. Over time, they create a habitus characterising large social units with shared conditions and inclinations. Bourdieu refers to 'a whole set of agents produced by similar conditions ... different conditions of existence produce different habitus' (Bourdieu [1984]2010: 166). In the context of taste and consumption, 'people who belong to the same social group and who thus occupy the same position in social space tend to share the same tastes across all forms of symbolic practice' (Bennett 2010: xix):

> The practices of the same agent, and, more generally, the practices of all agents of the same class, owe the stylistic affinity which makes each of them a metaphor of any of the others to the fact that they are the product of transfers of the same schemes of action from one field to another. (Bourdieu [1984]2010: 168)

This insight is striking for its resonance with consumer profiling techniques (discussed in Chapter 7), in which various aspects of behaviour are traced in order to predict (then retrace, and reinforce, through marketing) the kinds of goods and services people will buy. A given consumer group might, for example, prefer the same types of coffee, newspapers, travel destinations, leisure activities, home furnishings, food retailers and restaurants. Within an apparently 'infinite diversity of practices', Bourdieu finds a unity and specificity in them by breaking with 'linear thinking' and seeing instead the 'networks of interrelated relationships which are present in each of the factors' (Bourdieu [1984]2010: 101).

The 'field' and 'capital'

In the concept of 'the field', a 'structured social space' is characterised by inequality (Bourdieu 1998 cited in Laberge 2010: 774). Bourdieu looks at how people are positioned within a field given 'their access to power and resources', which are unequally distributed (Crossley 2005: 81, 83). Food itself constitutes a field (Bourdieu [1984]2010: 206). Though Bourdieu does not define what he means here, food provision and the way people interact with the food available to them are probably most typically considered a field in social and health research, as the resources people have to access, purchase and prepare food are investigated in the study of this field. Market research firms may not describe their analysis of food purchase data and behaviour as the study of a Bourdieuan 'field', but they are interested in how and where people interact with the food supply so that it can be ever more effectively produced, sited and targeted. Much of the social and health research which concerns itself with diet approaches it as food consumption and related behaviour. In this book, I approach the notion of food as a field primarily characterised by consumption patterns (alongside, perhaps, health effects) by relating consumption to the structural factors which shape the provision of food long before it arrives in supermarkets or appears in people's homes.

The competence required to operate in a given field flows from people's habitus – those acquired dispositions. So some will react to the continual expansion of snack food availability in public spaces by noticing it critically and ignoring it in terms of personal consumption; some will consume more of it, appreciating the convenience and perhaps unaware of the visual triggers to hunger. For Bourdieu, the term 'capital' encompassed cultural, social, symbolic and financial capital; these different categories of resources are not equally distributed or available (Crompton 2008b: 100).

Habitus, reflexivity and consumption

What convinces some people to defer gratification? Bourdieu proposes that they calculate whether the sacrifice of the pleasure of the moment will lead to future satisfactions, and whether the latter will be better than those sacrificed in the moment (Bourdieu [1984]2010: 176). Not everyone emerges from a habitus which would foster a 'yes' to that question. The capacity to defer gratification arises in the context of the 'practical materialism which is particularly manifested in the relation to food' (ibid.).

But how can we 'account for cases in which the same income is associated with totally different consumption patterns' (Bourdieu [1984]2010: 173)? When this happens, there must be different mediating forces at work: specifically, those relating to the multifaceted and lifelong experience of the habitus (ibid.: 377). Consumer marketing profiles assess this in some detail as a purely commercial matter. But how can it be explained? Bourdieu locates the rationale in the concept of cultural capital, which might not equate to economic capital.

Cultural practices, including food consumption, are the result of both educational level and social origin or 'home background' – he uses both terms (Bourdieu [1984]2010: xxiv–xxv). They are both dimensions of the habitus, and are thus interconnected. Together, they lead to either conscious or unconscious – he allows for both – 'implementation of explicit or implicit schemes of perception and appreciation' (ibid.: xxv).

Skeggs has argued that conscious reflexivity is characteristic not of agents in general, nor of one entire class, but of one *section* of the middle class, for whom education and the habits of acquiring information, questioning received wisdom, and making changes are part of their habitus. Similarly, food marketers observe a middle class subgroup interested in healthy foods, while other high status eaters remain susceptible to what marketers call 'indulgent' foods (see Chapter 7). The nutrition-conscious group is only one middle class consumer group; others might have adequate financial capital, but perhaps less cultural or social capital in terms of seeking out a healthy diet.

Webber, who originated consumer profiling for market research purposes several decades ago, describes middle class metropolitan groups based on quantitative data. Some are broadly conscious of diet and exercise: 'City Adventurers' (young, white, well paid private sector employees) are notable for their well researched consumer decisions (Webber 2007: 191–6). 'New Urban Colonists' (university educated, often working in media/public policy) are interested in food and its provenance, going to 'considerable trouble to shop at upmarket supermarkets offering variety and freshness' (ibid.: 196). There is, he concludes, 'a habitus under which people tend to huddle with people they identify as being like themselves' (ibid.: 106).

A 2012 study linked food cultures, commercial marketing and health outcomes among African and Hispanic Americans. The authors use the term 'foodways' to describe the practices and environments resulting from 'generations-old food preferences, preparation styles, and eating patterns', but they also trace how marketing interacts with these practices (Williams *et al.* 2012: 385). They conclude that foodways 'operate at the intersection of culture, marketing, and health disparities' (ibid.). Culture predisposes people to dietary types; marketing interacts with cultures to construct and target products for consumer groups; and over time, states of health may be affected – negatively, in the case of those studied by Williams *et al.* (2012).

Backett-Milburn *et al.* (2010) describe one middle class group – and the process of dietary reflexivity – in their research with middle class Scottish families. Wills *et al.* (2011) illustrate how differently working class and middle class families eat, and the distinct levels of social, cultural and economic capital necessary for and resulting from these eating practices. They interpret their data in a Bourdieuan framework, finding limits to reflexivity for families from different social classes. They also identify the low priority accorded the eating habits of teenagers in disadvantaged families. These are important insights for understanding the health of contemporary teenagers. However, this kind of research can reveal only a fraction of what market research – via commercial data – can teach the food industry about all population groups by intensive, continual tracking of consumption behaviour in both daytime and residential neighbourhoods. So studying the power of this commercial data, and how *it* shapes food production and consumption, is also a sociological task.

How food is classed

Bourdieu distinguished between the status of different foods, as do consumers, whose preferences are both tracked and then reinforced by food product design and marketing; this process is observed from an industry perspective in Chapter 8. Statistical studies do not always assess food quality, instead quantifying production and consumption of commodities such as grain or cereals, not acknowledging the ways in which these raw materials might be processed and consumed by different social groups (Bourdieu [1984]2010: 192). Yet 'most products only derive their social value from the social use that is made of them' (ibid.: 13).

There is an echo of this in a study by Fine *et al.* (1998) of consumption patterns. Examining National Food Survey statistics, the authors found that those in lower socio-economic groups persistently purchased sausages, even though sausage consumption overall was declining at the time (although speciality sausages have since grown in popularity, targeting higher status consumers). When measuring declining consumption of a given food, it is worth noticing if one group is actually increasing their consumption of it (ibid.: 106).

Bourdieu makes a distinction between two generative, internalised dimensions of the habitus: 'the capacity to produce classifiable practices and works, and the capacity to differentiate and appreciate these practices and products' (Bourdieu [1984]2010: 166). This seems a crucial distinction and could work in two ways in the context of eating: both expanding one's diet to include new and interesting foods, and/or making judgements, both positive and negative, about the kind of foods other people eat and what those choices say about those people as exemplars of social groups. In the latter case it would be possible to identify one's diet with one's own social group, yet to be aware in general terms that others eat differently (whether better or worse).

Bourdieu is sometimes criticised for an overly deterministic view of human action as characterised by a habitus seen as largely inherited. But he allowed for acquired aspects of the habitus, which influence subsequent practice. He objected to the portrayal of social experience as mechanistic, experienced without cognition, but also rejected 'the illusion of the spontaneous generation of consciousness' (Bourdieu [1984]2010: 168). The force of the past remains strong: 'it is yesterday's man who inevitably predominates in us, since the present amounts to little compared with the long past in the course of which we were formed' (Bourdieu 1977 cited in Scambler 2002: 74).

A key distinction in food consumption relates to income differences, which masks a secondary distinction between cultural and economic capital (Bourdieu [1984]2010: 172). Income is not the only factor where diet is concerned, though income does determine 'distance from necessity' (ibid.: 173).

But in a broader sense, 'necessity' can be understood in non-financial ways. For Bourdieu, across all social classes, there is 'the same fundamental relationship to necessity and to those who remain subject to it' (ibid.: 172). Certain consumer items are as *socially* 'necessary', or natural, to higher status groups, as others are to lower status groups; higher status consumers may not, of course, 'need' what they buy for survival, but their choices flow from their inclinations and expectations, which are shaped by both their habitus and the consumer environment. These increasingly pervade and interact with that habitus, much as happens for other social groups. Food – and the places we buy food – are powerfully influenced not only by income but also questions of status. Chapter 8 investigates these matters in some detail.

But does status, or class, influence freedom of choice? A Bourdieuan analysis could not conclude that 'some actors have a much greater autonomy to construct their identities than others' (Bunton and Burrows 1995: 211). Williams (1995) suggests that both freedom and constraint are present in daily life, influencing health behaviour. But Kelly and Charlton (1995: 89) insist that 'either we are all free or we are all socially determined'. Bourdieu might put this differently: an implicit understanding of classificatory systems generates practices 'adjusted to the regularities inherent in a condition' (Bourdieu [1984]2010: 171). Thus constraints become preferences; in this way, 'an agent has what he likes because he likes what he has' in the context of 'the properties ... legitimately assigned to him in the classifications' (ibid.). People develop 'a taste for what is available to them' or even 'what they are anyway condemned to' in an interplay of habitus and capital (Williams 1995: 590; Bourdieu [1984]2010: 173). This is also Bourdieu's answer to what he calls 'class racism', which finds that lower social classes make 'uninspired choices' and are therefore getting 'only what they deserve' (Bourdieu [1984]2010: 173–5).

But it is possible to overstate the degree to which people like to eat what they can afford: low income shoppers interviewed about food purchases have expressed dissatisfaction with the limited options they face (Hitchman *et al.* 2002). Dowler (2003, 2008a, 2008b) also challenges the notion that only higher income eaters have high expectations of food, citing evidence of low income consumers who desire nutritious food and are interested in sustainability. A further study examines small direct producer–consumer businesses which also serve customers who are on low incomes and state benefits (Dowler *et al.* 2009).

At the very least, 'choice' can be 'a forced choice, produced by conditions of existence which rule out all alternatives as mere daydreams' (Bourdieu [1984]2010: 173). And at a deeper level, there is another explanation for the poor quality of foods apparently popular with low income groups: 'it is possible to deduce popular tastes for the foods that are simultaneously most "filling" and most economical from the necessity of reproducing labour power at the lowest cost' (Bourdieu [1984]2010: 173).

Bourdieu and embodiment

Though Giddens referred to bodily aspects of reflexivity, he saw this as a conscious process of monitoring and caring for one's body. Bourdieu, by contrast, observed that habitus was manifested mostly *un*consciously, in body shape, size, weight, posture and style of movement. Embodiment was central to habitus, which he once defined as 'the social game embodied and turned into a second nature' (Bourdieu 1994 cited in Laberge 2010: 774). The taste in food typical of each class was related to their idea of how food affected the body in terms of strength, attractiveness and health (Bourdieu [1984]2010: 187). Taste, therefore, helps to shape the body – both its outer form and its inner health: 'the body is the most indisputable materialization of class taste', and attitudes towards the body reflect the 'deepest dispositions of the habitus' (ibid.: 188).

Food, work and leisure all contribute to the formation and health of the body in a 'classed distribution of body properties' (Bourdieu [1984]2010: 188). Lupton describes how food and nutrition are inscribed on the body – in 'skin tone, weight, strength of bones, condition of hair and nails, digestion' (Lupton 2003: 44). But individuals are only 'quasi-conscious' of deeply held ideas about the 'approved form' of the body (ibid.). Nevertheless, collectively, 'a universe of class bodies tends to reproduce in its specific logic the universe of the social structure' – an embodied social structure (Bourdieu [1984]2010: 191). As bodies manifest their class position, habitus is the 'hinge between agency and structure' (Crossley 2005: 112).

Conclusion

Bourdieu has been a lasting influence on health and diet research, but while benefiting from his insights into how and why we eat the way we do, we should also consider the role of the food industry and food marketing, as key forces which interact with and shape the habitus throughout our lives. Through food product development, food processing, packaging, advertising and marketing campaigns and retailing strategies, a range of images, cues and practices are continually absorbed by the habitus, altering it over time. Tracing how this process works is the task of Chapters 6–8.

Habermas analyses how a range of systems including politics, liberal capitalism, technical progress and even marketing interact with the social worlds of individuals. His thought illuminates the apparently paradoxical situation in which a habitus seemingly set in a given social context can nevertheless, over time, engage in altered social practices, including diet, with implications for bodyweight and health.

Habermas and the colonisation of food lifeworlds

Jürgen Habermas traces system manipulations which alter the experience of the 'lifeworld' while ensuring that class divisions and even the language of class do not arise to challenge the legitimacy of governments or markets. Habermas's thinking about structural forces, social class and human action addresses gaps in both Giddens and Bourdieu and supplies insights into the influence of marketing in food consumption. His work on the role of technology in politics and social life was also an advancement on Giddens and Bourdieu and can be set in the context of food processing and marketing technologies. But how can Habermas's concepts of system, lifeworld, and the colonisation of the latter by the former, help us to understand class-differentiated, diet-related health?

For Habermas, the lifeworld is intuitive, taken for granted; 'a complex world of practices and customs as well as ideas' (Outhwaite 1996: 117). The ethical dimension of the lifeworld is constituted by an idea of the good life, and any questions about the good life 'have *always already been answered*', as individuals perform duties which are 'inextricably tied to concrete habitual behaviour' (Habermas [1983]1996: 190; author's emphasis). Such understandings are cultural, given and unproblematic.

The lifeworld bears some resemblance to Bourdieu's habitus, and even to Giddens's acknowledgement of the unconscious or programmed nature of social action stemming from accumulated life histories (though he would ultimately conceive of social action as primarily a reflexive process).

However, the lifeworld is arguably seen more in the context of the present than the past, and in its broader societal dimension; it acknowledges that external forces and messages are absorbed into our lives. It is also centrally concerned with language in the form of what Habermas terms communicative action.

The structural influences flowing from market and administrative systems may not be *consciously* experienced by individuals in their lifeworlds; nevertheless they are present, and real. It is these potentially distorting influences on the lifeworld as it is 'colonised' that Habermas emphasises, rather than the continuities and coherence of the habitus as described by Bourdieu.

In liberal capitalism, the 'fusion of validity and social acceptance' characteristic of traditional lifeworlds sooner or later disintegrates (Habermas [1983]1996: 191). This process is arguably at work in the transformation of diets and their 'colonisation' by processed foods of varying types and quality, along with highly technical forms of food preparation in the home and even food technology training in schools. Such developments have an imposed, unreflective quality to them.

Lifeworlds are structured and experienced through language. A tacit acceptance of the daily experience of the lifeworld is expressed in terms which are shared among lifeworld participants. Communication would be meaningless and even impossible without these shared understandings and vocabularies (Habermas [1985]1996: 358). It is this role for shared language and understanding which skilled marketing seeks to tap into, building on existing tastes and concepts to introduce product innovations. At the same time, the discourses of healthy eating and individual responsibility for health are absorbed into the lifeworlds of those at whom such discourses are targeted.

But we only really become aware of our own lifeworlds when challenges arise which threaten their continued existence. Until that point, our lifeworlds are experienced as intuitive and unproblematic, but lifeworlds can fall apart (Habermas [1981]1996: 331). When this happens, we experience disintegration as aspects of the lifeworld are colonised by forces outside it. Societal developments regularly prompt such 'provocative threats' to the lifeworld (ibid.: 334). As problems make themselves felt, 'relevant components of such background knowledge are torn out of their unquestioned familiarity and brought to consciousness' (ibid.: 331). Then, ideally, 'processes of unlearning' can reveal how the lifeworld has been deformed (ibid.). Where food consumption is concerned, we would, in this scenario, become aware of the ways in which our food 'lifeworld' is constructed for and presented to us, and begin to see the forces and strategies behind it. Then we would be motivated to test alternatives to it by altering our previous, normal, unconscious routines. But what are the obstacles to this process?

A limited reflexivity

Food provision, whether at home, school, work or in leisure time outside these contexts, changes constantly, though with elements of continuity. Over time, new products and formats are introduced which build on our existing consumption, and we absorb these into our dietary practices or patterns. While health educators and alert consumers might perceive as a 'provocative threat' a drink like Sunny Delight, marketed as orange juice but in fact containing little juice and much sugar and water, it was initially successful with children and some consumer groups (BBC 2003). Because the low juice content was not highlighted (though it was on the label), and it was stocked in refrigerated cabinets (though it did not need to be), the product appealed to some parents as a fresh juice. Soon, however, the low juice/high sugar content became known, as well as the case of one child whose skin took on an orange tint after drinking large quantities of the beverage. Sales quickly declined (though Sunny Delight was later reformulated and remarketed) (BBC 2011a).

A degree of 'reflexivity' may take place when a product like this enters the market and is made known to its target consumers. The latter see it in a magazine or a TV advert, and it is made clear that this is a drink for people like them; families like theirs. Next time they are in a store selling it, they will, as a result, be 'primed' to notice it by its careful aisle and shelf placement, possibly with a price promotion, and – hopefully, for the manufacturer and retailer – purchase it. Reactions in the ever shifting consumer landscape take place with varying degrees of consciousness, related to lifelong habitus, including differing stocks of information capital which may be insufficient to prevent the lifeworld from being colonised by such tactics.

In short, some agents *do* have the capacity to reflect and make choices on the basis of thoughtful, critical reflection, some possess this capacity in some domains of choice and action, but not in others, and some do not possess it in any great degree.

Habermas's theory accounts for these variations by distinguishing between a cultural tradition which constitutes the lifeworld of a community and is experienced by individuals as pre-interpreted, and, alternatively, one which fosters among its members 'a reflective attitude toward cultural patterns of interpretation' (Habermas [1981]1996: 133). This is a distinction noted earlier by Skeggs, who observes the latter in some sections of the middle class. For Habermas, this reflective attitude happens when people are able to grasp 'information about lawlike connections' which have ideological underpinnings; this can begin to transform the 'unreflected consciousness' (Habermas [1968]1996: 99). Unmediated, unmanipulated communication is required for this to happen – but that is not always what we get when food is marketed or advertised to us. The lack of such communication can prevent a cognitive grasp of something that is hidden for strategic reasons. This is how the lifeworld is colonised – and distorted.

Giddens's thinking on reflexivity does not seem to acknowledge such distortion, and the resulting variable access to reflexivity. But the capacity for reflection is linked to an individual's knowledge and interests as constituted by the cultural tradition and social group inhabited by the individual; it must, therefore, be available to some groups, but not others, depending on the social constraints and influences – shared with others like them – inherent in one's habitus and lifeworld. Marmot, a leading epidemiologist, acknowledged this when he described the role 'for health and longevity of people's assessments of their placement and accomplishments *relative to those with whom they share their lifeworlds*' (Marmot 2006 cited in Scambler and Scambler 2013: 94, author's wording and emphasis).

Capitalism, the welfare state and the lifeworld

At one time, the lifeworld would have been a complete entity or structure, bounded by the practices and experiences of the social or cultural group. But as society developed, economic and administrative structures emerged which were distinct from those more indigenous structures and practices which previously governed the group. In this process, a pivotal point in human development is when the lifeworld is relieved of 'the tasks of material reproduction' (Habermas [1981]1996: 316), such as growing food. Even long after this point, the growing amounts of prepared and convenience foods throughout the twentieth century dramatically altered the lifeworlds of families.

With the emergence of capitalism, the economy rather than the state comes to attain primacy (ibid.). New structures emerge which Habermas calls the 'system'; he describes at length 'the uncoupling' of system from lifeworld and the dislocating effects of this process for our previous understanding of social classes:

> a class structure shifted out of the lifeworld into the system loses its historically palpable shape. The unequal distribution of social rewards reflects a structure of privilege that can no longer be traced back to class positions in any unqualified way ... The more the class conflict that is built into society through the private economic form of accumulation can be dammed up and kept latent, the more problems come to the fore that do not *directly* violate interest positions ascribable on a class-specific basis. (Habermas [1981]1996: 289)

So capitalism is able to 'use' the uncoupling of system and lifeworld to deflect attention from inequalities inherent in a capitalist system and from the very notion of classes themselves (Habermas [1981]1996: 288). Thus late modern capitalism has flourished alongside 'welfare state pacification of class conflict', in which conflicts regarding distribution of resources 'lose their explosive power' (ibid.: 288–9). The post-traditional 'classes' we are left with, then, are not what they were in previous societies.

The key difference is the intention that the welfare state 'intercepts the dysfunctional side effects of the economic process and renders them harm-less for the individual'; this is part of what weakens class identities (Habermas [1976]1996: 257). So monetary and housing benefits payments are available to those judged in need of them, for example (though such judgements have now, controversially, been reconsidered; these judgements have been harmful to some). Public healthcare, education and pensions additionally relieve the private (capitalist) economy of the responsibility for addressing these needs, and aim to lift all citizens out of the worst sufferings of pre-welfare eras (Habermas [1981]1996: 287).

Habermas traces the uncoupling of system from lifeworld without eluci-dating the implications for different social classes. Indeed, this uncoupling process is what makes it possible for class-based effects to be less obvious, while still deeply entrenched. But sociological debates over what consti-tutes class, and critiques of basing 'class' divisions on occupation, educa-tion or income, miss the point from a Habermasian perspective: these measurements are simply part of what has enabled the state to address the needs of those judged to be 'in need', so that they do not undermine the forces of capital and the wider social stability necessary for capital to flourish.

However, Scambler finds that Habermas has 'too hastily discarded a Marxian insistence on the continuing significance of relations of class' and the role of power elites in the uncoupling of system and lifeworld. For Scambler, class relations 'effectively underwrite' health inequalities (Scambler 2001: 87, 105, 108). Nevertheless, Habermas's understanding of the interplay between knowledge and interests, and how they influence capacities for reflection, reveals a differentiated social process resulting from lifeworld experiences and varying degrees of accumulated expertise.

Economy, state and lifeworld

While economic prosperity and the compensations of the welfare state may have blurred traditional understandings and experiences of social class, they have not removed status-related groupings, with some groups chronically lacking social, educational, occupational or economic power, capital or capability to transcend these deficits. This phenomenon is the result of an 'indissoluble tension' between capitalism and democracy itself, in which 'the propelling mechanism of the economic system has to be kept as free as possible from lifeworld restrictions as well as from the demands for legitimation directed to the administrative system' (Habermas [1981]1996: 285). In this view, capitalism and democracy are contrary systems which 'thwart and paralyze each other' (Offe 1984 cited by Habermas [1981]1996: 286).

This contrariness is detectable in the Coalition government's decision in 2010 to invite the food industry to fund health promotion campaigns, though the government would eventually resume its own contributions.[2] This was portrayed as placing some responsibility for dietary health on the industry's shoulders while avoiding further regulation. The language used by the food industry to communicate this point parallels that of health promotion discourse, described by one sociologist as being 'shot through with ... a language of choice – [insisting] that individuals have control over their health choices', and deflecting a focus on structural influences on health and 'choices' (Webster 2007: 96).

Technology, democracy and lifeworld

In *Toward a Rational Society* (1987), Habermas focused on the relationship between technology and the lifeworld in a way that is useful for examining the role of technology in dietary patterns. He included in his concept of technology manufacturing, management and administration but also – presciently – 'the manipulation of electoral, consumer, or leisure-time behavior' (ibid.: 55).

Challenging the notion of an unpoliticised and pure science, from which technology proceeds, he finds that instead, technological development often conceals 'unreflected social interests and pre-scientific decisions' (Habermas 1987: 59). So 'how can the relation between technical progress and the social life-world ... be reflected upon and brought under the control of rational discussion?' (ibid.: 53).

He distinguished between the 'capacity for control made possible by the empirical sciences' and the capacity for 'enlightened action' (Habermas 1987: 56). Thus his question becomes: 'how can the power of technical control be brought within the range of the consensus of acting and transacting citizens?' (ibid.: 47). There are two key problems: first, technological development often leads to unanticipated applications, with unacknowledged implications for the lifeworld; and second, achieving consensus among these 'acting and transacting citizens' requires a communicative openness and 'the redeeming power of reflection'. Mere technical knowledge is not the same thing (ibid.: 57–61). And there are many obstacles in the way of this communicative openness, as Habermas terms it.

Another problem is that political leaders have ceded power to science and technology (Habermas 1987: 64). This is reflected in the lack of political leadership in banking regulation, in part because the financial instruments which led to the 2008 credit crunch were beyond the comprehension of politicians and possibly even regulators (and indeed, some bankers). A broad parallel can be drawn with the food industry, where levels of both scientific and technical information regarding nutrition and technologies that process, site and market food operate at high levels of sophistication and complexity which may not be grasped by either politicians or consumers. With the construction (via food chemistry and the psychology of consumption) and marketing of food products high in fat, salt and sugar, and food industry colonisation of health promotion discourse, the public can be influenced in potentially distorting ways. The application of scientific information in strategic contexts (such as food or drug marketing) itself can contribute to 'a deformed public realm' (Lubbe 1962 cited in Habermas 1987: 70).

For Habermas, the conflict that has arisen between scientific progress and democratic decision-making prevents the realisation of 'the associated material and intellectual productive forces in the interest of the enjoyment and freedom of an emancipated society' (ibid.: 58). Instead, technical progress takes place 'without being reflected upon' in the reproduction of social life (Habermas 1987: 60). The result is that 'new technical capacities erupt without preparation into existing forms of life-activity and conduct' (ibid.). This is one answer to Giddens's critique of the 'absent core' in Habermas which, for Giddens, left the reproduction of social life unexplained (Giddens 1995: 256). The idea is developed more recently by Johnson as 'the adjacent possible' – the unanticipated results of continual scientific/technological developments ultimately resulting in major social change (Johnson 2010; discussed again in Chapter 6). Habermas sees dangers in this process.

What is the solution? Habermas finds an essential role for a 'politically effective discussion that rationally brings the social potential constituted by technical knowledge and ability into a defined and controlled relation to our practical knowledge and will' (Habermas 1987: 61). Only in this way can people become aware of the underlying interests at work, and decide how technical knowledge is to be developed in future (ibid.). Thus technical progress must be endowed with political consciousness; only then can its relation with the lifeworld be a legitimate one (ibid.). But this kind of discussion is difficult to achieve when there are powerful commercial and political forces shaping it.

The manipulation of communication

Habermas situates his analysis of economy and society in terms of how the lifeworld is affected and even distorted by developments in late modern capitalism. In this process the systems that intrude on the lifeworld become anchored and eventually institutionalised within it (Habermas [1981]1996: 279). Both state and market systems alter the character of the lifeworld in ways that cannot be mended by welfare state compensations, Habermas argues. Any negative impacts upon the lifeworld must be hidden, which invites distortion, deception and a reliance on false consciousness (ibid.: 282). In this context, 'communicative actions are increasingly detached from normative contexts' (ibid.: 292).

These negative impacts must be hidden because governments must foster economic growth, ensure that processes of production address collective needs, and initiate social reforms to address the destabilisation and inequalities inherent in capitalist growth (Habermas [1976]1996: 258–59). But it must carry out the latter while not risking further problems in the economy – 'without violating the complementarity relations that exclude the state from the economic system' and yet which render it dependent on the well functioning of that system (ibid.: 258). Thus the state must use subversive techniques such as manipulation and 'indirect control', with all the disadvantages these terms imply (ibid.: 259). The state will try to conceal the close relations it has with the capitalist economy, while convincing us that capitalism is, nevertheless, the best way of satisfying 'generalizable interests' (ibid.). This might describe the broadly neoliberal approach of successive UK governments in recent decades as they sought to allow 'the market' the freedom it wished to expand and grow.

Habermas is sometimes criticised for an idealistic view of the potential for public communicative democracy. Only emancipated societies could engender 'non-authoritarian and universally practiced dialogue', leading to true consensus (Habermas [1968]1996: 102). Yet an open, rigorous pursuit of knowledge and understanding confronts many obstacles, even in supposedly emancipated societies. This problem contributed to the rise of critical discourse analysis, which aims to reveal the deficits in modern democracies by analysing what discourses conceal.

But Habermas's idealistic notions still constitute a useful standard for clear, transparent communication and informed public debate. Habermas decried the 'staged or manipulated publicity' which takes the place of true debate and information-sharing (Habermas [1969]1996: 29), and which we sometimes see reflected in the language and tactics of marketing and advertising, as well as political discourse. In opposition to the conformity and submission cultivated by both the welfare state and market forces, he believed autonomous public spheres should be fostered, with greater citizen participation and restrictions on the media (Outhwaite 1996: 217). By comparison, the mediatised public debate on many issues of late modernity, taking place within a weakened public sphere and influenced by the media's own ideological/financial interests (Habermas [1962]1989: 29), falls very short of what we should be aiming for. For example, Scambler and Scambler critique policies to address health inequalities in a Habermasian framework, arguing that they represent

> forms of distorted, or systematically distorted, communication. In other words, they are primarily strategic: it is more important politically that they demonstrate a 'compassionate', legitimating and vote-culling responsiveness to the lifeworld than that they actually reduce health inequalities. (Scambler and Scambler 2013: 96)

How have such communicative distortions happened? For Habermas, the public sphere has been weakened by the rise of 'societal organisations' which are economic in nature, but different from those owned by individual autonomous owners or property holders in the past. The organisations which have replaced such private individuals must 'obtain and defend a private status granted to them by social legislation', defending 'private autonomy by means of political autonomy' (Habermas [1969]1996: 28). In this process, organisations must negotiate with the state, 'as much as possible to the exclusion of the public' (ibid.: 29). Periodically, contentious issues must be resolved and in the political arena, elections must be held. Yet even in these processes, information and communication takes the form of 'staged or manipulated publicity' (ibid.).

Alongside this development stands the state's commitment to social welfare. But there is no possibility of open public communication regarding social policies because there are no unmediated channels or forms of communication left; any debate that does emerge is influenced by 'the very organizations that mediatize it' (Habermas [1969]1996: 29).

Citizen and consumer

As clients of the state, we are in receipt of benefits or services, but this is split off from the citizen's potential for political participation; similarly, the alienation of labour is alleviated as labourers become consumers (Habermas [1981]1996: 290). The compensations of a prospering economy are redistributed in some degree by the state and 'channelled into the roles of consumer and client'; private households become units of mass consumption (ibid.: 291). This is a systematised form of material reproduction of the lifeworld, with food production, for example, taken out of the hands of individual households. This process, while natural and beneficial in many ways, can engender 'pathologies in the lifeworld' (ibid.: 317). The changes in diet in recent decades and the omnipresence of non-nutritious food arguably constitute just such a 'pathology'; a radical redesigning of the food supply with implications for public health.

Habermas did not theorise food consumption, but he acknowledges the rise of the consumer in the context of the compromises of the welfare state, which alter the relationships between system and lifeworld, and therefore the roles we all have as employees, clients of the state, citizens – and consumers (Habermas [1981]1996: 289). This still results in alienation, which Marx associated with industrialisation, but it is of a different order (ibid.).

In the highly empirical world of food production, processing, distribution, consumption and regulation, we can see how these developments are manifested: the individual farmers of the past are the agribusinesses of the present, often subsidised in distorting ways by governments; the small grocers of traditional societies are today's large food retailers; the bakers or butchers are the food processing conglomerates (though small specialist food shops catering to a high status clientele continue to flourish, under-scoring the 'classing' of food discussed subsequently).

Collectively, large food production/retail organisations are significant employers and major economic forces. They are regulated by government agencies, with the usual concerns about regulatory capture which have been identified in late modernity in various domains.[3] In the case of the UK's Food Standards Agency (FSA), the White Paper which established it in 2000 proposed that the board should include those with a food industry background, with the proviso that their interests should be declared (Millstone and Lang 2008: 94). Gradually the number of such board members increased until a 'preponderance' of them had food industry interests (ibid.: 95).

Alongside food producers and retailers, promotional organisations have emerged to inform us which foods are available where, and to present them to us in ways which appeal to our emotions and lifeworlds. Alongside these in turn are state organisations/campaigns which encourage healthful eating, an idea co-opted by the food industry and its promotional operations, which can distort the legitimacy of public health advice (Herrick 2009). In Chapter 6, marketing research into the paradoxical effect of low fat foods marketed alongside health images is discussed: essentially, people tend to *over*consume these foods *because* they are described as low fat, and this may contribute to weight gain.

Foodscape and lifeworld

To bolster market research, firms have emerged which track our purchases quantitatively, interview consumers for qualitative insights, and advise client firms where to site their products. These organisational activities shape the nature and location of food retail outlets. The surrounding food-scape on high streets and other public spaces is constituted by growing numbers of fast food outlets. This expanding foodscape was quantified in a Canadian context, where it was interpreted as an illustration of the 'hyper colonization by pseudo food corporations of the wider societal foodscape' (Winson 2004: 308; he defines pseudo foods as those high in fat and sugar but low in nutrients including 'protein, minerals and vitamins' (ibid.: 302)). Yet the obesogenic foodscape in which we live retains what Habermas might call the 'subjective and accidental character of uncomprehended events' (Habermas [1981]1996: 312). Constantly spreading into previously non-food areas, it is arguably not fully grasped by anyone – not by research-ers, not by public health experts, nor governments. As the concept of the foodscape has been raised repeatedly in this book, and can be interpreted as a key and evolving feature of the lifeworld, it is worth investigating in more detail in the present discussion.

In the introductory chapter, I noted the use of the term by Winson (2004). He defined the foodscape as 'the multiplicity of sites where food is displayed for purchase, and where it may also be consumed' (Winson 2004: 301). He lists its differing manifestations in supermarket chains, fast food outlets, independent supermarkets, restaurants, speciality food shops, local (though increasingly corporate-controlled) convenience stores, farmers' markets and street food (ibid.: 302). But the list is not and cannot be exhaustive, as the foodscape is constantly expanding, a theme explored in Chapters 6–8. Winson also notes the expansion of corporate food into public spaces such as hospitals, schools and transport hubs.

By 2011, Mikkelson describes 'foodscape studies' as a vital tool 'to improve our understanding of the impact of food environments on our behaviour' (Mikkelson 2011: 206). The foodscape has two 'trajectories': the commercial, encountered in food service outlets, and the 'public yet captive trajectory that we meet in schools, hospitals and workplaces' (ibid.). Methodologies for tracking what is going on in the foodscape, including ethnography, photography and GIS (geographic information systems) are continually improving (see Chapters 6–8).

Most academic studies of the foodscape have been qualitative but Mikkelson finds scope for quantitative research in identifying determinants and predicting behaviour (ibid.). However, quantitative research which could track the rate and type of expansion of the food supply in all its dimensions is still lacking. I note dimensions of its expansion in London, where the increase in vending machines and hutch-style food outlets in public spaces and non-food shops which did not previously have them has been striking in recent years (see Chapters 6–8). There are also examples of fast food companies announcing expansion plans. But these are random samples of an observed phenomenon which has not yet been accurately tracked in its totality (though food company and market research firms doubtless possess much relevant data). Such data would provide useful insights into the relationship between an increase in the food supply and food consumption patterns. The presentation of food provides the visual cues for the desire for foods so vital to their purchase, as described in discussions of psychology and food marketing in Chapters 7 and 8. If the food supply is expanding, how can the voluntary effort by food providers to reduce the calorie content of food be assessed? Increasing the number of food outlets and displays expands the cues or 'nudges' to purchase; such 'nudging' is a strategy long pursued by food marketers, as they acknowledge (see Chapter 1).

In Habermasian terms, the expansion of the foodscape, especially by foods high in fat, salt and sugar into previously non-food spaces, is one way in which food lifeworlds can be colonised.

Resisting lifeworld colonisation

Following the original dislocating experience of lifeworld colonisation, and the absorption of these dislocations into the lifeworld, how can people perceive the activities or effects of systems which have become so embedded that their origins or predecessors are forgotten? How can they become conscious of these distorting systems, communicate about them, or seek to change them? The deception inherent in these systems engenders *self-deception*, which 'can gain an objective power in an everyday practice' (Habermas [1981]1996: 313). The issue then becomes how to defend and restore 'endangered ways of life' (ibid.: 323).

Attempts to colonise the lifeworld have not gone unchallenged. In *The Theory of Communicative Action*, Habermas traced the 'revaluation of ... decentralized forms of commerce ... [which are] meant to foster the revitalization of possibilities for expression and communication which have been buried alive' (Habermas [1981]1996: 326). He lists social movements during the past 200 years which were a response to attempts to colonise the lifeworld (ibid.: 325). In the context of food, the popularity of organic foods, farmers' markets, box delivery schemes, local food movements, anti-GM protests, the campaign to improve school meals, some academic research and an array of popular books critiquing the food industry can all be seen as challenges to the colonisation of food lifeworlds by agribusiness and corporate food retailing.

Those who challenge supermarket/food industry provision have become, in Habermasian terms, 'drastically aware of standards of liveability, of inflexible limits to the deprivation of sensual-aesthetic background needs' (Habermas [1981]1996: 325). This notion of how colonisation of the lifeworld can be resisted recalls Foucault's idea that even a dominant discourse does not block out opposing voices, but can actually give rise to them. The image of the lifeworld penetrated by systems which create a degree of dissonance sufficient to provoke opposition illustrates how even hegemonic discourses can be opposed and, over time, their hold weakened. However, alternatives to supermarkets and processed foods remain minor players in overall food consumption and can themselves be colonised as emerging trends with sales potential (see Chapter 6).

Conclusion

In theorising health inequalities, no new theory is required, but rather a 'reflexive revisiting of what is already known'; in other words, 'meta-reflections, or thoughtful, independent-minded and critical reassessments of the received theoretical and empirical wisdom delivered by today's dominant paradigm' (Scambler and Scambler 2013: 99). In this and the foregoing chapter, I have attempted to do just this, testing differing theories of class, human agency, consciousness and consumption in the context of food consumption and its implications for health and society.

In sifting through theoretical perspectives to illuminate understandings of food consumption, that of Giddens offered much insight into the process of human consciousness, but did not consider the structuring power of food production, though he acknowledged the 'forces of commodification' in shaping consumption in general (Giddens 1994: 101). The food industry and food marketing are key influences, alongside class, on individual 'choice', even if we are not aware of their activities, hence unable to engage with them with full, conscious reflexivity.

Giddens's ideas arguably lend weight to the lifestyles/personal responsibility discourse without illuminating the underlying structural and psychosocial reality. For a more nuanced picture, which considers the roles of social class and habit, and how habitual behaviour can be altered, Bourdieu's and Habermas's ideas of habitus and lifeworld respectively provided greater depth of analysis. Habermas's theorising of the colonisation by distorting, disembedding forces can be set and tested in the context of health, food production and consumption, and social inequality.

Bourdieu's theoretical work was closely linked to his empirical investigations of how people of differing social backgrounds live, eat and work, and the ways in which our food practices throughout life are shaped by our social and geographic environments. Habermas revealed the power of manipulation and the linked role of technology in distorting the clear communication of information as this would unfold in an ideal democracy, although he was more focused on manipulation by the state than by capital. Nevertheless, his ideas come closest to theorising the power of marketing and help to explain the paradox in which a society which insists on individual responsibility for diet and health is also able to trace food consumption patterns and their bodyweight and health consequences via social strata amid a dramatically altered food supply in recent decades. In focusing on the distorting effect of manipulated communication, Habermas's work also serves to guide us to critical discourse analysis to uncover how this might be happening with diet.

In the debate over the nature of social class, including conflicts over the term itself and even dismissal of the concept of class, perhaps the one that best articulates the way ahead for consumption and health research is a definition of habitus proposed by Atkinson:

> the complex of durable cognitive and corporeal dispositions, tastes and schemes of perception possessed by each agent ... generated out of the particular class of conditions of existence ... associated with one's relative position in social space as measured by the level of economic and cultural capital they hold. Those possessing similar levels and types of capital are subject to similar conditions of existence and, therefore, possess similar habitus and lifestyles. (Atkinson 2007: 545)

This definition takes in the role of cultural practices as well as economic and social resources and constraints, and outlines one vision of what class has become, how it is produced in a neoliberal age, and how it can lead to inequalities. In subsequent chapters Atkinson's definition will be uncannily reflected in marketing and food science analyses of how tastes and consumption patterns are formed. But food marketing *itself* is part of what shapes our habitus, a constant background influence on our tastes and perceptions. From the location of the food supply to its promotion and styling, it is aimed at social groups in different ways.

Shared social backgrounds, resources and conditions of existence – even inequality itself – are all functions of the role of capital in consumption and governance, influencing the degree of both receptivity and exposure to certain types of information, and the varying capacity of individuals and groups to use that information to change their lives. In this sense, socio-economic status is not merely a way of measuring social class effects; it is a *product* of social class, which in turn is a product of capital and those who control and regulate it in a political and global context (to paraphrase Scambler 2012, citing Coburn 2009).

An exploration of the theoretical basis for this claim underlies the challenge to explanations of individual responsibility for one's social position, development and achievements (Savage 2000: 44); it is also resonant in the context of healthy eating discourse, in which the term 'choice' is prominent and people are urged – for the most part, ineffectively – to adopt a healthy diet.

How can researchers seek out mechanisms which help to explain 'not only capitalism's deepest contradictions but the contradictory ways in which different classes, groups and individuals understand, forage and subsist in its lifeworlds' (Scambler and Scambler 2013: 92)? In the present research, the next step is to examine the empirical evidence for the diet–class–health link, the subject of the following chapter. Examples are also given of academic research which finds an audience beyond the academy and reinforces the predominant individual responsibility discourse where diet is concerned, influencing both public policy and public understanding.

In later chapters, the food industry's attempts, via market research, food product development, and food marketing, to segment and serve distinct consumption patterns will be described. In this way, the effects of both the 'demand' side via food consumption, and its 'supply' side via production by the food industry – and the ways in which they interact – can be explored and brought together.

Notes

1 *Distinction* was first published in English in 1984. The 2010 edition cited here uses the same translation but a new introduction.
2 'Lansley said that big food and drinks companies would not face new regulation in return for helping meet the cost of Change4Life, the biggest ever healthy eating and fitness campaign' (*Guardian* 30/12/10; also see *Observer* 24/04/11). Government funding later resumed, and a firm which also promotes snack foods and soft drinks was hired to promote Change4Life (*Guardian* 20/12/11).

Change4Life's The Great Swapathon allowed shoppers to exchange vouchers for food items promoted as healthier choices (www.change4lifewm.org.uk/resources/The_Great_Swapathon_Resource.pdf).

3 For example, a firm lobbying on behalf of agribusiness in favour of GM foods was found to have made changes to a draft report by the government's food regulatory body, the Food Standards Agency (*Observer* 06/06/10). These changes influenced the final report, describing the role for GM foods in keeping food prices down. Two food regulators subsequently resigned, criticising the close relationship between the FSA and the lobbying firm. This was a case of regulatory capture, although these two regulators had resisted capture themselves.

5 The evidence for a diet–health–class link

Introduction

In challenging the personal choice/individual responsibility discourse where diet is concerned, various social theories have illuminated the role of social class in shaping patterns of food consumption, and the intricate relationship between state, capital, food producers/marketers, and the shaping of individual lifeworlds. Widely varying capabilities, resources and behaviours result from these interacting influences.

What is the outcome for health? In general terms, socio-economic position 'shapes people's experience of and exposure to virtually all psycho-social and environmental risk factors for health – past, present and future' (House and Williams 2000 cited in Graham 2007: 112). More particularly:

> Poor diet is known to influence the risk of cancer, heart disease and other conditions ... around 70,000 fewer people would die prematurely each year in the UK if diets matched the national guidelines on fruit and vegetable consumption, and saturated fat, sugar and salt intake. (Cabinet Office 2008: ES.11)

In this chapter many studies of food consumption, its interaction with social class and its impact on health are investigated.

Because the relationship between obesity and health risk has dominated discourses regarding food consumption in both the media and public policy, I focus initially on the evidence for the obesity–health link, as well as the social gradient for obesity. However, non-obese diet-related health problems and the social gradient of such outcomes will also be examined.

Some academic research has crossed over to a wider audience via popular books and widespread media coverage, such as that by Christakis and Fowler and their work linking obesity to social networks. It and other popular/academic works such as *Nudge* by Thaler and Sunstein (2009; see Chapter 1), and a popular but highly ideological review of academic research on social behaviour by Brooks (2011) have all been embraced by British politicians and, as cited in Chapter 1, even the Department of Health itself.

They are clearly an influence on public policy and as such merit discussion in the present context.

Finally, research in an international context showing links between political ideology, history and health outcomes is cited here for its capacity to challenge the individual responsibility discourse by revealing underlying structural factors. This chapter, then, gives a comprehensive empirical grounding to the foregoing theoretical insights and challenges the discourse of healthy eating as a matter of individual responsibility by making clear the ideological and class-mediated nature of food consumption patterns.

While there is a strong relationship between obesity and deprivation, obesity is significantly present in all social classes, according to various measurements, including the National Obesity Observatory (NOO 2010). As Skeggs proposed, reflexivity is characteristic of only a section of the population – indeed, only a section of the middle class. In subsequent chapters, food marketers describe the conflicted nature of affluent consumers, who say they are interested in healthy eating, but also consume 'indulgent' foods (marketing-speak for foods high in fat, salt and sugar (HFSS)). Along the lines of Skeggs's proposition, marketers identify only a subset of consistent health-seeking behaviour.

Many studies cited in this chapter speak uncritically of measuring reported food intake, bodyweight, body mass, exercise levels, levels of body fat, blood sugar, blood lipids, etc. Some sociologists have critiqued these approaches, building on Foucault's analysis of surveillance and the clinical gaze (Annandale 1998); sociologists who challenge obesity discourse do so forcefully. Clinical assessment and categorisation by bodyweight can be viewed and experienced as intrusive. New technologies which bypass the need for sometimes unreliable subject reporting of food intake will only strengthen these critiques. While acknowledging the validity of these critiques, it is not possible to enter into a discussion of public health surveillance of food consumption in this book, for reasons of space and remit. However, it is reflected in my analysis of the obesity critique.

Although much research continues to be devoted to detecting the biological pathways for illnesses which might be diet related, a growing resistance to the association between obesity and ill health has been mounted by sociologists. The discourse of obesity as a health risk is pervasive; it dominates health discourse in the media and in politics. But if there are truly gaps in the evidence base, as some critics allege (Rich *et al.* 2011, Monaghan 2005, Aphramor 2005, Rich and Evans 2005, Jutel 2006), then this needs to be addressed at the outset.

Challenging the weight–health link

The challenge posed by these researchers takes place in the context of an emerging size acceptance movement, both inside and outside of the academy. This movement mobilises efforts to defend fat people against stigma and discrimination, critiques the manipulations of the weight-loss industry and develops the idea of fatness as a legitimate choice and bodily experience. Two British sociologists argued this case eloquently at the 2011 British Sociology Association conference (White 2011; Cooper 2011). A number of books on the subject indicate the popularity of this critique (Bacon 2008; Harding and Kirby 2009; Wann 1998; Braziel and LeBesco 2001; Gaesser 2002; Campos 2004; Bovey 2000; Cooper 1998).

Even among those who acknowledge the validity of obesity health warnings, some concede that 'strategies for dealing with it [the obesity epidemic] are not working and may be counterproductive' (Blair, unnumbered introductory page, endorsing Bacon 2008). Blair, a professor of public health and preventive cardiology, suggests size acceptance might be more effective, alongside exercise and healthier diets.

Monaghan, a sociologist, questions warnings of the dangers of overweight and obesity, believing them to be the result of the social construction of fatness as a public health issue (Monaghan 2005: 303). He is highly critical of the crisis nature of the discourse, which 'legitimates potentially harmful calls to action' (ibid.: 304).

Monaghan detects a misuse of power, both by medicine and the weight-loss industry, with its gym memberships, low fat foods and diet clubs; together they have a vested interest in continued warnings of the health risks of obesity (Monaghan 2005: 312). It is a significant industry in the UK, worth £3.92 billion by March 2013, with a membership of 7.9 million; growth has been steady in recent years (Leisure Database Company 2013). Recent guidance from NICE recommended a range of 'behavioural weight management programmes', including commercial ones, with the caveat that they should be based on a healthy diet, exercise and moderate rate of weight loss (NICE 2014a). Under the rubric of 'lifestyle weight management' guidance, healthcare professionals have a role in assessing this and making referrals to appropriate groups or organisations (NICE 2014b).[1] Yet between one-third and two-thirds of dieters more than regain the weight they have lost, according to a 2007 review of long-term studies (Mann *et al.* 2007; actual regaining rates may be even higher since studies tend to be biased towards weight-loss maintenance).

Monaghan does not mention the use of drugs to treat obesity, yet this, too, has been a notable trend:

> In 2006, 1.06 million prescription items were dispensed for the treatment of obesity ... more than eight times the number prescribed in 1999 ... In 2006, around 73% of prescriptions were for Orlistat and 25% prescriptions were for Sibutramine, the two main drugs used for treatment of obesity. (NHS 2008: iii)

That increase in prescriptions since 1999 was rather steeper than the rate of increase in obesity, which raises the questions about whether these drugs work.

If so, why hasn't obesity decreased and why are obesity-related diseases predicted to continue to increase? Were the drugs being overprescribed? In fact the prescribing trend subsequently changed, decreasing for the first time in seven years (by 24 per cent) between 2009 and 2010. This probably reflects the withdrawal of two obesity drugs, Sibutramine and Rimonabant, by European regulators, following concerns over an increased risk of heart attacks and strokes (NHS 2012: 52).

Bariatric surgery as an obesity treatment has also increased, nearly doubling from just over 4,200 procedures in 2008/09 to just over 8,000 in 2010/11 (NCEPOD 2012: 5); it could now also be available for obese people with Type 2 diabetes following proposals by NICE (NICE 2014e).

Yet Monaghan points out weaknesses in the research on which health warnings over obesity rest, concluding that the science on disease–weight links is equivocal (Monaghan 2005: 204). Given increased life expectancy during the past 30 years in many developed countries, a period in which overweight and obesity increased dramatically, populations are living longer on the whole – and longer than leaner people did 30-plus years ago (Gregg *et al.* 2005 cited in Monaghan 2005: 308).

For obesity discourse critics, it is not that a higher than optimal weight (even by contested BMI measurements) does not have the potential to affect health beyond a certain point, which may vary for individuals; but rather, the way it is assessed may result in inappropriate recommendations to groups not well measured by BMI categorisations. These may include not only older people and fit 'overweight' people but also some ethnic groups (Munro-Wild and Fellows 2009).

Obesity research since Monaghan's 2005 analysis shows that there is continuing uncertainty in the epidemiology. While obesity is still thought to constitute a heightened health risk, there are several exceptions to this. Epidemiologists regularly admit that there is much to be learned about the relationship between bodyweight and disease risk. A series of systematic reviews in *Obesity Reviews*, the journal of the International Association for the Study of Obesity, has found that:

- Mortality rates are lower in aerobically fit individuals with a high BMI than in normal weight people with low levels of fitness (Fogelholm 2010). However, a high BMI is associated with a higher risk and prevalence of Type 2 diabetes (ibid.).
- Overweight people aged 70–75 were found to have lower mortality risk than those of normal or low weight (Flicker *et al.* 2010: 234). Overweight may offer some protection in old age even for those with chronic illnesses, possibly because of the 'metabolic and nutritional reserves' it gives them (ibid.: 238). A subsequent review of 312 studies confirms that finding; BMI standards for younger adults cannot be meaningfully applied to older people (Donini *et al.* 2012: 96).

- An increase in BMI *can* indicate an increase in lean body mass rather than an increase in fat (Canoy and Buchan 2007: 3).
- Obese people *can* be metabolically healthy. It is excess central adiposity (fat around the waist) that is associated with a significant increase in heart disease risk (Iacobellis and Sharma 2007).

The World Cancer Research Fund has acknowledged the role of body composition and body fatness as distinct from BMI, and notes that internationally, 'healthy ranges of BMI varied between populations' (WCRF 2007: 212). By contrast, waist circumference measures both subcutaneous and intra-abdominal fat stores: the size of the latter predicts the risk of chronic diseases such as metabolic disorders and cardiovascular disease better than overall indicators of body fatness, such as BMI (WCRF 2007: 213). In the UK, NICE guidelines advise that waist circumference should be measured along with BMI in assessing weight-related health risks (NICE 2006, 2010).

Jutel is critical of the health value placed on thinness and, suspicious of the overweight–disease link, shows via a content analysis of medical articles that overweight is itself becoming a disease entity (Jutel 2006: 2268–70). She speculates that BMI measurement may have contributed to this phenomenon and traces its emergence in nineteenth century practice and ideas; a quantitative 'certainty', it enabled doctors to disregard unreliable patient reports of diet/exercise (ibid.: 2272), a purpose it could still serve, as unreliability on this point remains a concern. Like Monaghan, she critiques the medical and social construction of the ideal body, which 'underpin[s] a multi-billion dollar diet, gym, self-help, television and pharmaceutical approach to weight maintenance' (Jutel 2006: 2275).

Monaghan finds the medical profession guilty of 'fat bigotry', especially against those of 'inferior social status' and argues that fitness levels achieved by overweight and obese people should be acknowledged (Monaghan 2005: 308). Aphramor, a research dietician, critiques the evidence base for clinical guidelines on obesity and urges governments to address underlying social injustices rather than focusing on weight (Aphramor 2005 cited by Monaghan 2005: 308). Huizinga *et al.* (2009) found that physicians were less respectful of patients with a high BMI, and ask whether this affects quality of care.

Jutel urges healthcare practitioners to help people to change their diets and to exercise, but without focusing on weight loss per se (Jutel 2006: 2275). Gaesser points to the health risks of dieting (and the tendency of diets to fail) and believes people should be encouraged to adjust their diets and exercise moderately to improve metabolic health – not to lose weight (Gaesser 2002 cited in Monaghan 2005: 310–11). This view contrasts sharply with the fitness–weight-loss discourse; the relationship between the two is thus worth investigating in some detail.

Fitness, obesity and health

One way of understanding the implications of large bodyweights is by examining the costs of associated health conditions. A recent study ranked physical inactivity lower than poor diet, high alcohol consumption and smoking in terms of its cost impact on the NHS. The authors estimated that 'the largest economic burden to the NHS is due to poor diet [£5.8bn] and much of this food-related burden is due to overweight and obesity. Physical inactivity asserts a considerable burden on the NHS [£0.9bn], but not as high as other behavioural risk factors' (Scarborough *et al.* 2011: 531).

Research by Metcalf and colleagues has shown that exercise was not effective in achieving weight loss among 200 children in a longitudinal study (Metcalf *et al.* 2008, 2011). They did, however, find that exercise improved the children's metabolic health.

What do large-scale studies say about fitness, obesity and health? A study of 115,000 US nurses (Hu *et al.* 2004) found that obese but active women had a lower mortality rate than obese but inactive women, but higher than normal weight, active women. Lean, inactive women were also at higher risk than lean, active women. 'This data does not support the hypothesis that if you are physically active, you don't have to worry about your weight' (Hu cited in *Guardian* 09/03/10). However, exercise does reduce mortality risk even among the overweight.

Sui *et al.* (2007) carried out treadmill fitness tests on 2,600 people aged 60 and over rather than using self-reported fitness levels. Results showed no definitive link between overweight and higher mortality, though an inverse relationship was observed between levels of fitness and obesity. As weight increases, there is a decreasing tendency for people to be fit, but 'among class II obese individuals (BMI 35–39.9), about 40–45% are still fit' (Blair,[2] a contributing author to Sui *et al.* 2007, cited in *Guardian* 09/03/10). Despite 'higher rates of mortality, chronic diseases, heart attacks and the like, in people with high BMI … when we look at these mortality rates in fat people who are fit … the harmful effect of fat just disappears' (ibid.). Hu *et al.* would dispute this, citing several studies which disprove such claims (Hu *et al.* 2004: 9). Sui *et al.* note that their study participants were mostly white, educated and middle class or higher, and that this might have skewed their findings (Sui *et al.* 2007: 2515). They were also unable to track diet or medication (ibid.). They do, however, rely on a more objective measurement of fitness (treadmill tests) than the Hu study, which based its findings on self-reported exercise. Such data may be unreliable. Nevertheless, both studies find significant value for exercise in reducing illness and mortality risks, even if bodyweight is not affected.

A 2008 study of 39,000 women, none of whom had coronary heart disease at the outset, found that overweight active women were 54 per cent more likely to develop heart disease, and obese active women had an 87 per cent greater risk, compared to normal weight active women over a ten-year period (Weinstein *et al.* 2008; fitness was self-reported). They concluded that 'the risk of CHD associated with elevated body mass index is considerably reduced by increased physical activity levels. However, the risk is not completely eliminated' (ibid.: 884).

If physical activity is effective in lowering health risks even among the overweight, how likely is it that this group does exercise? The Health Survey for England 2008 shows that self-reported levels of physical activity were higher for those of normal BMI than those classed (according to BMI measurements) as overweight or obese (HSE 2008: 21). The 2012 survey found similar trends, as well as an increase in aerobic activities as household incomes increased (HSE 2012a: 1). There is also an association between low levels of physical activity and a 'raised waist circumference' (>102cm in men, >88cm in women (HSE 2008: 100)). This in turn is associated with a higher risk of metabolic syndrome,[3] including heightened risk for Type 2 diabetes and heart disease (HSE 2008: 184).

Devices which record exercise are beginning to allow researchers to verify self-reported fitness efforts, and they are found to be much lower in actuality. A Canadian study which fitted accelerometers onto nearly 2,800 adolescents found that all participants over-reported their exercise activities; those who were the most inactive were also more likely to over-report exercise (Leblanc and Janssen 2010). Similarly, the WCRF has found that self-assessed bodyweight tends to be underestimated (WCRF 2007: 214).

There is some dispute over the extent of the mitigating effect of fitness on bodyweight. However, there is clear potential for public health discourse and practice to shift the focus away from weight loss on its own and towards the health benefits of exercise.

Evidence for obesity and disease risk

Much of the academic literature reviewed for this book, as well as health charities' research and advice, links obesity with ill health. Monaghan (2005) targets the taken-for-granted nature of a problem which he believes needs to be much more intensively researched before specific aetiologies can be established. Even then caution is indicated. He notes that many risks, illnesses and deaths are '*attributed*' to excess weight (author's emphasis) yet such assessments are 'scientifically indeterminable' (Monaghan 2005: 304). In fact, much (though not all) clinical and statistical research and many recommendations from health charities speak of obesity as *a* risk factor rather than *the* cause of illness or death; or studies note correlations or associations between obesity and disease. Epidemiologists regularly admit to the limitations of the data and the need for further research, though these reservations do not always find their way into the broader discourse on obesity. But even though they acknowledge the potential for inconsistencies in the data, many links have been established between bodyweight and illness risk.

For example, Huda *et al.* (2006), reviewing 289 studies, find that obesity is linked to a higher incidence of Type 2 diabetes. Narkiewicz's review of 53 studies finds that most patients with hypertension are obese, and that assessing blood pressure and organ damage in obese patients with hypertension is more difficult than in those of normal weight (Narkiewicz 2006). Obese hypertensives respond less well to treatment than those of normal weight, with blood pressure harder to control (Narkiewicz 2006: 155, 160). Obesity 'appears to be the most important risk factor for hypertension' (ibid.: 160); prevalence of hypertension increases with age and increase in BMI. This is backed up by McNaughton *et al.* (2008), who also found an association between adult diet and BMI, waist measurement and blood pressure.

Canoy and Buchan's review finds that 'BMI correlates reasonably well with body fat mass and the risks of obesity-related diseases' (Canoy and Buchan 2007: 1). Previously the WCRF (2007) linked low levels of physical activity, raised waist circumference and diabetes; Narkiewicz (2006) additionally notes the association between central (waist) obesity and both cardiovascular and metabolic risk factors. A later WCRF report (2010) reaffirmed the cancer risks (bowel, breast, endometrium and pancreatic) associated with larger waistlines; in England 44 per cent of women and 32 per cent of men have raised waist measurements, placing them at increased risk.

In 2011 the WCRF warned that about 43 per cent of the UK's bowel cancers (17,000 cases per year) could be avoided with lower consumption of meat and alcohol, sufficient activity and healthy bodyweights (*Guardian* 23/05/11). A review of studies that same year, collectively tracking over a million people, found little connection between fruit and vegetable consumption and cancer risk among those who were well nourished, though the author acknowledged that the studies were retrospective, perhaps weakening recall of past diets (Key 2011). There *was* some potential benefit of increasing intake among those with the lowest intakes, though the conclusion was that obesity was a more important risk factor. The study recommended at least five portions of fruit/vegetables per day to assist weight loss and as substitutes for unhealthy foods. The benefits for overall health were also noted (Key 2011).

Even those of normal weight who have hypertension are eventually more likely to gain weight; the obesity–hypertension association is a 'two-way street' (Narkiewicz 2006: 156). His review concludes that weight reduction is linked to reduced blood pressure, possibly because of accompanying reductions in sodium intake. Even if weight loss is not achieved, decreasing saturated fat intake will lower blood pressure.

Canoy and Buchan note an increase in soft drink consumption in the USA between the 1970s and 1990s, which is associated with an increase in obesity (Canoy and Buchan 2007: 3); this is confirmed by the 2004 Nurses Health Study and a study by the Harvard School of Public Health

(Malik *et al.* 2010), which further associate soft drink consumption with an increased risk of Type 2 diabetes. In the UK, 14.5 billion litres of soft drinks were consumed in 2013, with a market value of £15.6 billion (BSDA 2014: 4).

A National Heart Forum report analyses Health Survey for England data (1993–2007), and warns of significant increases in obesity-related diseases among adults, especially vascular disorders but also 'arthritis, coronary heart disease, diabetes, gall bladder disease, hypertension, stroke and the following cancers: breast, colorectal, endometrial, kidney, oesophageal and liver' (Brown *et al.* 2010: 1, 2). This is in line with the prediction of an increase in obesity overall, morbid obesity, and a decline in normal weight in the adult population (Brown *et al.* 2010). The authors conclude:

> the number of normal weight individuals is inexorably falling, those overweight remaining broadly steady and those obese rising. Of equal concern is a significant rise in rates of morbid obesity BMI > 40 which have extremely high associated disease risks. These predicted levels of obesity will lead to significant rises in the levels of vascular diseases. (Brown *et al.* 2010: 15)

It is worth examining these disease rates in greater detail. The cases of CHD, diabetes and hypertension numbered approximately 2,000, 3,200 and 5,800 (approximately 11,000 in total) respectively per 100,000 in 2010 (Brown *et al.* 2010: 9). All these disease rates, along with the others the authors investigated, are expected to continue to increase; the three selected for highest incidence are predicted to (collectively) reach approximately 18,000 per 100,000 by 2050. Together with the other diseases investigated, nearly 20 per cent of the population could have a 'BMI-related disease' by 2050. This is obviously highly significant, but these figures are below the overall incidence of obesity both now and in terms of future predictions. By 2020, 41 per cent of men and 36 per cent of women aged 20–65 are expected to be obese; another 40 per cent of men and 32 per cent of women are expected to be overweight. Even the much increased combined disease rate of 20 per cent by 2050 is somewhat lower than even those 2020 obesity predictions. While a time lag in disease experience and diagnosis will be a major factor, it seems that weight beyond the BMI normal range is a risk factor but not a determinant of such disease.

Nevertheless, research continues to identify risks for a range of additional health problems linked to obesity. For example:

- Pregnancy/birth risks: a systematic review of 84 studies of over 1 million women concluded that obese mothers have an increased risk of early pre-term birth and even in full-term births, and an increased risk of extremely low birthweight babies (McDonald *et al.* 2010).

- Arthritis: obesity is a major risk factor in osteoarthritis of the knee (Arthritis Care 2010). For every pound of weight lost by overweight or obese people with knee osteoarthritis, there is a four-pound reduction in 'knee stress' (ibid.). Even moderate overweight can strain weight-bearing joints, worsening osteoarthritis after it has developed. Wearing *et al.* (2006) recommend more research into the effect of childhood obesity on the musculo-skeletal system, given the findings to date regarding risk of injury and functional impairments.
- Liver disease: obesity is one of three main factors in liver disease (after alcohol consumption and hepatitis B and C (Moore and Sheron 2009)). Public health efforts should tackle all three, given a six-fold rise in liver disease in the past 35 years (ibid.: 31).
- Cancer: in addition to the National Heart Forum research which found a cancer–obesity link, a (2007) WCRF review of 950 studies concluded that alcohol consumption, sedentary lifestyles and over-weight increased breast cancer risk. There was convincing evidence that 'greater body fatness is a cause of cancers of the oesophagus (adenocarcinoma), pancreas, colorectum, breast (postmenopause), endometrium, and kidney ... [and] probably a cause of gallbladder cancer, both directly, and indirectly through the formation of gall-stones. There is also limited evidence suggesting that greater body fatness is a cause of liver cancer.'

Greater body fatness may protect against pre-menopausal breast cancer (WCRF 2007: 228), though a subsequent study found higher 'circulating concentrations of oestrogens and androgens' present in post-menopausal obese women; this is thought to account for higher levels of breast cancer in this group (Key *et al.* 2011: 709).

It seems unwise to dismiss the evidence linking obesity with a range of illness risks, given the epidemiological evidence to date. But why and how has obesity grown so dramatically in recent decades? In the next section evidence for increased bodyweights is examined.

Obesity, gender, age and class

Progress in understanding the mechanisms underlying illness risk and body-weight should be seen in the context of the increase in obesity prevalence. The 2014 global obesity study, citing regional and national estimates, finds about 25 per cent of both men and women (aged 20 and over) to be obese in the UK (Ng *et al.* 2014: 9). In England, it 'rose three- to fourfold across the two decades from 1980' among adults (Bajekal *et al.* 1999 cited in Canoy and Buchan 2007: 2). The graphs in Chapter 1 show its trajectory for England between 1993 and 2011 for both adults and children. Obesity rates increased among children of both manual and non-manual parental employment categories, but the increase was sharper in those in manual households (ibid.). This is reflected in the National Child Measurement Programme graph. Canoy and Buchan find an association between low socio-economic status in childhood and higher BMI in adulthood (ibid.).

Obesity rates have increased for both men and women of all social classes since 1997, but the gap between social classes is clearest among women; the increase for professional women, for example, is minimal (Marmot *et al.* 2010: 58, full report). The rate of growth of obesity among men is similar across all social classes, and the lack of a clear social gradient or pattern among men holds true for household income and occupation. But when occupational categories are combined into manual and non-manual groups there is a general trend: obesity rises when educational attainment is lower among both men and women (NOO 2010: 4).

Educational attainment and manual/non-manual occupational group may be the best way of tracking men at risk of obesity and, given the clear social gradient for circulatory disease and cancer, seeing what the illness patterns of obese men might be by social class. This dimension of obesity may be missed by critics of obesity discourse. For women, adolescents and children, the social gradient is clear, but unless patterns among younger people change, a stronger social gradient could emerge for obesity among men in years to come.

Poor women and children are most likely to be overweight or obese. In London's poorest local authority, obesity rates are two-thirds higher than in London's most affluent one (Munro-Wild and Fellows 2009). Among the 1958 birth cohort, those with a 'less advantaged social position' had a greater likelihood of higher BMI in childhood, and a higher risk of cardio-vascular disease in adulthood (Elliott and Vaitilingam 2008: 36). Those who are less advantaged also reported poorer general health in adulthood (ibid.: 19). The pattern of lower prenatal growth, shorter child-to-adult height and greater risk of obesity associated with the least advantaged social position is also associated with higher blood pressure, blood lipids and blood glucose levels in mid-adulthood (ibid.: 36). A review of 138 studies noted emerging associations between childhood obesity, adult obesity and cardiovascular risk (Wearing *et al.* 2006).

In the UK, the National Child Measurement Programme report found that nearly 10 per cent of four and five year olds and 18.7 per cent of 10 and 11 year olds were obese (DoH 2010b: 7). For both groups there is a strong association between area deprivation and obesity (ibid.); and a further association between area deprivation and a high proportion of non-white ethnic groups (ibid.: 32). The report observed that

> obesity prevalence increase[s] as socio-economic deprivation increases; for both school years, the four most deprived groups have obesity prevalence that is significantly higher than the national average; for both school years, the five least deprived groups have obesity prevalence that is significantly lower than the national average. (DoH 2010b: 29)

By 2015, obesity rates are predicted to fall for girls 'from professional back-grounds', but rise for boys in this group; for lower social classes a more marked rise is predicted for both boys and girls (Marmot *et al.* 2010: 146, full report).

Despite major area variations, overall life expectancy is improving in the UK, along with treatments for illnesses associated with poor diet. But the experience of chronic and long-term illness, endured at significant cost to individuals, families and the state, should not be underestimated. Research linking social class and health has tended to focus more on mortality risk than on morbidity, even though 'health differences between classes may be more clearly illustrated by health and illness experiences than by life expectancy' (Borooah 1999 and Blaxter 1989 cited in Veenstra 2006: 117).

Even so, there is a seven-year life expectancy difference between those in the richest and the poorest neighbourhoods. And examining obesity only in the context of mortality risk does not portray the morbidity dimension adequately, particularly in its varying class profile: there is a 17-year aver-age difference between income areas in disability-free life expectancy (Marmot *et al.* 2010: 10, executive summary). Many health problems asso-ciated with persistently high bodyweights, particularly if accompanied by poor diet and sedentariness, are chronic and disabling.

Figures for children indicate that the gap between bodyweights for differ-ing social classes is widening. The future for children at increased risk of obesity implies an increased risk of illness. The obesity critique risks under-estimating both the social gradient in bodyweight and the future disease risk for today's obese children.

In the following section, the social network approach to obesity studies is explored because of its contribution to strengthening obesity discourse as a matter of behaviour (in this case, spread by individuals in groups) and the ways in which it has been popularised outside the academy. Little attention is paid to social class dimensions when analysing the role of social networks on obesity. Its proponents have written a bestselling book and their work is cited by politicians and even the UK's Department of Health.

Obesity and social networks

An influential book by a popular American thinker addressed social class, if only to negate its importance. David Brooks (2011) writes: 'Society isn't defined by classes, as the Marxists believe. It's not defined by racial iden-tity. And it's not a collection of rugged individualists, as some economic and social libertarians believe. Instead ... society is a layering of networks' (2011: 155). Here class is not considered a dimension of social networks. This book has been popular with British politicians; Brooks met both David Cameron and Ed Miliband during a UK book tour (*Guardian* 04/06/11). Anthony Seldon, a Tory, calls Brooks, along with Thaler and

Sunstein (who wrote *Nudge*), 'micro thinkers' and chastises the government for overlooking more significant thinkers (Seldon 2012).

Research by Christakis and Fowler (2007) revealing the links between obesity and social networks was so striking that their work became a popular book published a few years later (2010) and was cited by a British health minister (see Chapter 1). They used unique longitudinal datasets drawn from the US Framingham Heart Study, in which 12,000 study participants underwent physical examinations and completed written questionnaires between 1971 and 2003. For the study, a BMI of 30 or more was considered obese.

Participants, aged between 21 and 70, were studied not as individuals but in the context of their social relationships, ranging from siblings to spouses and friends of varying degrees of closeness. Results were then compared to results from random BMI networks and found to be significantly higher for social networks, even across geographic distances. The authors speculated that perhaps obesity was increasing in part because there had been a change in the 'general perception of the social norms regarding the acceptability of obesity' (Christakis and Fowler 2007: 377).

The only class-related indicator available in the study data was educational attainment, and the authors only mentioned a mean educational level of 13.6 years (approximating completion of secondary school) out of a range of zero to more than 17 years. They noted the presence of obesity among all socio-economic groups without acknowledging any social gradient (2007: 371); but in a subsequent book, they accepted that friendship networks are constrained by several factors including socio-economic status (2009: xi).

In the US, obesity is significantly present even among higher status groups; paradoxically, this may be decreasing associations between inequality and large bodyweights among US adults, though not among children or adolescents (Singh *et al.* 2011). Perhaps the *incidence* of obesity among adults is accounted for or at least reflected in some measure by social networks; but overweight and obesity in children as young as five is disproportionately prevalent among those from lower socio-economic backgrounds. These children are likely to be obese in adolescence and beyond (ibid.). Furthermore, the obesity–inequality gap has widened among US children and adolescents since 2002 (Frederick *et al.* 2014; Singh *et al.* 2011).

Neighbourhood location often reflects socio-economic status, but Christakis and Fowler conclude that because immediate neighbours did not influence weight gain (unless they were friends), 'common exposure to local environmental factors' could be ruled out as an explanation for the spread of obesity (2007: 377). Yet many neighbourhoods, certainly in the UK, contain people representing different socio-economic backgrounds, and high streets featuring both lower and higher status shops and food retailers (my own included). Consumption patterns can remain distinct among different socio-economic groups, and, presumably, the networks that emerge within them, within the same neighbourhood. Christakis and Fowler may dismiss local environment too quickly. Additionally, their study was not able to address the role of the daytime/working environment in food provision and consumption.

The Christakis and Fowler study is criticised from a health economics perspective by Cohen-Cole and Fletcher (2008a). Their study reworks the data using econometric techniques, citing weaknesses in the models used, and finds a reduced social network effect for obesity, at least in terms of 'induction and person-to-person spread – though peer support might well be useful in addressing weight loss' (ibid.: 1386). Their study suggests that 'shared environmental factors can cause the appearance of social network effects' (ibid.). Fowler and Christakis (2008) later critiqued this data and analysis; Cohen-Cole and Fletcher (2008b) further challenged the social network approach by applying it to what they deemed non-socially related physical features and health issues. They warn that the social network effect could be 'implausible'.

In both food consumption studies and UK marketing profiles for different consumer groups, patterns of food consumption are similar among social groups, whether those patterns are healthy or unhealthy (or somewhere in between); this is so even without noting a network effect. The rise in obesity is also vitally connected to the changes in the food *supply* itself in the latter half of the twentieth century.

But the social network–obesity link has taken root. A DoH report stated that 'through social networks, obesity can actually be "spread" by person-to-person interaction' (DoH 2010a: 19) with a similar lack of contextualisation. In embracing social network explanations along the lines of Christakis and Fowler, little account is taken of the social *class* effect. Yet there are clear associations in countless studies of obesity and social class, both in the UK and abroad. In the UK, particularly among women and children, measurements of socio-economic status show obesity prevalence along a social gradient (NOO 2010: 8). Area-level indicators (e.g. Index of Multiple Deprivation) also illuminate obesity risk (ibid.).

Social networks among lower status people may themselves be more limited, given the findings of Savage *et al.* (2013) discussed in Chapter 3. They found that the lowest-ranking group in terms of economic capital (the precariat, 15 per cent of the population) also had the lowest number of social contacts (an average of seven); other low ranking groups also had comparatively few social contacts (ibid.: 230).

A study by Crossley addressed social network analysis and the 'small world problem' for sociology in general (Crossley 2008: 266). In 'small world' theorising since the 1960s, 'analysing chains of acquaintances allows us to explore the significance of, for example, status differences ... upon this pattern of relationships. It affords us a perspective upon group closure, segregation and stratification' (ibid.: 262). Christakis and Fowler's work was not able to explore social structure in these terms, or reveal whether these social networks reflected social structures and stratifications. However, they did improve on previous research into small world networks, which were orchestrated rather than naturally occurring, and which did not distinguish between different types and degrees of social relationships (Christakis and Fowler 2008: 268).

But Crossley critiques the 'new social physicists' who 'ignore the meaning of social relations, the time-space relations that are central for social organisations, the role of technology and transport in human relations, and key issues of inequality, conflict and exclusion' (Crossley 2008: 266). These all play a role in food consumption, bodyweight trends and health. Even weak social ties are shaped by social life and events 'and by variously distributed resources, dispositions and social positions that enable, incline or otherwise lead us to partake in them. They are not random' (Crossley 2008: 265).

The media also plays a role in extending social networks and 'shrinking the world' (Crossley 2008: 271). Advertising and marketing, as well as the increasing use of social networking via computer and mobile technologies, influence consumer purchases. Consumer research can collect this data, communicate the likes and dislikes of friends, inform retailers of potential consumers, and predict where consumer interest is heading. Retailers which track customers, informing them by smartphone of marketing offers when they are in the vicinity of one of their outlets, can also communicate the purchases of consumers to their friends (*Observer* 09/01/11). One marketer noted the proliferation of brand-based Facebook groups with games, offers and discussions to keep consumers in touch with each other and with the brand itself, fostering peer-to-peer recommendations:

> The more details I put on my profile, the more it [Facebook] knows ... if I 'like' a new soft drink, then they'll go to friends with the same likes and interests as me and market the product using my endorsement ... [so] brands are not doing the advertising, but your friends are. (Romano cited in *Guardian* 15/11/10)

The Christakis and Fowler research was done before this kind of food advertising via social networks was happening on any great scale; such techniques seem destined to further the patterns of food consumption observed in social network research (although word-of-mouth among friends and acquaintances long predates social media).

Christakis and Fowler suggest that the dynamics of social networks could be harnessed to address obesity and stop it spreading, with interventions that feature peer support – 'that is, that modify the person's social network' – designed to encourage weight loss (Christakis and Fowler 2007: 378). They propose that their findings could address social inequalities. Since their interest is in behavioural rather than structural matters, this would presumably involve dietary/weight loss interventions designed with socio-economic status in mind. A UK health behaviours study also recommends targeting such interventions at those with the lowest levels of education and income, among whom 'unhealthy behaviours' are increasing (Buck and Frosini 2012).

These insights may helpfully inform future health promotion approaches. However, thus far, interventions which focus on behaviours have not been successful in reversing population bodyweight and diet-related illness trends; arguably the power of a highly palatable, omnipresent, large-portioned and targeted food supply is simply too great. Nevertheless, social network research has made a strong impact, and in this process has reinforced the focus on human behaviour, but in a decontextualised manner – divorced from either social structures or the nature, supply and marketing of food itself.

Obesity and inequality in a global context

Studies which examine obesity in an international context contribute unique perspectives on the relationship between socio-economic structures, political ideology, and obesity levels. Another academic work which had a wide impact outside academia was *The Spirit Level: Why More Equal Societies Almost Always Do Better* (Wilkinson and Pickett 2009). In it, social epidemiologists Wilkinson and Pickett reported on long-observed relationships between the degree of income inequality in a country and a range of issues including obesity.

The UK has a very large gap between the highest and lowest incomes, and comparatively high rates of obesity (Wilkinson and Pickett 2009: 82). Wilkinson and Pickett speculate that the chronic stress and anxiety associated with living in unequal societies prompts an increase in food intake and makes it more likely for those under long-term stress to accumulate fat around the waist, increasing the risk of illness (ibid.: 95). Pregnant mothers who are stressed tend to have low birthweight babies with a slower metabolism, who are prone to weight gain later in life (ibid.: 100).

Given the presence of overweight and obesity even among those in higher socio-economic categories, they note studies which found that subjective social status was more indicative of health status than income or education (ibid.: 101) – if people *felt* as though they were struggling, their health suffered.

This general line of investigation is followed by Offer *et al.* (2010), who trace obesity prevalence in 16 affluent countries. They distinguish between six 'market-liberal welfare regimes', with a higher prevalence of obesity, and ten 'co-ordinated market economies' (Offer *et al.* 2010: 298), with lower prevalence. The authors note that 'since the 1980s, there has been a movement away from social democratic policy norms, towards more market-friendly policies. This matches the timing of the emergence of obesity as a mass social phenomenon' (ibid.).

But obesity has grown faster and is more prevalent in market-liberal countries, where market freedoms have led to lower prices for fast foods, because of lower wages and taxes; this price effect has been accompanied by intensive marketing (Offer *et al.* 2010: 301). Income inequality and less extensive social safety nets are also a cause of insecurity, the most influential factor in obesity levels in the study (ibid.: 306). Offer *et al.* trace the psychological effects of employment-based insecurity to decreasing unionisation, a decrease in bargaining power, and the link with obesity in market-liberal countries (ibid.: 304).

Monaghan suggested that social inequalities, stress and anti-fat discrimination may provide better explanations of ill health among overweight people than the weight itself. Marmot's Whitehall study linking social status and states of health all the way up the social scale, as well as more recent research on health inequalities, provides some evidence for psychological/stress explanations for ill health unassociated with weight. But it is also possible to trace broadly structural pathways or mechanisms for ill health which manifest themselves in bodyweight: for example, low birthweight due to poor maternal diet, as mentioned previously, or early life experiences of deprivation which can limit growth in infancy and affect lipid levels in midlife (Skidmore *et al.* 2007).

Offer *et al.* do not explore the possibility that food regulatory regimes might be associated with varying levels of obesity. Cutler *et al.* (2003: 110) found food regulatory data lacking but cite 'proxies' – regulations regarding tariff and non-tariff barriers to agriculture, packaging, labelling, use of preservatives and pesticides, and time requirements for registering new food businesses (where it takes longer there is less obesity). In nine countries studied, those with more food laws have less obesity (ibid.).

The World Bank (2010) assesses a much larger range of countries on a variety of governance indicators, including overall regulatory 'quality' (defined as 'the ability of the government to provide sound policies and regulations that enable and promote private sector development' (Kaufmann *et al.* 2009)). The World Bank does not assess regulation in a food–health context, but the capacity to quantify regulatory quality raises the prospect of quantifying the impact of food regulation on public health.

The historical dimensions of current trends are reflected in the analysis of Ferguson, a historian, as he traces the consumption of sugar in England in the context of what he calls 'Anglobalization' (Ferguson 2002: xxvi). The largest import to Britain from the 1750s to the 1820s, average sugar consumption at 20lbs a year was ten times what it was in France by the late eighteenth century (ibid.: 14). British sugar consumption (along with diabetes and obesity rates) remains far above that of other European countries.

The influence of agriculture and agricultural subsidies on nutrition is not a major focus in social science periodical literature. However, in 1993 it was suggested that since

> the CAP largely controls the type, volume and price of food produced in the [European] Community … it would be quite feasible to increase

the supply and lower the price of healthier foods such as fruit and vegetables, in order to encourage greater consumption, and conversely to discourage the consumption of tobacco, sugar and fats (especially saturated fat). (Joffe 1993: 60)

Others have proposed that Europe's CAP be regularly assessed for its influence on health and nutrition, and subsidies used to increase consumption of fruit and vegetables (Hautvast *et al.* 2000).

The WHO's study of saturated fat production/consumption in Europe found that a substantial portion of cardiovascular disease could be attributed to the CAP (Lloyd-Williams *et al.* 2008). Most policy and food industry representatives interviewed for the (2006) Porgrow study thought that the CAP might be influencing overconsumption of unhealthy foods 'but there was little confidence that the CAP will be reformed in ways directly beneficial to public health in the short- to medium-terms' (Lobstein *et al.* 2006: 9).

These studies, drawn from diverse research programmes and disciplines, show the role played by public policy and the ideology which shapes it, for public health problems such as obesity. But even these innovative investigations have not been able to seriously challenge the discourse of personal responsibility and a focus on behaviour which continues to prevail in the context of dietary health and bodyweight. Christakis and Fowler's work on social networks and Brooks's stance on the power of the individual were both embraced by Britain's leading political parties; neither addressed structural forces of any kind.

Non-obese diet-related ill health

In recent years, there has been a shift in food and nutrition policy from an interest in nutrition and health to a focus on obesity (Dowler and O'Connor 2012: 48). I set out in this book not to limit my search to obesity or even overweight. As we have seen, large bodyweights do not always indicate increased health risk, particularly in the presence of high levels of physical fitness. People of normal weight can also experience ill health which may be influenced by diet. As Lustig, an endocrinologist, notes, 'Twenty percent of the obese population have a normal metabolic profile whereas up to 40 percent of normal-weight people have an abnormal metabolic profile' (Lustig 2014: 93). Subcutaneous fat does not increase health risk as visceral fat does, and the latter may not always be obvious – but it surrounds our organs, increasing the risk of circulatory and metabolic disease (ibid.: 125, 306).

In a US study, 500 overweight and lean people were asked about their responses to food – particularly feelings of loss of control, not being satisfied after eating, and being preoccupied by food. The author noted 'a sizable minority of lean people with features of conditioned hypereating' (Kessler 2009: 160). These people had limited their food intake thus far, but Kessler speculates this might be difficult to maintain over the long term (ibid.). Conditioned hypereating is spurred by 'environmental exposure' – an omnipresent foodscape – and constitutes 'a psychological adaptation to the environment that occurs among certain susceptible individuals' (ibid.: 162).

A look at the diet–health link independent of obesity will broaden our understanding of how food consumption relates to health. The health implications of raised salt intake are discussed separately from obesity per se, and reviewed in some detail below because they are often missed in an obesity-dominated nutritional health discourse.

Salt and health

The risks of high salt consumption have been researched and documented by the health charity Consensus Action on Salt and Health (CASH 2010 and 2012). The main health risk is high blood pressure. It is not necessary to be overweight to have this health problem or indeed to suffer a stroke. The range of health risks (based on CASH analysis) are summarised below:

- Salt is the major factor increasing blood pressure, a greater risk than low fruit/vegetable intake, obesity, sedentariness or high alcohol intake.
- High blood pressure (HBP) causes 62 per cent of strokes in the UK. There is increasing evidence that salt is independently associated with stroke. Older people, those with HBP, diabetics, smokers and those who smoke *and* have a high salt intake are more likely to be from lower socio-economic groups.
- A 2009 meta-analysis of 19 cohort samples totalling 177,000 participants demonstrated a link between high salt intake, stroke risk and cardiovascular disease. HBP is responsible for 40 per cent of cardiovascular disease.
- There is evidence of a link between salt consumption and kidney disease; high salt intake increases protein in urine (a risk factor for kidney malfunction) and HBP also increases the risk of kidney disease.
- There is a link between high salt intake and cardiovascular disease and diabetes; people with hypertension are 2.5 times more likely to develop diabetes.
- High salt intake causes thirst and may increase sugary drink consumption, which may contribute to both obesity and diabetes.
- Salt intake may contribute to osteoporosis via calcium excretion. This association has also been observed among teenage girls; lowered salt consumption among this group could reduce their risk of osteoporosis later in life.
- High salt intake raises the risk of stomach cancer. This risk is higher for those in the most deprived social groups, for men overall and for the over-55s.

- For most of the UK population, 80 per cent of salt consumed is in processed foods; for Africans living in the UK, most salt consumed is added during cooking and at the table, suggesting a need for culturally targeted health information on salt intake.

The Scientific Advisory Committee on Nutrition, FSA, and NICE all recommend a maximum salt intake of 6g per day, less for children (CASH 2012). This would be a substantial reduction from high levels registered in a 2008 National Centre for Social Research/MRC study (9.7g for men and 7.7g for women on average). NICE calls for a further reduction of salt intake to a maximum of 3g per day by 2025 (NICE 2010).

Further nutrition and health links

Barker's foetal programming hypothesis illustrated how health is influenced in utero. Marmot cites Barker's finding that

> when human foetuses have to adapt to a limited supply of nutrients, they permanently change their structure and metabolism: these 'programmed' changes may be the origins of a number of diseases in later life, including coronary heart disease and the related disorders of stroke, diabetes and hypertension. (Barker 1998 cited in Marmot *et al.* 2010: 60, full report)

Marmot also cites a range of birth cohort studies showing the influence of early life on subsequent states of health (Marmot 2004: 55). Weight is not necessarily a factor.

A 2008 study analysing Whitehall II data found that a diet characterised by processed foods high in fat, salt and sugar was associated with both insulin resistance and, prospectively, with Type 2 diabetes; the study was not primarily concerned with bodyweight, though the authors noted evidence that those who drank diet soft drinks tended to be overweight (McNaughton *et al.* 2008: 1346).

The WCRF systematic review cited previously found evidence that 'some types of vegetables and fruits in general probably protect against a number of cancers' (WCRF 2007: 114 full report). This finding is unrelated to obesity per se.

A study of nearly 3,000 UK adults (Shaheen *et al.* 2010) tested for links between dietary patterns and lung disease as reported in questionnaires, rather than the consumption of individual foods. The authors found that a pattern they described as 'prudent', containing a high degree of fruit, vegetables, fish and wholemeal cereals, may offer some protection against impaired lung function (ibid.: 277). Again, weight is not mentioned.

A study commissioned by the FSA and the Department of Health described teenage girls' diets as the worst of all population groups. While consuming too much sugar and fat, they lack key nutrients. Nearly half did not consume minimum recommended levels of iron or magnesium, and only 7 per cent ate five portions of fruit and vegetables per day (FSA/DoH 2008/09: points 5.5.2 and 5.3). Overall, this group does not eat enough, according to the FSA's head of nutritional research – the opposite of obesity, but still a problematic diet with the potential to harm health (*Guardian* 09/02/10). The report further noted that only about a third of adults eat their 'five a day' and that all population groups are eating too much saturated fat, although mean levels have dropped as a percentage of overall food intake (FSA/DoH 2008/09: points 5.3 and 5.4.7).

Other illnesses relating to poor diet include anaemia due to lack of iron, a particular risk during pregnancy; mothers with inadequate nutrition giving birth to low-weight babies (low birthweight in turn carrying future health risks); dental problems; eczema; asthma; cataracts – all connected to poor nutrition (Lobstein cited in Lawrence 2008c).

One study predicted that a diet containing more fruit, vegetables and fibre, and less salt and fat, could save 33,000 lives per year (Scarborough *et al.* 2012: 420). The study assesses the differing role these nutrients could have in saving lives:

> The modelled reduction in deaths for coronary heart disease was 20,800 ... for stroke 5,876 and for cancer 6,481. Over 15,000 of the avoided deaths would be due to increased consumption of fruit and vegetables ... Achieving UK dietary recommendations for fruit and vegetable consumption (five portions a day) would result in substantial health benefits. Equivalent benefits would be achieved if salt intakes were lowered to 3.5g per day or saturated fat intakes were lowered to 3% of total energy. (Scarborough *et al.* 2012: 420)

Nutrition, health and class

In their review of 196 studies across developed countries, including the UK, on the relationship between social class and diet, Darmon and Drewnowski (2008) bring together associations between diet and health, and between diet, health and class. They find that 'whole grains, lean meats, fish, low-fat dairy products and fresh vegetables and fruit are more likely to be consumed by groups of higher SES' whereas 'the consumption of refined grains and added fats has been associated with lower SES' (Darmon and Drewnowski 2008: 1107). The latter group experiences a greater incidence of health problems related to diet: obesity, diabetes, cardiovascular disease, osteoporosis, dental caries and some cancers (ibid.). These relationships were observed for a range of SES indicators including occupation, education and income, and several measures of diet quality, including 'fiber and nutrient intakes and selected plasma biomarkers' in many developed countries (ibid.: 1112).

There is evidence that fruit and vegetables have seen higher cost increases than foods high in fat and sugar. Greater food availability in general, and 'ongoing marketing incentives to consume large quantities of low-cost energy-dense foods' may be especially damaging for lower status groups (Darmon and Drewnowski 2008: 1113). In the UK in 2010, fruit and vegetable purchases (excluding potatoes) had declined to 2005–06 levels, particularly among low income households, where the reduction since 2006 was 30 per cent (2.7 daily portions per person): 'low income is associated with lower levels of fruit, vegetables and fibre, and with higher levels of NMES (non-milk extrinsic sugars)' (Defra 2011: 1). There is also a greater consumption of refined cereals as incomes decrease (Darmon and Drewnowski 2008: 1112). Those with a high income and higher education tend to have less energy-dense diets and to eat more fruit and vegetables (ibid.: 1110).

The type of fat consumed appears to differ by socio-economic group, but this was discussed by only one study out of 196. Five studies found lower status groups using more 'added fats' but did not always distinguish between animal and vegetable fats (ibid.: 1109). There may be some scope for assessing the type and quality of fats consumed by different social groups, as well as quantities. This might help to account for the significant presence of obesity, yet better health prospects, among some higher status groups, who may be consuming higher quality fats in both prepared foods and vegetable/cooking oils.

Kantar Worldpanel data shows that while the volume of take-home food grew by 0.5 per cent in 2011, the purchase of saturated fats grew by 4.8 per cent. Kantar data also shows a social gradient in saturated fat consumption, with ABC1s purchasing less and C2DEs purchasing more (these marketing classifications are discussed in Chapter 8) (Kantar 2011). Dorling and colleagues suggest that globalisation has increased fat production and consumption overall, while broadening choice and variety for affluent consumers, who can afford healthy but more expensive fats such as olive and fish oils (Pitts *et al.* 2007: 16, 28). They conclude that 'further distinctions need to be drawn between the conscious choice of fats and oils for cooking within the household, and the consumption of lipids that have been already incorporated into processed fare by the food industry' (ibid.: 30).

In studying fat consumption by low income people, the UK Low Income Diet and Nutrition Survey found that 'mean intakes of saturated fatty acids exceeded the dietary recommendation ... in all age groups, but most notice-ably in adults aged 65 and over and children aged 2–10' (FSA 2007b: 165). Intakes of 'good' fats – mono- and poly-unsaturated fatty acids were *below* recommended levels (ibid.).

Research into nutrition and health will become increasingly accurate with the growing use of metabolic testing (blood and urine tests for nutritional markers), addressing the under-reporting of food intake thought to be so common in dietary surveys (Darmon and Drewnowski 2008: 1110). Metabolic tests have hitherto been carried out mainly on 'at risk' groups, including pregnant women and older people (ibid.). Findings include an SES gradient for vitamins C and B12, riboflavin, carotenoids and potassium. Seven studies have found that iron deficiencies are more likely among children in lower SES families (ibid.: 1111). A subsequent US study in which Drewnowski participated found that consuming key nutrients vital for health led to higher overall dietary costs (Aggarwal *et al.* 2012). Conversely, diets high in saturated and transfats as well as added sugars cost less to purchase; and those consuming such diets were more likely to be found among those of low socio-economic status (ibid.).

The Marmot review of health inequalities (Marmot *et al.* 2010, full report) reviewed nearly 600 studies on all aspects of health inequality and found that:

- Internationally, 'among low income groups, price is the greatest motivating factor in food choice' (ibid.: 132). Robust evidence of the link between problematic access to healthy food and obesity or malnutrition is lacking; but shops that locate in deprived areas do not tend to sell healthy food and especially fresh produce (ibid.: 133).
- 'Low income groups are more likely to consume fat spreads, non-diet soft drinks, meat dishes, pizzas, processed meats, whole milk and table sugar than the better-off' (ibid.: 133).
- Obesity seems to be declining among girls from professional households, rising slightly for boys from this background, but rising faster for boys and girls from lower social classes.
- Adults' fitness levels rise by socio-economic group and 'children from high income households participate in nearly twice as much sport as children from low income households'. Higher income adolescents play more sport but 'participate less in active transport' (ibid.: 146).
- 'Improving the availability of and access to healthier food choices among low income groups involves population-wide interventions, such as reducing salt and saturated fat in products ... interventions may be needed to target particular groups' (ibid.: 146).

Marmot questions whether the social gradient in ill health is really as unavoidable as it seems, noting its variance for different health problems, and from one region or society to another. The most plausible explanation for differences in disease rates from one area of the country to another is 'characteristics of the social environment' (Marmot 2004: 46). Gradients for some diseases, including heart disease, have become steeper in recent decades (ibid.: 41). If these gradients can vary for reasons which governments did not intend, could they not be *induced* to vary to public health benefit by adopting policies which *aim* to do so (ibid.)? For example, if people stop smoking or achieve lower cholesterol or blood pressure rates, their CHD risk alters within five years (ibid.: 55).

Conclusion

This chapter has taken an empirical look at what is proposed in this book: that diet affects our health; that much more than individual choice is involved; that the discourse of personal responsibility obscures both social gradients in diet-related illness and the real suffering experienced in such illnesses, often over many years. By tracing the links between particular aspects of poor diet and specific health problems, and drawing further links with social structure and even governance as a factor in experiencing both poor diet and illness, the material discussed in this chapter clarified the firm empirical grounds for addressing the health and social consequences of the modern diet.

Poor quality foods, consumed disproportionately to healthy foods, and in the context of sedentary lives, are associated with chronic diseases, with or without the presence of overweight or obesity. The mortality risks of obesity may not be as pronounced as obesity discourse would imply, though they are higher for those of lower social class. Joint, circulatory, metabolic and other categories of health risk can also be heightened by the quantity and type of food we eat – and these risks are more likely to be experienced by those of lower social class. Our dietary options are shaped by the social and physical worlds we inhabit, and some social groups are eating a substantially less healthy diet than others.

The risk of disease varies significantly according to fitness level, disease category, ethnicity, class and age. There is a consensus on the value of exercise for metabolic health, but reservations about its effectiveness for losing weight, and an acknowledgement of the health risks for older people of losing weight. These nuances do not seem to have permeated the obesity discourse of a weight-obsessed society. But there is much rigorous, balanced epidemiological analysis of the links between obesity and the major disease groups discussed in this chapter. This work is characteristically open about areas of uncertainty and the scope for future clarification.

Overly rigid bodyweight measurements, moral judgements, exhortations to lose weight and the blaming and stigmatisation of fat people are worthy of attention and critique by social scientists. Scholars from a range of disciplines addressed these problems forcefully in a 2011 collection, under the rubric of critical weight studies (Rich *et al.* 2011). The activities of both weight loss and pharmaceutical industries in addressing obesity are also deserving of critical investigation. Based on the evidence that weight loss is difficult and usually unsustainable, and to address the stigma suffered by those with large bodyweights, Bacon and Aphramor (2011) make a powerful case for a Health at Every Size approach for improving health, rather than weight loss per se.

But social scientists should not be diverted from investigating the role of the food industry in shaping dramatically different patterns of food consumption – and their health and bodyweight consequences. As one of Monaghan's fellow critics of obesity discourse observed: 'Should we … be unconcerned that fast food multinational companies target poorer communities in order to sell more low quality food?' (Gard 2009: 34).

This chapter has given empirical substance to the theoretical analysis of class, capital, governance, consumption and health in the previous two. In the following three chapters, various dimensions of the food industry will be examined for their understanding of and engagement with these matters. There is much surprisingly common ground, with food scientists acknowledging health concerns and food marketing offering a highly operationalised, commercial, empirical grounding for the theoretical analysis in Chapters 3 and 4.

Before discussing how food marketing engages with notions of social class and helps to shape dietary patterns, I will outline the broader context from which food marketing strategies emerge, beginning with agricultural production, the processing and merchandising of foods, and industry's understanding of both health and limitations to the consumer's capacity to choose freely.

Notes

1 Effectiveness of these programmes varies: the longer people persist with them, the more effective they are (NICE 2014c). However, 'the weight difference with untreated comparison groups diminishes over time' (NICE 2014d: 7). No studies examined the effectiveness of such weight-loss programmes by socio-economic status; and 'there is a lack of high quality reviews on the effectiveness of weight-loss maintenance interventions' (NICE 2014c: 19). If the weight were to be regained in the long run, then the effectiveness of these programmes would be seriously challenged; but at the moment this cannot be known.

2 Blair acknowledges that he has received honoraria for board membership and research grants from US fitness company Jenny Craig (Sui *et al.* 2007: 2515)

3 Metabolic syndrome: 'a combination of medical disorders that increase the risk of developing cardiovascular disease and diabetes. Abnormal fat levels in the blood can lead to arteriosclerosis (fatty plaques) on the walls of blood vessels, high blood pressure and insulin resistance or glucose intolerance' (HSE 2008: 19). Differing criteria had developed under the metabolic syndrome label, provoking much debate (Nichols 2006). But by 2009, a harmonisation of the two most widely used definitions required three out of five criteria to be met (in the categories of 'population and country-specific waist circumference, triglycerides, HDL cholesterol, blood pressure and fasting blood glucose') (Thankamony *et al.* 2011: 301).

6 How the agri-food industry shapes our diets and influences our health

Introduction

> I serve the same to everyone, for when I invite guests it is for a meal, not to make class distinctions. (Pliny the Younger, cited in Steele 2009: 221)

> There are many [consumer] segments and subsegments, each with different motivations, different need states and different purchase drivers ... age, income, family status, ethnicity, education, employment ... and other factors shape consumers' beliefs, goals and purchases. (Schmidt 2009: 222; advice to food marketers)

These statements were made two millennia apart but each observes the concept of social ranks and distinctions where food consumption is concerned. In fact, Pliny's dismissal of class did not reflect the typical Roman view – in ancient Rome, as now, class distinctions *did* emerge at mealtimes (Steele 2009: 221). The marketing advice in the second quotation reflects how food products are conceived and segmented for marketing, with social rank denoted by the use of terms such as status, education, employment and income.

The previous chapter traced the health implications of qualitatively different diets and their link to socio-economic position – a manifestation of the role of social class in driving not only food consumption but also the varied nature of the food supply. Political and historical forces were also identified as factors influencing food consumption. The current and subsequent two chapters take a further step back from the act of eating and the social factors which influence it in order to examine the changing nature of the food supply and how it is financed, structured, processed, distributed and marketed. I discuss critiques of these activities, explore how the food industry understands consumption, and investigate concerns revealed by industry regarding human health.

The way agriculture has developed since the mid twentieth century has dramatically changed the nature, quality, quantity, availability and pricing of the food supply. But there are also historical continuities in the ways industry, forms of governance and technology have engaged with the food supply, altering consumption practices – and health – in class-specific ways. These continuities are also traced in this chapter.

Having reviewed the evidence in Chapter 5 for a link between social class, diet and health, and even political ideology and bodyweight trends, these insights need to be situated within the context from which they emerge: namely, that of agriculture and, subsequently, the way food is designed, processed and retailed. In this chapter, industry texts which discuss these technical and scientific matters reveal an almost Bourdieuan grasp of how food 'choices' arise, and they raise concerns about the food supply resulting from industrial processes and the health of those who routinely eat the poorest quality processed foods.

There are opportunities in this discussion to link the role of agricultural and food industry strategies with the theories of both Bourdieu and Habermas: agricultural and food industry trends and practices are forces interacting with and shaping the habitus, and altering the lifeworld, in terms of dietary practice. Concrete examples of the effects of the food chain from agriculture to arteries – from the changing ways food is grown to the health implications of the way it is processed, retailed, consumed and digested – link theoretical insights with the empirical world of food production and the way industry understands its health effects.

While it is certainly possible to prepare food from original ingredients, and to eat outside the norms for our social group or consumer segment, much of our diet is processed, consumed both in and outside of the home in an omnipresent foodscape, and targeted at us based on population tracking and segmenting techniques. Chapters 7 and 8 analyse these processes in detail. However, food marketing is one of the later stages in a process that begins much farther upstream. So it is useful to get an overview of the globalised, agro-industrial context in which food is produced and consumed so that food product development and marketing are fully contextualised.

The blanketing of British foodscapes with highly processed foods and the rise of bodyweights accompanied the growth in production of key commodity crops which are the basis, along with additives, for an array of snack foods, both sweet and savoury. The food and agriculture writer and journalist Felicity Lawrence describes this process: 'The same half-dozen heavily subsidised commodities – soya, rapeseed, palm oil, corn, sugar and rice – are broken down into their individual parts and endlessly reconstituted. They are sold back to us as processed food or turned into animal feed' (Lawrence 2008b).

Trade and investment policies play a major role in a globalised agriculture, food processing and food merchandising industry, and are traced in this chapter. The changing nature of British supermarkets and their role in shaping the food supply has in turn influenced consumption patterns, and is discussed here. Finally, the health effects of processed food as discussed by food industry scientists and others will be analysed. These reflect the epidemiological linkage between food consumption and health made in the previous chapter, and Bourdieuan ideas about how food tastes and habits are formed, but further concerns are revealed about processed foods which food scientists have identified.

Agricultural developments and changes in the food supply

Despite the importance of agriculture for health, there is little overlap or sectoral co-operation between agriculture and public health (Hawkes and Ruel 2006: 985). Yet changes in agricultural production in recent decades have dramatically increased production of the constituent ingredients of snack and other processed foods, altered consumption patterns, and accompanied an increase in obesity and diet-related illnesses. Neoliberalism, technological advancements and globalisation have been key to agricultural developments, but diet-related illness has not become central to international negotiations, which have liberalised trade and investment in agriculture, food processing and retailing. Instead, 'human health remains marginalized as a supply chain issue ... in contrast to the environmental and labor issues now perceived as supply chain issues' (Hawkes 2009: 338–9). Tracking the complete chain reveals gaps between 'processes and actors' where change could be introduced to alter supply chain dynamics and the nature of the food itself (ibid.: 340).

Changes at the agricultural level, whether because of technological advances, subsidies or market liberalisation, or some combination of these, can lead to the substitution of cheaper food items or ingredients for more costly ones (Hawkes *et al.* 2012). This can lower costs for agricultural components in processed food products. For example, switching from sugar to high fructose corn syrup means that the cost of the sweetener in US soft drinks is just 3.5 per cent of the total (Hawkes *et al.* 2012: 348).

Increased apple production can reflect not an increase in apple eating, but the use of apples and apple juice concentrate as sweeteners in highly processed foods and drinks (though they may be promoted as healthier products because of the apple content) (Hawkes *et al.* 2012: 349). Hawkes *et al.* identify 'food consuming industries' or FCIs as crucial actors in the food supply chain. Providing stable markets for growers, they have the power to influence what is produced (ibid.: 350). With product innovation and marketing constituting value added, and driving growth, FCIs buy basic agricultural commodities relatively cheaply and differentiate them into innumerable products (Hatanaka *et al.* 2006 cited in Hawkes *et al.* 2012: 349). These products are then targeted at appropriate consumer groups. This basic process applies to a range of foods: the processing of vegetables into prepared salad ingredients, chicken into fried chicken, corn into high fructose corn syrup and then soft drinks, or apple juice concentrate into cakes or soft drinks (ibid.: 349–50). Thus promoting healthy eating, even at the agricultural level, will not be effective unless the entire supply chain is taken into account, including processing and marketing. Investing in local agricultural production would need to ensure a direct producer to consumer distribution, without the intervention of FCIs (ibid.: 350).

But FCIs will remain dominant and continue to 'meet, mobilise and create consumer demand' (Hawkes *et al.* 2012: 350). If improving the nutritional quality of foods became a public policy objective, then 'a coherent framework of consumer-end standards and regulations to discourage the production and sale of energy-dense, nutrient poor foods' would be required (ibid.). Clearer global standards for the development and marketing of 'healthy' foods should also be set (ibid.: 351). In short, 'policymakers and suppliers need to ask and be asked: what would a food supply system and agriculture look like if they were responding to public health concerns?' (ibid.: 351).

The food industry texts analysed in this and the following two chapters reveal the challenges for policymakers should they try to set such standards. These texts portray the ideas and concerns of those working much further down the chain from agriculture, as commodities, processing technologies and market research and targeting techniques are mobilised in the service of company profits and shareholder returns. In this context public health is a concern for some in the industry, but for others it may be relevant only if identified by their target consumers. There are also varying interpretations of what 'healthy' foods are from an FCI perspective, reflecting consumer confusion on the same point.

But how is it that we find ourselves with a food production process which leverages agricultural commodities into so many unhealthy foods, and by such powerful intermediaries? Burch and Lawrence, sociologists studying shifts in global food systems, observe that in the twentieth century, the capitalist state began developing policies and incentives to 'fuse both agribusiness input-manufacturing firms (providing equipment, fertilisers and pesticides) and agribusiness output-processing firms (storing, packaging and selling farm products) ... [which] enhanced the role of corporate capital in the sourcing and in the delivery of foods to consumers' (Burch and Lawrence 2005: 11). Several studies have traced the use of science and technology 'to establish tight, usually vertical control over seeds, planting, tending, harvesting and processing specifications, and increasing centralisation of considerable commercial and intellectual power in transnational corporations' (Lang and Heasman 2004, Tansey and Rajotte 2008, McMichael 2009 all cited in Dowler *et al.* 2009: 201).

Agriculture has been in the process of globalisation and liberalisation since the 1970s, but received a major impetus with the international agreement on agriculture in 1994 as part of the General Agreement on Tariffs and Trade. This agreement reduced subsidies and tariffs, although some forms of protection remain (Hawkes 2006: 3). Agricultural liberalisation increased foreign investment and these forces spurred the growth of transnational food companies via 'vertical integration and sourcing', encompassing production, distribution, sales, outsourced inputs, and advantageous global siting arrangements (ibid.). Hawkes describes the integration of the global soybean market (soybean oil is used in many processed foods) across Brazil, Argentina, China, India and the US. Health concerns regarding trans fats have prompted the development of healthier forms of soybean oil for affluent markets, alongside continuing production of the basic soybean oil, with implications for health inequalities globally (ibid.: 5).

In the past 25 years, trade in processed foods – predominantly branded products produced by transnational corporations – has increased faster than the trade in unprocessed foods. This reflects a shift in foreign direct investment (FDI) from a focus on exporting raw materials to financing food processing within target markets, including the processing of products for sale in supermarket chains and fast food outlets (Hawkes 2006: 6). In this process, purchasing and marketing/advertising costs can be streamlined and foods sold at lower prices, all of which has increased sales. Essentially, then, FDI is 'making more processed foods available to more people', initially in developed country markets but increasingly in developing countries (ibid.: 7). FDI has influenced trends in agriculture and food processing via investment in everything from 'seeds, fertilisers and pesticides, to grain silos, milling equipment, refrigeration and packaging plants, to shipping containers and runways to move product to global markets' (Hawkes and Murphy 2010: 17).

But FDI has also influenced the expansion of food retailing and food service outlets (Hawkes and Murphy 2010: 24). By purchasing foreign affiliates, transnational corporations are able to bypass the costs and complexities of exporting while getting closer to customers around the world and lowering costs, because trade liberalisation has meant they can source the cheapest ingredients for their products (Hawkes 2010: 50–2). The growth of high volume supermarket chains has driven demand for processed foods, and made their distribution highly efficient: 'due to economies of scale in storage and distribution and technological advancements in supply logistics, they [supermarkets] are also able to sell processed foods at lower prices, while still maintaining profits' (Reardon *et al.* 2003 cited in Hawkes 2010: 52). Supermarkets use incentives to attract consumers to this proliferating array of foods, not least through promotional pricing (see Chapter 8). It is an interwoven pattern of developments in agriculture, trade, investment and retailing, to which food product development, food science, market research, marketing and advertising have also contributed. In the process, the entire food supply chain has been affected and sales have increased (Hawkes 2006: 7; 2010: 36).

These interlinked developments can be viewed within a Bourdieuan framework, as forces shaping the habitus. The end result, the increasing consumption of an increasing supply of highly palatable processed foods, many of them high in fat, salt and sugar, has its beginning in global forces in agricultural science and technology, alongside the global financial forces and techniques which have emerged in the neoliberal era. Bourdieu's focus is on social, structural factors such as social class, education and income, but the activities of the food industry, beginning with agriculture and including financing and retailing strategies, also affect the habitus, influencing 'behaviour' and 'choices'. Several examples of this are explored in the present and subsequent chapters. Habermas's ideas about technology, capital and the colonisation of the lifeworld provide a framework for linking diverse, global, agro-scientific trends and strategies, with their capacity to influence both food retailing and the dietary experience of individuals and social groups in the UK.

Liberalised trade and foreign investment have made processed and especially fast foods more available, alongside increased advertising and promotion of such foods (Hawkes 2010: 52). FDI and the increased trade in 'the inputs to processed energy-dense foods (refined grains, sugar cane and corn sweeteners and vegetable oils)' have markedly decreased the cost of such foods, not least through technical innovation (Drewnowski *et al.* 2010: 78–9). The global supply of vegetable oils such as 'corn, palm, palm kernel, rapeseed, soya bean and sunflower oil' was over 100 million tons by 2005, 'more than twice the amount produced in 1991 and more than 13 times world production in 1961' (ibid.: 79). How did this happen? To give three examples of shifting trends:

- Agricultural subsidies on corn led to overproduction dating back to the 1970s, which led to a search for alternative uses for it. High fructose corn syrup was one result; cheaper than sugar, it is used in many processed foods.
- Palm oil consumption grew as export taxes in Malaysia and Indonesia (the main producers of palm oil) decreased, and import barriers declined in key importing markets China and India (Hawkes 2007: S317–18).
- Soybean yields grew dramatically from the 1960s, when a tropical strain was developed in Brazil, where it is now the main vegetable oil produced. It is exported worldwide (Hawkes 2007: S317).

To address the health implications of the shift in diet brought about by these global developments, public health bodies should undertake stronger advocacy and monitoring of the food chain – but to do that, they would need 'new expertise, resources and, critically, imagination and political will' (Rayner *et al.* 2007: 72–3). All this requires an understanding of global agriculture, trade and investment activities. Other analysts suggest that given the implications for human health, governments should conduct health impact assessments of trade arrangements (Rigby *et al.* 2004: 426), ideally jointly carried out by economists and health and agricultural experts (Hawkes 2007: S319).

Agricultural oversupply and industrial foods

As a result of subsidies and agricultural innovation, excess calories began to be produced. The food industry sells these calories using various strategies:

> packaging foods in larger portions, increasing inducements for buying more food (package meals, etc), intensifying advertising, targeting new groups for sales (youth, minorities, etc), developing new sites for selling food (schools, drugstores, gas stations, etc), engineering foods to maximize taste (enhancing flavours, adding sugar and fat), reducing prices. (Brownell and Horgen 2004: 200–1)

This list renders how a Bourdieuan habitus can be permeated by developments in both food science and retailing. Existing tastes and practices are studied for clues to how to expand consumption where possible without altering consumers' routines and established behaviours.

Consumption must be expanded, though it can be difficult to track in terms of overall food consumption and health. To give a random set of examples of food retail expansion in the UK:

- In 2011 planning permission had been granted to more than 16,000 supermarkets, a 50 per cent increase (*Guardian* 22/12/11).
- Starbucks planned to open 300 new stores, including 200 drive-through outlets, in the next five years (*Guardian* 01/12/11).
- Greggs bakery planned 90 more stores in 2012 (*Guardian* 14/03/12); it already had 1,500 shops and was aiming for 2,000, according to *Marketing Magazine* (24/08/11a).
- Krispy Kreme has 46 outlets and 400 'branded cabinets' in other UK shops and planned to double outlets by 2015 (*Guardian* 07/03/12).
- Subway is to nearly double its UK and Ireland outlets (to 3,000) in the six years from 2014, creating 13,000 additional jobs (*Guardian* 22/01/14).
- The UK has 47,000 takeaway food outlets (Local Data Company) of which nearly half are independent. This varies by area: in London's Tower Hamlets, 89 per cent of takeaways are independent, most serving fried chicken (Bagwell 2011).

Gard, a critic of obesity discourse observing such trends, queries the conclusions of nutritionists

> who argue that human brains are 'hard wired' to crave sugar, fat and salt [when] there is no convincing evidence that the amount of sugar, fat and salt in modern fats and convenience foods is anything other than the product of successful marketing and the global over-production of these substances. (Gard 2009: 34)

In fact, both of these trends are real: we do crave these macronutrients, but they had never been supplied in such omnipresent and affordable quantities before the late twentieth century. This has in turn cued food consumption, increasing it along with the increase in the food supply.

The former Coca-Cola executive interviewed by Kessler seems to substantiate Gard's point, suggesting that the low cost of fats and sugars is at least partly responsible for the prevalence of fast/convenience foods:

> If McDonald's could sell anything and make money at the same rate that they're doing now, they couldn't care less whether it was fat- or sugar-laden. It just happens to be that fats and sugars and flours are some of the least expensive food items we have in the world. (Kessler 2009: 129)

This comment pithily exposes one dimension of food industry thinking, illustrating the journey ingredients make from agriculture to food processing to food retailing.

But how does an enhanced agricultural supply translate into palatable foods? Healthy eating messages have succeeded in reducing consumption of sugar added at the table, but the sugar that is produced must be consumed. Thus it is used as 'an industrial ingredient – particularly in carbonated drinks but also in a wide range of processed foods' including savoury foods (Fine *et al.* 1996: 274). The success of skimmed and semi-skimmed milk products has generated large quantities of leftover cream, which is then used as an industrial ingredient in processed foods or other dairy products (ibid.).

Europe's Common Agricultural Policy (CAP) guarantees minimum prices for producers. When prices fall below this level, 'the EU buys the product … and disposes of the surplus stocks' (Hawkes 2007: S315). Butter fat, for example, is resold to the food industry at lower prices and is used in processed foods, whereas 'surplus' fruit and vegetables are destroyed (ibid.).

The changing role of supermarkets

Sociologists and food regimes analysts Burch and Lawrence (2005) trace structural shifts throughout the supply chain. Nothing less than a 'restructuring of the capitalist agri-food system' is under way, they conclude, with Britain the primary site for its development, via supermarkets and distribution systems (Burch and Lawrence 2005: 1–2, 10). Examining the dominant role of processed food in contemporary diets, they argue that the decisive power in the food system has shifted from food manufacturers to food retailers. Ready meals are now routinely processed by manufacturers who have emerged merely as processors for retailer-branded products. Supermarkets are physically closer to their customers, and have developed a high degree of technological and marketing sophistication in tracking customer behaviour and inclinations. This has resulted in an increasingly segmented, targeted range of products which supermarkets are uniquely placed to deliver (Hawkes 2008: 668). Even by 1998, a food industry text noted that 'scanners give food retailers greater leverage with market information' (Michman and Mazze 1998: 27).

While contracting out the preparation of own-brand foods to manufacturers – many of whom prepare such foods for a range of stores, from elite to discount, and to a range of standards *within* stores – supermarkets are able to pressure suppliers and processors to keep costs low. They can also insist on up-to-the-minute changes in orders. Technology and especially logistics also play a vital role in this process, with deliveries organised to tight schedules and tracked by GPS systems (Burch and Lawrence 2005: 9).

At the same time, state sovereignty in terms of food governance has declined, with authority and market power shifting to supermarkets (Richards *et al.* 2013). The state continues to set basic standards for food safety, but since the UK's Food Safety Act of 1990, food retailers must observe 'due diligence' in ensuring the foods they sell are safe (Fulponi 2006 cited in Richards *et al.* 2013: 237). Food governance has effectively been privatised, with food retailers deriving their power 'through the neoliberalisation of regulation and uneven market relationships, which further serve to consolidate their power' (Richards *et al.* 2013: 237).

There has also been a shift in their influence over consumption. Food retailers have assumed the role of dietary authority, conferring legitimacy on new food products and formats while – contrary to food industry discourse – reducing consumer sovereignty (Burch and Lawrence 2005: 4). Retailers often speak of their commitment to satisfying consumer demand, but they are also active in shaping that demand via their capacity to leverage the food supply, carry out continual consumer research and encourage repeat purchases via loyalty schemes and special offers. Loyalty cards track the type, location and timing of purchases, alongside consumer addresses and credit ratings – invaluable for marketers and product developers (Fuller 2005: 120). Loyalty cards have thereby enabled 'a steady transition from mass marketing to targeted marketing' (Carrefour 2004b cited in Hawkes 2008: 679). In sociological terms, tracking customer practices provides insights into the habitus, so that new products can be targeted in ways which fit the existing habitus.

Fostering the loyalty of existing customers is worthwhile, since 'it is five times as expensive to recruit a new customer as it is to retain an old one' (Blythe 2006: 63). The logic of learning what consumers like in order to serve their needs well is unassailable in commercial terms. The effect is to reinforce consumption patterns for all types of diet, even as food products themselves are continually developed.

Benefits to consumers from the shift in power to retailers might include higher quality from suppliers for supermarket own-brand products, many of which now aim for 'restaurant quality' standard, as well as a high degree of manufacturing flexibility in delivering a growing range of 'home meal replacements' (ready meals) (Burch and Lawrence 2005: 5). In portraying themselves as 'the moral guardians of consumer sovereignty', food retailers have certainly purported to deliver high standards in their food provision (ibid.: 6, 14). In such cases the food industry meets and reinforces consumer expectations of freshness and novelty in their food products (ibid.: 6). Yet inspections of supermarket own brands have uncovered revealing variations in industry standards (see Chapter 8).

The transformation in the food system is characterised by food retailers 'operating under the same impulses to accumulation that has driven manufacturing capital in the past ... As globalisation proceeded, corporate capital in the agri-manufacturing sector proved to be highly mobile, moving around the world to source the cheapest inputs to the food manufacturing industry' (Burch and Rickson 2001 cited in Burch and Lawrence 2005: 12).

Opting out of the mainstream food industry: alternative producers and eaters

The permeation of consumption practices and food cultures by a globalised, highly technologised, marketing-oriented food industry is central to understanding the sociology of food. Through these processes, human health and well-being can be powerfully affected, a Bourdieuan habitus permeated and altered, a Habermasian lifeworld colonised, and a class structure and system enacted and reproduced.

But some social groups pursue alternative methods of food production, purchase and consumption: 'as individuals rebel against being confined to the role of simple consumers, as purchasers, some will inevitably escape from preoccupation with intrinsically constructing their own identity and extrinsically engage with the more distant determinants of consumption' (Fine 2006: 305). This is taking place with 'green' and local consumption, nowhere more evident than in the category of food. Extending the discourse of consumption from the practices of individual consumers to questions of 'provision, power and conflict' could help to expand the identity of the consumer to 'the realm of the citizen ... so the engaged consumer becomes the politicized citizen' (ibid.). Yet activists committed to alternative food supplies and networks can be insufficiently engaged politically: 'agro-food activism is often quite removed from a politics that names and addresses actually existing neoliberalizations of the food system' (Guthman 2008: 1180).

Alternative systems of food provision have received much academic attention, but have been inconsistently defined (Holloway *et al.* 2007: 2). While they offer useful insights for challenging existing systems of food production, alternative approaches remain marginal in terms of overall UK food consumption. Supporters of alternative approaches can also be colonised in ways they may not realise:

signs of resistance and revolt are quickly absorbed and commodified by capital. Rather than threatening the market, consumer boycotts, resistance to material acquisition, revolutionary consumers, and use of consumption for political expression rejuvenate the market. (Holt 2002 cited in Cherrier and Murray 2004: 511)

So what begins as defiance can become absorbed by consumer culture (Cherrier and Murray 2004: 511). Reflecting this tendency, one US entrepreneur in the 1970s argued that

> mass production requires consumer education which limits the concept of social change and progress to the 'commodified answers rolling off American conveyor belts' (Ewen 1976) ... freedom and liberty should be confined to the marketplace ... what needs to be emphasized regarding responsible citizenry is consumer choice, not political action in a public sphere. (cited in Cherrier and Murray 2004: 517)

An undergraduate marketing textbook describes how the 'giants of the global food industry have embraced the [green/fairtrade] movement, reflecting the growing interest in ethical trading by consumer and major retail chains' (Dibb and Simkin 2009: 86). Firms like Nestle and Kraft have introduced ethically traded product lines, or products with a percentage of ethically traded ingredients, reflecting 'their alert scanning of market trends' (ibid.). This seems a positive step, though a prosaic one when compared with Fine's hopes for an engaged citizenry demanding market transformation.

While fairtrade issues have surged ahead in consumer and corporate awareness, the same cannot be said for food–health concerns in a supply chain context. An illustration of this phenomenon is pictured in Figure 6.1: fair trade as a concept is embraced and promoted in these vending machine products.

These machines are also an example of the spread of snack foods into locations where they did not previously exist. In February 2013, the Academy of Medical Royal Colleges issued ten recommendations to address obesity, including an appeal to local councils to limit the number of fast food outlets near places where children gather, including leisure centres (AMRC 2013: 10). Yet these snack and drinks machines like the ones pictured here are located inside such centres.

Alert food providers and marketers track challenges to the corporate food system and create products and services to meet emerging green/ethical/quality/provenance demands. This *can* produce high quality foods, fairly traded, with concern shown for the environment. But that is not necessarily the case for all apparently 'ethical' products; consumers need to remain alert to ensure that this is what they are getting. Nor are these industry practices immune to larger economic conditions: organic food sales declined by 3.7 per cent in 2011 in the UK, decreasing by 5 per cent in supermarkets,

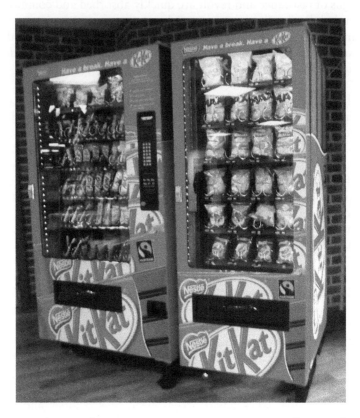

Figure 6.1 Vending machines in a community sports centre sell Fairtrade crisps and chocolate (Fairtrade stickers are on the machines). Photograph by Melanie Jervis.

where 71.4 per cent of organic food is sold (Soil Association 2012).[1] Ethical considerations may not have the same appeal during times of austerity (*Marketing Magazine* 14/03/12). Only 29 per cent of consumers said social responsibility figures in their purchases, down from 43 per cent in 2008 (Ipsos MORI poll cited in ibid.). So while a sense of social responsibility had been absorbed into the habitus of some consumers, financial pressures stemming from the economic crisis pushed this consideration regarding food consumption back out again. It is another illustration of how the habitus can be influenced by events external to the individual or social group.

The process of processing food

Food processing can be considered a form of predigestion of raw biological materials prior to consumption. (Watzke and German 2009: 153)

This description of processed food, by food product developers, is in stark contrast to the expertly packaged, temptingly described ready meals available in supermarkets, and is a pointed reminder of the unseen and highly industrialised dimensions of the retail food industry. Given the significance of processed food in the foodscapes and diets of all social groups, whether consumed at home, in schools and workplaces, or as takeaway or restaurant meals and snacks, it is useful to understand how such foods are produced, why they have become so successful and the implications for health. Epidemiological studies on this point have already been discussed; in this section the views of food industry figures will be traced via their published work. Their conclusions are naturally generous towards the intentions and achievements of the industry, but there are concerns about the problems associated with an industrialised, highly processed diet.

Historical context

The earliest techniques and tools for harvesting, processing and preserving foods appeared after 11,000 BC, mostly to allow consumption of wild cereals in the Fertile Crescent (Diamond 1999: 110–11). Fermentation of foods dates back 9,000 years; cured meats, salt cod, sausages and marmalade have a long history (Saberi 2011). Food processing was the result of natural developments (animal extinctions, climate change); domestication of wild plants; new technologies (cutting, grinding, roasting, storage); a rise in population as food production increased; and displacement of hunter-gatherers by food producers (Diamond 1999: 111–12). Diamond identifies an 'autocatalytic process' in an accelerating cycle of positive feedback as food production expands (ibid.). This is one illustration of what another analyst has termed the 'adjacent possible': it is what happens when technological and scientific progress collide with cultural and societal forces to produce incremental but ultimately decisive change (Johnson 2010). This process is now happening so rapidly and at such high levels of technical complexity that the implications of changes taking place may not be grasped while they are unfolding. Arguably, this is what has happened with the predominance and merchandising of foods high in fat, salt and sugar. As Habermas noted previously, such progress takes place 'without being reflected upon' in societies lacking political consciousness.

Interlocking technological and social developments define food production and consumption at any stage in history. In eighteenth century British towns, little food preparation was carried out in many households. Instead, 'there was a large market in ready-cooked food, both take-away and pub food' and 'a multiplicity of cookshops' serving the urban poor (Laurence 2002: 149–50). Technology, housing and market conditions combined to produce prepared food for the home in this very public way.

In another example of the 'adjacent possible', by the late nineteenth century, technological and transport advances meant that Britain was the world's major importer of preserved and processed foods, primarily tinned fruit, meat and condensed milk (Steel 2009: 92). This was quite apart from massive imports of wheat and sugar by that time. Prepared foods made locally were also popular in the nineteenth century. Many industrial workers, living in cramped housing without cooking facilities, survived on bread, tea and small amounts of cheese, salted fish and meat (Burnett 1989: 28). Many town-dwellers had no hot food unless they took it to a bakeshop for cooking or bought pies, bacon or baked potatoes from cookshops (Steel 2009: 164–7; Gaskell [1848]1970). Wilson's study of food adulteration in the nineteenth century shows that the quality of foods for the poor was low, with meat often past its best, and they were victims of swindling more than other social groups (Wilson 2009: 100–1). This gives some historical contextualisation to the role of societal structures and practices in determining the type and quality of foods consumed.

Yet a newspaper report from 1864 bemoans the lack of cooking skills among working-class girls, who, in adulthood, supposedly become reliant on prepared foods such as 'relishes, cooked meat from the shop' and beer or spirits (*Guardian* [1864]16/01/07). A similar criticism in 1901 describes 'the combination of careless methods and downright waste which passes for cookery among the poorer classes' (*Guardian* [1901]03/09/10). These are early illustrations of a tendency to blame the poor for their own predicament.

Experience of land enclosures in the nineteenth century had seen traditions of foraging and peasant cooking lost, changing dietary habitus and altering lifeworlds in an alienating way. During industrialisation, workers' inadequate diets and limited cooking facilities were of little concern to most employers or authorities (Wilson 2009: 21).

Britain's industrialised palate had made it a ready market for American processed foods long before the rest of Europe (Steel 2009: 237). From 1860 to 1960, British consumption of sugar doubled, fat consumption increased by 40 per cent, and 90 per cent less fibre was consumed (Porter 1999: 559), a dramatic illustration of how, over a 100-year period, dietary practices were altered by a changing food supply fuelled by developments in technology and trade. The dietary practices emerging from the habitus of the time were highly permeable to such change. Nor were these changes all palatable ones: recalling Bourdieu's observation that people develop a taste 'for what they are anyway condemned to' (Bourdieu [1984]2010), by the 1930s many British people apparently preferred tinned milk, peas and fish to fresh versions (Orwell 1937 cited in Steel 2009: 237). Friedmann contextualises today's poor quality diets by finding their origins during the 1930s:

> had the poor been able to purchase enough horticulture and meats from local farms beginning in the 1930s, their purchases would have strengthened regional fresh markets in 'advanced' countries, leaving major grains and livestock to industrial agriculture. Instead, those

farmers and markets were decimated by half a century of industrializa-
tion of food and farming, and the poor (in the US) were given surplus
industrial food, which came to dominate the diets of the poor in the
[global] North. (Friedmann 2009: 341)

She finds this process now happening in the global south, as food supply
chains there are colonised by transnational companies, affecting farmers,
markets and consumers alike. Thus 'the growing masses of the poor who
can no longer access fresh foods find that if they can afford any commercial
food at all, it is the least healthy and most durable commodities' (Friedmann
2009: 341).

Food processing today: combining technology and psychology

Processed foods today are the result of disassembling constituent commodities in order to 'separate the biological tissues into their biomaterial components, proteins, carbohydrates, oils, etc.' (Watzke and German 2009: 136).
Once these ingredients have been 'purified' in this way, they are used in a
range of food products 'most of which are unrecognizable as the original
commodity' (ibid.). This is in contrast to the origins of food processing, which
aimed to stabilise foods during storage (ibid.; Burch and Lawrence 2005: 11).
Today even the most glamorous ready meals are the product of highly industrialised processes. But technology is not the only driver of changes in food
processing. This section looks at how industry expertise in both technology
and psychology shapes the development and processing of foods.

   Food products are developed 'from concept to marketplace': consumer
researchers uncover the 'perceived needs' of potential consumers and relay
this information via product statements to food technologists, who in turn
develop prototypes which are subsequently tested and refined (Fuller 2005).
Food product development involves 'a continuing interplay of market
research, technology and financial efforts of companies' so that a new product will make its mark with targeted consumers (ibid.: 31).

   Key steps in food product development are set out in another industry
text which advises food industry managers to categorise both consumers
and food products:

> analyze the socioeconomic developments in specified markets, translate
> consumer preferences and perceptions into consumer categories, trans-
> late consumer categories into product assortments, group product assort-
> ments in product groups at different stages of the food supply chain ...
> match specified state of the art processing technologies with future needs.
> (Jongen and Meulenberg 1998 cited in Van Boekel 2009: 41)

In a consumer-centred model of food processing, 'the industry does not
formulate products per se, but rather targets the consumer and the eating

opportunities to provide a wide variety of benefits, using foods as the vehi-cles of those benefits' (Watzke and German 2009: 139). This is a flexible model which enables the industry to address changing consumer needs and lifestyles.

The need for food itself might be accompanied by the need for conveni-ence in terms of time, purchase location and ease of preparation; the need for affordability; and the need for comfort. So technological capacity is brought together with insights into the lives of consumers, and into their psychological states and the 'needs' which derive from those states. This is in effect a commercial attempt to understand the habitus in order to engage with it when introducing new or modified products, and then, through the successful marketing of the products that emerge from this research, gradu-ally changing the habitus, perhaps without the consciousness of the indi-vidual ever having been fully engaged. Lanier, an architect and analyst of digital capitalism, concludes that 'Advertising counter-balances the tendency of people to adhere to familiar habits' (cited in *Guardian* 02/03/13). This is one way the food lifeworld is altered, with some individuals consuming an ever more industrialised diet, having seen it attractively portrayed in adver-tisements being consumed by people like them.

Corporate food science is dependent on a good understanding of 'how people respond to products at a basic, sensory, subjective level, [and] are by necessity grounded in the measurement of perception' (Cox and Delaney 2009: 278). In order to develop this sort of understanding, food industry scientists need to work closely with marketers and, via them, consumers (ibid.: 278).

Hyperpalatability of processed food

Dr David Kessler, former commissioner (head) of the US Food and Drug Administration, used his FDA contacts to interview food industry repre-sentatives anonymously (Kessler 2009). One described how his firm designed food for 'hedonic' or pleasurable appeal: 'sugar, fat and salt are either loaded onto a core ingredient' (ibid.: 19). The resulting 'fat-on-sugar-on-fat-on-salt-on-fat combinations generate multiple sensory effects' (ibid.: 91). The industry also uses chemical flavourings 'to drive consumer desire' (ibid.: 119). These are examples of how advances in food technology are driven by insights into consumer psychology.

Kessler's interview with an industry expert in sensory enhancement reveals the range of stimuli foods can provide: 'flavour ... aroma ... oral texture ... visual texture ... manual texture ... creaminess ... firmness ... melt ... viscosity ... tooth stick ... mouth coating ... particle size ... adhe-siveness ... moisture absorption' (Kessler 2009: 90). These technical terms are linked to psychological responses to foods.

An innovation in pizza stylings – the stuffed pizza crust – illustrates the point. While currently widely available from several pizza chains, Pizza Hut apparently introduced a cheese-filled crust in 1995, which became instantly popular (*Business Week* 01/02/13). The Pizza Hut website in June 2014 notes the return of its cheese-filled crust (though it had by then been available for at least a few years), now with a garlic butter finish.

This kind of innovation can cue the psychological response which hyper-palatable foods aim for. It adds fat and calories to a product category not short of these elements and is one way in which consumption can be subtly steered. Some people who already eat pizzas from pizza chains – for whom regular pizza consumption is part of their Bourdieuan habitus – will be open to product innovations that add known elements to a tried and tested product. In food design and marketing terms, because it builds on existing, successful products, it is not a big risk. Crusts stuffed with cheese are still widely available in the UK and many other countries, from a variety of pizza restaurant chains (see Figure 6.2).

A twist on the cheese-filled crust was the crust filled with a circular hot dog, introduced by Domino's. The company attributed its positive results in the first quarter of 2013 to the popularity of this new pizza (*Independent* 04/04/13). A version of it also became available at Pizza Hut, though neither appeared to stock it as of June 2014 (see Chapter 7, 'The power – and weaknesses – of marketing: a critique', for a discussion of the fast-moving consumer goods product cycle).

How could these product innovations find consumers? The idea that the pizza crust could provide extra value by being stuffed with something other than dough was already established. A variation on the cheese stuffing was

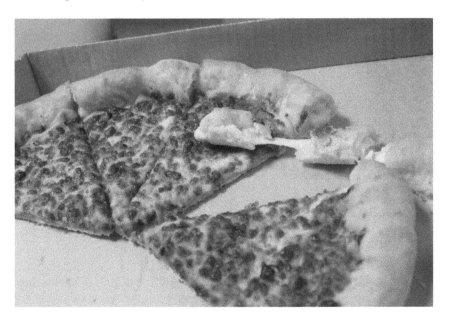

Figure 6.2 Cheese-filled pizza crust. Photograph by Eric Davidson.

the hot dog filling in the crust. Pizza Hut followed this with a pizza surrounded by 'hot dog pizza bites': instead of one curved hot dog in the surrounding crust, several smaller hot dogs in rolls of dough served as the outer edge of the pizza, with pizza toppings in the centre. This pizza was designed so that it was easy to pull apart – possibly less messy than the hot dog pizza above. While not currently available, another similar innovation is a cheesy bites 'crust': 28 cheese-filled rolls topped with garlic butter, surrounding a large pizza.

It is one illustration of how food companies continually refresh product categories by altering formats or ingredients while building on a product that is already familiar to consumers – and how the convenience/snack food habitus of target consumers is gradually expanded in new directions. It encapsulates the 'fat-on-salt-on-fat' characterisation of food designed for hedonic appeal, as described by Kessler's food industry informant.

Thus an already calorie-dense and hyperpalatable food becomes even more so. Pizza eating has been transformed from its origin as a simple tomato sauce and cheese on a plain crust into this hyperpalatable dish, featuring an ever increasing variety of layered flavours and ingredients. How can this process of continual product innovation of hyperpalatable foods fit with the government's expectation that the food industry will be removing calories from the food supply?

A key dimension (and appeal) of much processed food is the ease of chewing. Foods which are crispy on the outside may be soft inside and quickly chewed (Kessler 2009: 69). This is achieved by replacing water content with fat, the use of binders, chopping techniques and 'autolyzed yeast extract, sodium phosphate and soy protein concentrate' (ibid.). A restaurant concept designer describes the results of such processing as 'adult baby food' (Kessler 2009: 95). Thus shredded cabbage and carrot become coleslaw in a high fat dressing; apples become apple sauce; brown bread and brown rice become their whitened versions, with the bran milled away from them (ibid.). A Big Mac burger bun contains 'high-fructose corn syrup, soybean oil, canola oil, and partially hydrogenated soybean oil', although the partially hydrogenated oil was scheduled for removal (Kessler 2009: 86). Many baked products are made with 'a chemical mix of preservatives and oil', according to a former Coca-Cola executive (ibid.: 129).

Kessler concludes: 'by eliminating the need to chew, modern food processing techniques allow us to eat faster ... refined food simply melts in the mouth' (ibid.). Technology will always aim at increased efficiency and lowered production costs, but in the case of food products, the technology will also serve the psychological dimension of eating. It is not necessary to embrace the notion of consuming chemical preservatives and enhancers in order to enjoy food products; indeed, few people will be aware of these chemical constituents even as they permeate our diets. Hence no conscious change to the habitus, in the context of dietary practice, is required. But the lifeworld is nevertheless altered as consumers understand less about their food, which is portrayed in ways which divert attention from the industrialised nature of it.

Kessler's book emphasises the role of palatability and even hyperpalatability in obesity, citing dozens of psychology studies on the subject, but does not consider the social gradient in obesity or what might modify these seemingly universal tendencies in some eaters. Yet there is much evidence for the link between social inequality, obesity and other diet-related health problems in the US (see Lee 2011; Wang *et al.* 2008; Kant and Graubard 2013; Singh *et al.* 2011; Cunningham *et al.* 2014; Su *et al.* 2012; Bambra *et al.* 2012; Aggarwal *et al.* 2012).

Wilson's historical study of adulterations does make modern comparisons in a class context, noting the persistence of adulterations in the form of additives and chemical/industrial substances, which are more likely to be found in foods purchased by those on low incomes. Addressing such consumers directly, she writes:

> Your meat is more likely to come pumped with hormones and water. Your bread is more likely to be bleached ... Your fat is more likely to be hydrogenated. Juice is too expensive, so your children drink squash laced with colourings and sweeteners. (Wilson 2009: 100)

The industrialised nature of such products is not apparent in images or language used in marketing them. These foods are designed to appeal to those at whom they are aimed. In order to afford a healthy diet, Wilson suggests, those on low incomes would need to grow vegetables, find a local market or co-op, or shops selling rice and lentils economically, 'but the disparity is still there. The rich can eat unadulterated food without much bother, whereas for most of the poor, it is a constant effort' (Wilson 2009: 100). This link between food and poverty is made by several studies (for example, Dowler *et al.* 2001; Hitchman *et al.* 2002; Dowler 2008a, 2008b; Dowler and O'Connor 2012; Ashton *et al.* 2014).

'Health' foods, food science and food product development

> Obesity is now one of the biggest drivers of food-based scientific research. It seems to me that consumers have decided to blame the food and drink companies for making their products taste so good. (Former industry food scientist cited in *Guardian* 19/01/10)

The satiety research being carried out by the scientist cited above aims to curb appetite via 'an aqueous solution that gels into a solid structure in the stomach' (*Guardian* 19/01/10). But having made processed foods 'taste so good', industry scientists must now turn their attention to more functional matters, such as the manner and speed at which food is transported through the digestive system, for those who are trying to lose weight. Other research is looking into the functionality of food components, food structure, taste, texture and flavour. The food industry's development of healthy products naturally focuses on technological processes used in food processing. This section highlights industry activities and commentary which focus on the potential for technology to address consumer interest in healthy eating.

Guthman and DuPuis set these activities in a neoliberal context, describing industry responses to consumer concerns about weight. One approach is to create functional products like the ones described above – 'food products that do not act like food' (Guthman and Dupuis 2006: 441). Thus

> the substance used as fat in low-fat ice cream or ... the new low-calorie sugar, break right through the problem of inelastic demand ... the commodity simply passes through the body, enabling the product to be consumed with no weight-gaining effect ... New pharmaceuticals ... and nutritional supplements designed to reduce the body's absorption of fat (along with essential vitamins and minerals) fulfill a similar function. By thwarting the body's metabolizing functions, these products allow producers to sell much more of these products per person. (Guthman and Dupuis 2006: 441)

Another strategy is to commodify dieting itself, with low fat products targeted at concerned eaters, even while foods such as fruit and vegetables are neglected (Guthman and DuPuis 2006: 441). Fruit and vegetables are important in a healthy diet, but it is expensive to chop and prepare them: 'that's why it's so hard to run a business that sells fresh and healthy foods on a mass scale' (Kessler 2009: 122). So in Habermasian terms, the food lifeworld of those targeted with diet foods is disrupted as emerging health concerns are colonised not by overtly healthy foods, but by industrialised foods which themselves constitute a growing market for individuals worried about their weight.

Food industry scientists note a growing interest in healthy eating, as 'poor choices in foods have been damaging the health of the average consumer' (Watzke and German 2009: 148). Yet public food intake data and consumer research data show that healthy eating is increasingly appealing to some, but not all, population groups. Nevertheless, the greatest growth area in the food industry is in foods considered (by consumers, according to industry research) to be health-promoting (ibid.: 149). But this notion hinges on perceptions of healthy products: 'If we can understand the consumer's lifestyle and perception of health we can develop products with functional ingredients that will address these needs and create value for the consumer – from the consumer's perspective – as well as the food industry' (Wennstrom and Mellentin 2002: 31). Industry needs to

> build sufficient knowledge on the relations between personal health and appropriate diets to create a new marketplace reality. The opportunities to capture consumers and market share are massive. Growing

scientific knowledge and technological advances will race to meet these needs and opportunities. (Watzke and German 2009: 149)

Science and technology are central to the development of health-promoting foods for health-seeking consumers, providing both challenges and opportunities for the food industry.

Food industry research shows that people define health in positive terms, and feeling energetic: 'that's why one of the fastest growing areas of the functional foods market is energy-boosting products' including snack bars, sports beverages, and drinks containing caffeine. These are not technically healthy drinks, 'but those who buy it don't see it that way. Companies need to understand that' (Wennstrom and Mellentin 2002: 16). Consumer *perceptions* are key, then, whether they are accurate or not. Thus some people will be making choices they believe are healthy, or at least not harmful, when this may not be the case.

Energy drinks: a case in point

The health status of 'energy' drinks is problematic. A systematic review of studies of the health effects of such beverages on young people notes a link with obesity (Seifert *et al.* 2011). Energy drinks containing caffeine are not regulated because they are described as 'natural dietary supplements' (ibid.: 520) and are not therefore subject to the same caffeine limits as other soft drinks. The authors conclude:

> Energy drinks have no therapeutic benefit, and many ingredients are understudied … The known and unknown pharmacology of agents included in such drinks, combined with reports of toxicity, raises concern for potentially serious adverse effects in association with energy drink use. In the short-term, paediatricians need to be aware of the possible effects of energy drinks in vulnerable populations and screen for consumption to educate families. (Seifert *et al.* 2011: 511)

Consumption of energy drinks has increased markedly. In the UK in 2010, consumption of take-home glucose and stimulant beverages rose 19 per cent in quantity and value, according to an industry report (*Guardian* 23/03/11). In 2011, growth was 17 per cent (*Marketing Magazine* 25/04/12). The energy drinks market in the UK was worth £1,400 million in 2012, a 12.8 per cent increase over 2011 (volume increased by 9.7 per cent) (BSDA 2013: 16). In Figure 6.3, energy drinks machines are located in a neighbourhood sports centre. The beverages are aimed at those on their way to the fitness studio and are described in terms associated with physical strength (power, muscle, etc.).

Despite the health risks, particularly as consumption increases, such drinks continue to be described and understood as energy products, and

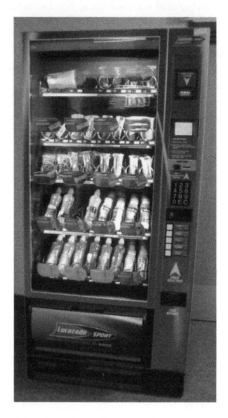

Figure 6.3 Energy drinks and snack vending machine in a community sports centre, occupying previously empty spaces. Photograph by Melanie Jervis.

linked to ideas of health and strength. Studies challenging these linkages have not permeated the production or consumption of such products; the language used diverts attention from health concerns to a more positive interpretation of the drink's action on the human body.

Retailers are advised in marketing literature that 'designing and positioning functional products so that they fit readily within the consumer's lifestyle without major behavioural change, or even enhance that lifestyle, is already well established as a critical success factor for functional foods' (Wennstrom and Mellentin 2002: 16). This recalls a Bourdieuan concept of habitus: established eating patterns cannot easily be dislodged, so new products should build on those which are already part of consumers' lives. Understanding consumer psychology and lifestyles is vital: retail success relies 'not only [on] the excellence of your science but the excellence of your understanding of the consumers' lifestyle, needs, beliefs, values and psychology' (ibid.: 5). Thus, tapping into well-studied patterns of behaviour and preferences, one energy drink brand, targeting 16 to 24 year olds, invited social network users to a web page where they could access music content aimed at this age group (*Marketing Magazine* 02/03/11b). While energy drinks might not have previously been part of their dietary habitus, by targeting this group through music they already listen to, and associating the energy drinks with the kinds of people who listen to such music, the habitus is subtly permeated. The blackcurrant variant of this drink was being launched with a £1 million marketing campaign (ibid.).

Since new products are commercially risky, a popular strategy for expanding sales is to modify existing products (Wennstrom and Mellentin 2002: 4). In Bourdieuan terms, it is possible for outside agents to alter the habitus, but it is easier to sell products which are similar enough to those already consumed by the target group – already a part of their dietary habitus – that a major change in habitus is not required. Thus food manu- facturers should 'increase value-added by using the new nutrition science to add health benefits to products in the food categories in which they are already competing' (ibid.: 16).

Consumers have widely differing understandings of what constitutes healthy foods, because of 'the massive increase in the amount of media coverage of food and health and the increasing advertising of products which offer health – and the apparently contradictory nature of many of the messages consumers receive' (Wennstrom and Mellentin 2002: 5). 'Healthy' eating can range from 'low-carb high-protein diets to the wheat-free diets or low-fat foods, energy drinks and so on' (ibid.). With fragmented consumer understanding of healthy foods, mass market success is difficult: 'most functional brands perform as niche products' (ibid.). However, it is possible to 'evolve brands from the niche towards the mainstream' and firms are encouraged to do so (ibid.). Previously cited sales figures for energy drinks marked growth in product use; these products are now a normal feature of sports centres and the practice – and habitus – of many of those who engage in sport and fitness.

Low fat products and health

Not all 'healthy' fast food and snack products are this successful, yet they may still be worth manufacturing and retailing for other reasons. Kessler asked a food industry executive if low calorie/low fat products sell well. The executive responded: 'Who cares? You're going to build your image' – i.e. that the company is addressing health issues (Kessler 2009: 131). In the UK, many fast food restaurants offer low calorie/low fat options. But do they appeal to their customers? Noting fast food customers' traditionally stronger attraction to palatable food, one marketer writes, 'It's no coinci- dence that fast food companies often launch healthy products that custom- ers don't actually buy' (Graves 2010: 18–19). He cites skinless chicken at KFC, low calorie pizza at Pizza Hut and the reduced fat McDonald's McLean burger as having failed (ibid.). So some fast food retailers do respond to pressures (if not from their own customers) to produce healthy versions of their products, a justifiable strategy even if not commercially successful. While providing healthy items, firms can continue to develop and market products for their main customer base, who may not be attracted or diverted by healthier alternatives. From the examples discussed in this chapter, it seems easier to divert an already unhealthy dietary habitus towards similar new products than to try and convince this group to eat healthy versions of products they already consume. Those who are interested in healthy eating presumably purchase food elsewhere and may be sceptical – if they are aware at all – of healthier versions of fried chicken, pizza and hamburgers from fast food retailers. This activity may ultimately be a distraction from the larger, core commitment to producing calorie-dense foods for their main target group.

What about the health status of low fat products? This too is controversial. People tend to 'overconsume' such products and this may contribute to weight gain (Wansink and Chandon 2006: 605). Everyone, but especially those who are already overweight, consumes greater quantities of snack food labelled as low fat (ibid.: 606). Ingredients which replace fat in low fat foods can have an unsatisfying taste, 'which consumers may try to offset by consuming more' (ibid.: 616).

People tend to confuse the low fat designation with low cholesterol and low calorie (Wansink and Chandon 2006). Yet 'low-fat foods typically compensate for the reduction in fat by an increase in carbohydrates' (Burros 2004 cited in Wansink and Chandon 2006: 607). Sugar is frequently used to mask unpalatable tastes (although a lower calorie sweetener is being developed; company representative cited in *Marketing Magazine* 11/01/11).

Consumers are not able to track accurately the calories they are consuming (Wansink and Chandon 2006: 607). Even products with nearly 60 per cent less fat had only 15 per cent fewer calories than the standard version of the same product (ibid.: 609). Calorie estimates were markedly lower among overweight eaters, who ate more low fat products (ibid.); the nutrients used in place of fat seem to make people feel more hungry (Nestle 2002 cited by Wansink and Chandon 2006: 607). Consumers experience confusion when faced with the terms '"reduced calorie" or "low carbohydrates" and labels such as "Sensible Snacking" (Nabisco/Kraft), "Smart Spot" (PepsiCo) and "Healthy Living" (Unilever) – all of which lend a "health halo effect"' (Wansink and Chandon 2006: 614). In adopting a critical perspective on healthy eating discourse, it is clear that consumers need to be wary of these terms. Even food industry voices acknowledge that consumers can be confused about what constitutes healthy foods, and that products can sometimes be portrayed as healthier than they are.

Reformulated processed foods may be an improvement on their predecessors, but how 'healthy' are they? Referring to the replacement of fat by sugars, grains or starches in low fat foods, the Harvard School of Public Health (2012) describes the result: 'our bodies digest these refined carbohydrates and starches very quickly, causing blood sugar and insulin levels to spike and then dip, which in turn leads to hunger, overeating and weight gain'. Furthermore, in cutting back on fat, people might 'stop eating fats that are good for the heart along with those that are bad for it' (ibid.).

A further, paradoxical problem with the marketing of 'healthy' foods was identified by marketing academics who tested implicit health references and images ('primes') in the purchase or consumption environment (Geyskens *et al.* 2007: 118). They found that background health messages increased consumption, lowered risk perceptions and encouraged people to think they are closer to their ideal weight than they are. This also increases consumption: 'consumers may believe that they can devote less effort to their diets than in situations without health primes' (ibid.: 122). These find-ings build on earlier research which found that healthy product images and thin models in food advertising may lead people to consume more because, identifying with these healthy looking models, they temporarily distance themselves from their goal to restrict food intake' (ibid.: 119–20). Alternatively, overconsumption may become a coping mechanism: 'health references may induce consumers to realize that they are not healthy at all, which may demotivate them to stay with their plan' (ibid.: 123).

Among people who stockpile low fat foods, not perceiving a risk of weight gain from eating them, and influenced by the healthy references on these products, overconsumption would result: 'stockpiling makes people consume convenience products at a faster rate' (Chandon and Wansink 2002 cited in Geyskens *et al.* 2007: 123). The same could happen with 'virtue' convenience foods. The authors urge public policy regarding obesity to take account of these phenomena (ibid.). The government's request to the food industry to make processed foods healthier – a strategy supported by the WHO in 2004 for tackling obesity (Geyskens *et al.* 2007: 118) – needs to be seen in this light. Lowering fat content and using health-promoting images and language have some paradoxical effects.

This section has revealed the insights of food and marketing industry practitioners and academic marketers in either promoting or critiquing the use of 'health' concepts in formulating and marketing food and drink prod-ucts. The terminology and images used to portray food as healthy can add to consumer confusion and increase consumption of products that are problematic for health (particularly as consumption increases, which is what the marketing of these products is designed to achieve).

Food, habit, consciousness and consumer 'choice': industry perspectives

> We become who we are by copying others ... through the interaction of copycat individuals, a crowd (or market) can develop strikingly consis-tent behaviour without any agreed or planned intention to do so. (Earls, a marketer, 2009: 14, 41)

> Over 85 per cent of consumer buying behaviour is driven by the non-conscious. (Buyology Inc. cited in *Economist* 2011)

The underlying assumption of healthy eating discourse – that one's diet is a matter of choice – is frequently cited by the food industry in defence of its activities, but challenged by the quotations above. If an understanding of human psychology is so central to developing and selling consumer products, as marketing literature often emphasises, how 'free' is the consumption activity which emerges from psychological states? How effectively can industry engage with those states to shape them? And what do industry figures say about the nature of choice? As with their acknowledgement of the role of socio-economic status in food consumption, there is a nuanced understanding of choice in industry texts which acknowledge that food choice is shaped by biological/psychological factors, social background and environmental cues.

Food and consumption research, whether by food scientists, psychologists or marketers, in industry or in academia – and there is some movement back and forth between these two worlds, amid extensive food industry funding of academic research – does not hesitate to use the term 'choice' in the context of diet. However, much research interest is focused on consumer behaviour, and it is acknowledged that food 'choice' is not always conscious. Indeed, the fact that it is habit-based influences how foods are positioned, in terms of both marketing and location – so that target consumers will encounter and purchase them in a manner which does not challenge their habitus. For food retail companies, location is a 'transcendental decision' in terms of supply logistics and because of the need to serve the socio-economic group in the catchment area of the store (Gonzalez-Benito and Gonzalez-Benito 2005: 295).

Even those who express an interest in healthy eating do not buy foods simply for their 'nutritional quality, healthfulness, convenience or price. These factors undoubtedly affect our food purchases, but we are still constrained in our choices by the routines, habits and associations that have surrounded our interactions with food throughout our lifetimes' (Sims 1998 cited in Wennstrom and Mellentin 2002: 67). People will only be alert to matters such as nutritional quality if these things have been part of their 'habits and associations'. Underlining the habit-based, indeed habitus-based nature of eating, 'most of us eat foods from a core group of about 100 basic food items ... [choosing] our evening meal from a repertoire of around 8–10 recipes' (Wennstrom and Mellentin 2002: 67).

Another marketing author describes consumer choice of brand or store as emerging naturally from previous experiences. This determines

> the detailed influence of the situation on his or her behaviour. It is the combined effect of the personal and environmental factors ... summarized in the BPM (behavioural perspective model of marketing), that

transform the general setting into a situation of immediate personal relevance to the consumer. (Foxall 2010: 8)

According to this model, each consumer has a 'learning history' based on their accumulated experience of the product category (Foxall 2010). Such experiences are reinforced as they are repeated in a given setting (for example, a restaurant/food outlet or supermarket): 'It is that learning history that determines what can act as a reinforcer or punisher for that individual and thus the probability of his or her behaving in such a way as to produce those consequences' (ibid.: 78). So consumption experiences influence subsequent food choices, as shown by studies relating patterns of consumption behaviour to 'reinforcement schedules' (ibid.: 19–23). Thus industry is able to shape what, for Bourdieu, emerged naturally in human practice. Consumer products, strategically marketed, can, over time, influence purchasing behaviour through the capacity to tap into existing practice and psychological states or needs.

Lang, a food policy academic and critic, concludes that 'democratic access to health-enhancing diets is mediated by price structures, income, class, location, culture, which all warp the fabled level playing field in which consumer votes drive markets' (Lang 2009: 328). Instead, 'choice-editing' takes place, as food retailers pre-choose the range of products to present to target consumers along with appropriate presentation styles (ibid.: 329). Health concerns are part of this process only if they fit the profile of the target purchasers. While we often hear of consumer choice or healthy choices in general terms, 'no advertiser … takes such a simplistic position; marketers and the entire consciousness industry wants to know what determines choice, how extensive it is and whether everyone exerts this in the same way, and how and when behaviour changes' (Lang *et al.* 2009: 224).

Marketing influences consumer tastes and has the power to alter norms based on what is learned from the food industry's sensory research, resulting in the highly processed, highly palatable diet consumed by many of us, and in the pervasive siting and bundling of such products. Koster, a food industry psychologist, insists that conscious choice is a fallacy in dietary matters, where habit, instinct and emotion are pivotal: food consumption is 'not available to introspection' (Koster 2009: 76), much as psychology researchers pointed out decades ago (see Chapter 7), and as 'nudge' thinking now appears to accept. Referring to pioneering marketing work in the 1950s, Stanford University's director of marketing management said, 'We've come back full circle … emotion is back in, the unconscious is back in' (*Economist* 2011).

Social psychologists, reporting to the previous UK government in the Foresight report on obesity, spoke of the unconscious, habitual nature of much consumption behaviour (Maio *et al.* 2007: 3). Marketing textbooks describe the often subconscious nature of consumer motivation, and the need for market research to avail itself of indirect research techniques; thus focus groups should be led by 'motivation researchers' trained in clinical psychology (Dibb and Simkin 2009: 119). 'Projective techniques' require participants to perform a task which is then analysed for unconscious motivations (ibid.: 119). Lessons from such research help to 'position' products, giving them a distinct image which, it is hoped, will be lodged in the minds of target consumers (ibid.: 193).

Food products have long been designed to deliver 'essential nutrients through various fortification methods. The result is nutritionally adequate diets to populations (sic). But this strategy is neither designed nor able to achieve optimal diets for individuals within populations' (Watzke and German 2009: 134). The problem of sub-optimal diets, as these industry scientists see it, is that, faced with ever greater choice, individuals 'are pursuing widely different dietary intakes of nutrients, caloric content and macronutrient compositions. These are all in conspicuously diverse foods that vary in structure [and] complexity' (ibid.: 142).

In describing their understanding of choice, there are echoes of a Bourdieuan habitus: 'the development of preferences for sensory attributes of foods – principally olfactory preferences – persists through much of an individual's life, guiding his or her lifelong food choices' (Watzke and German 2009: 143). So palatability is not an objective, scientific property; it is based on our experience of tasting food when young.

> The imprinting of sensory preference is perhaps the least understood but most influential in the conditioning of modern humans to their habitual diets ... olfactory preference is the process by which positive and negative preferences for particular flavors are acquired (German *et al.* 2007 cited in Watzke and German 2009: 143) ... Flavor preferences for foods with poor nutrient quality, if acquired by an individual early in life, will guide a lifelong habit of poor food choices. (Watzke and German 2009: 143)

If these preferences are acquired in childhood, and guide us throughout our lives, are we really exercising 'choice'? The concept of sensory-linked 'acquired food preferences' lends weight to the theoretical proposition regarding the habitus-based nature of food preferences and their implications for lifelong health, and situates these phenomena in the highly empirical and market-driven world of processed food.

In 2011, the House of Lords Science and Technology committee on behaviour change called expert witnesses from the food industry, who acknowledged the tensions between consumer health, food 'behaviour' and commercial interests in food retailing:

> Richard Wright, Director of Sensation, Perception and Behaviour at Unilever, told us that 'the reality ... is that any business is in business

to make money' and that opportunities to influence behaviour will be taken if they are a means to selling more products. Mr King [Chief Executive, Sainsbury's] said that decisions taken by Sainsbury's that might discourage consumption of unhealthy products, for example removing confectionery from their checkouts in some stores, were taken when they were what the customer wanted rather than on the basis of any judgement about improving the health of consumers. Mr Letwin [Cabinet Office minister then responsible for co-ordinating government policy] ... said that working with businesses through voluntary agreements involved thinking about whether the agreement was 'possibly in their commercial interest'. (House of Lords 2011: 40)

Wright, King and Letwin articulate the commercial interests logically central to business decisions. The lessons of product siting are discussed by food marketers (see Chapter 7) and criticised by health campaigners (NCC, see Chapter 8).

Alongside commercial interests where food consumption is concerned, health is also at stake. In the developed world, an ageing, sedentary population is gaining weight and experiencing a greater incidence of hypertension and diabetes, conditions which are 'propelled by poor diets' (Alberti 2001 cited in Watzke and German 2009: 148). Other health problems, 'including atherosclerosis, obesity, diabetes, hypertension, and osteoporosis are attributed at least in part to food choices' (Watzke and German 2009: 167). These are the authors who described the decisive role of olfactory preferences on diet throughout life; so 'choice' would appear to be somewhat circumscribed.

How food structure can affect metabolism

If food choice is acknowledged to be less than completely conscious, even by some industry scientists, how do they understand food–health risks? This section explores the science and technology of food processing and nutrition, and how health and bodyweight can be influenced. Even where risks cannot be known with certainty, important areas of *uncertainty* among both industry and non-industry scientists and researchers are acknowledged.

Improved understanding of the function of diet in altering 'physiology, metabolism and immunological functions' has led to greater concerns about safety in food (Watzke and German 2009: 134). Maternal diet affects the future health of children: 'adipocyte hyperplasia'[2] during childhood development can predispose overweight children to obesity in adulthood (Ailhaud *et al.* 2008 cited in Watzke and German 2009: 143). Further links are made between the role of diet, especially protein content, and muscle mass, with its influence on metabolism. The condition of muscle mass could alter an individual's response to health and diet (Peterson *et al.* 2007 cited in Watzke and German 2009: 143).

Food industry solutions to overweight/overeating focus on reducing fat and calories in processed foods, including 'reduction or replacement of the fat in the food by substituting, wholly or in part, some less calorically dense material (fat extender)' (Fuller 2005: 298). But there is particular concern about fat digestion and the role of 'multiphase mixtures' on the digestion process and 'postprandial lipid state' (Watzke and German 2009: 156). Little is known about this or how the effects of multiphase mixtures might influence overall health (ibid.).

Scientists do not yet understand in detail how food structure affects nutrition, metabolism and physiology, but 'the fact that food products with the same composition but different structures generate different postprandial metabolism' indicates a link between food structure and metabolism (Watzke and German 2009: 157). Whatever the original ingredients or commodities in a food product, the way it is altered in the manufacturing process can affect digestion and health.

Most people are not deficient in vitamins and minerals, according to these food industry scientists, but diets are often unbalanced:

> Research is only beginning to recognize that macronutrient imbalances lead to chronic disregulation of normal metabolism within susceptible individuals. Such metabolic disorders are eventually devastating to the health of the population … [fostering] an epidemic of endogenous, noncommunicable diseases. (Quam *et al.* 2006 cited in Watzke and German 2009: 149)

Yet Ames, a biochemist who has researched nutrition-related disease, finds micronutrient shortage to be widespread, and investigates the outcome of diets in which convenience foods dominate. He proposes that in the overconsumption of high energy, high fat foods, a kind of metabolic 'triage' or emergency response to the missing micronutrients is at work (Ames 2006: 17591). In this process, the body allocates scarce resources, or nutrients, to ensure short-term survival at the cost of long-term health risk. While such diets are themselves linked to metabolic disorders, the drive to consume them continues in an acute yet chronic reaction to the lack of nutrients: 'Suboptimal consumption of micronutrients often accompanies caloric excess and may be the norm among the obese and contribute to the pathologies associated with obesity' (ibid.: 17589). Satiety is not achieved with moderate consumption of high energy, high fat foods and should be considered alongside psychological insights regarding satiety and overconsumption of food. Ames suggests overeating may be an attempt by the body to ingest necessary micronutrients.

This pattern of 'episodic deficiencies' must have characterised human life during periods when essential nutrients were unavailable or insufficient because of food shortages. We may experience them now, paradoxically, because of overconsumption of inadequately nutritious food. Concluding a review of 156 studies, Ames proposes that those at risk of micronutrient deficiencies – especially the poor, teenagers and obese people – should take a multi-vitamin and mineral supplement, a strategy he believes is more likely to improve health among these groups than exhortations to eat more healthily (Ames 2006: 17592–3).

Making foods from a variety of components has allowed industry to add essential nutrients, enriching food products. This has given the impression 'that the population was well nourished, and yet wider choices meant that subsets of the population could easily place themselves at risk, simply, of unbalanced diets' (Watzke and German 2009: 137). This is particularly true for those eating lower priced processed foods, they observe. In manufacturing such foods, the food industry is under pressure to lower the costs of inputs and manufacturing processes, but the outcome is that 'the products emerging from this enterprise are neither designed for nor consistent with the optimum health of consumers' (ibid.: 136).

Yet lower priced processed foods, often of low nutritional quality, are produced in enormous quantities, in all food/meal categories. Earlier in this chapter, industry voices acknowledged that consumers are confused about what constitutes a healthy diet, and that food 'choice' is not fully conscious. Additionally, some groups have developed suboptimal diets. The food scientists cited above linked food consumption to an array of illnesses and concluded that nutrition research must try to solve these problems. They expressed particular concern about the role of emulsifiers.

Emulsifiers, toxicity and overeating: how is health affected?

Much remains unknown about how the human body responds to the altered structures of processed foods. Some health implications of food processing have not been fully understood by either policymakers or consumers themselves. But the texts discussed below indicate that scientists do not fully understand them either. Technical progress in food processing may have implications for health which were not foreseen, and which may take years to detect.

It was food safety considerations – the need to eliminate 'microbial and chemical toxicities' – which originally led to the separate processing of individual food components (Watzke and German 2009: 137). As processed foods have become safer and more convenient, consumers are 'freed' from the obligation to prepare their own meals (ibid.). The additional goal of making foods more palatable was achieved through processing: 'Gels, fibers, emulsions, and foams are complex food structures ... formed during food processing and preparation ... to contribute to the desired stability, shape, texture and taste/flavour of the final foods' (Watzke and German 2009: 137). Consumer panels for palatability testing are held during product development 'to figure out what proportion of which elements will be acceptable to a consumer' (former food industry executive cited in Kessler 2009: 98).

But there may be a problem with emulsifiers. Millstone has speculated on a relationship between emulsifiers and obesity:

> Emulsifiers are used to suspend oils and fats in aqueous solutions, and *vice versa* (Whitehurst 2004). In recent decades, the quantities of emulsifiers used in the food supply have risen markedly, and so too has the fat content of consumers' diets ... The incidence of obesity in all industrialised countries is also rising rapidly, so if the use of emulsifiers was more tightly restricted, that might make a significant contribution to combating the obesity epidemic ... While emulsifiers may well be toxicologically innocuous, they may nonetheless be exerting a significant and collective adverse impact on public health nutrition, but that issue is currently outside the scope of official risk assessment. (Millstone 2009: 632)

The food industry's concern is to avoid acute toxicity in which cause and effect is clear, usually in the short term. But is there a longer term, chronic sense in which foods can be considered 'toxic'? Alongside Millstone's concern with emulsifiers and obesity, Lustig, a paediatric endocrinologist, raises similar points about sugar: sugar (and his particular research interest, high fructose corn syrup) is not toxic in the short term and is not therefore regulated. But could it be a chronic toxin, taking some years and a high degree of consumption to alter our biochemistry and increase the risk of metabolic syndrome, due to the way it is metabolised (Lustig 2014: 30)? Lustig is convinced that it is (ibid.: 127).

Cancer researchers Parkin and Boyd estimate a ten-year span between low fruit and vegetable intake and the appearance of cancers, and a similar latency for cancers related to red and processed meat consumption (the ten-year latency is 'the average interval between "exposure" and the appropriate increase in risk of the cancers concerned') (Parkin and Boyd 2011, Parkin 2011a, 2011b: S4). Parkin notes that 'detailed quantification of risk is not available for most exposures' and that categories of risk for population groups would be impossible to establish (2011b: S4). Nevertheless, the ten-year period gives some shape to the notion of extending concepts of toxicity to encompass longer timespans.

Food scientists note the influence on metabolism of 'even small changes in food structure': food materials 'containing large-sized emulsion particles ... produced a more rapid appearance of lipids in blood than the same quantity of dietary fat in smaller sized emulsions' (Armand *et al.* 1999 cited in Watzke and German 2009: 157). This study by Armand *et al.* found that fat globule size influenced digestion and assimilation of fat in the body: 'Fat emulsions behave differently in the digestive tract depending on their initial physicochemical properties' (Armand *et al.* 1999: 1096). By July 2014, this article had been cited 152 times. I trawled these articles for reviews of the research.

Eleven years after Armand *et al.*'s study, a review of 144 studies (Golding and Wooster 2010) found that there remained 'surprisingly little consideration ... given as to how food structure impacts on fat digestion and metabolism'. Yet there was a 'pressing need for the food industry to develop strategies to combat obesity' (ibid.: 93). The review concluded that 'quite profound differences in lipid digestion can be observed based on emulsion design'. But this has been seen only in highly modelled (in vitro) systems; the challenge was to replicate these findings in actual foods (ibid.: 99).

Another review assessed 240 studies on fat digestion to reveal ways in which food industry engineers 'can adjust the digestive behavior of emulsified fat, focusing on food structuring, for example to change the digestibility or to make it more satiating' (Van Aken 2010: 259). This review concurs with the Armand study but concludes:

> It is not obvious if a special structuring, emulsification or protection of the fat can also be used to induce a long-term reduction of food (and fat) intake. Several patents claim to achieve a reduction in food intake, suggesting the involvement of the ileal brake mechanism. However, this explanation is not supported by fundamental studies in literature (Van Aken 2010: 279–80)

Additionally, there is evidence of 'fat-induced adaptation of the digestive system to high fat intake, leading to increased preference of fatty food and including abnormalities of the pancreas ... leading to metabolic syndrome' (Van Aken 2010: 280). Furthermore, 'even when eating has stopped by physiological satiety processes, *the introduction of a new food type can restart eating, showing that satiety is to some extent "sensory-specific"'* (Van Aken 2010: 269; emphasis added).

Among scientists in the food industry and beyond there is a clear desire to address the possible contribution of emulsifiers in processed foods to obesity, but since Armand *et al.*'s 1999 observations, solutions have apparently not yet been found. Food science aims to reformulate food products which prompt fat absorption and delay satiety. But if consumers find they can be satisfied with lesser quantities, this could lower consumption – and sales. On the other hand, even if emulsions can be modified so as to stimulate satiety and slow food intake, Van Aken finds that this effect is weakened if another type of food is subsequently eaten. Those who have already adapted to a high fat intake, with an increased capacity to eat fatty foods, may have damaged satiety mechanisms.

Food scientists also acknowledge that food structures alter digestive processes beyond the satiety mechanism, influencing bacteria in the colon, for example:

> The complexity of the gut and its myriad physiological, immunological, metabolic and neurological processes makes it clear that the postprandial

state is sensitive to more than the simple composition and energy density of the food. The structural dimensions of the food influence the amount of the nutrients and the time and location in which they are solubilized and absorbed into the body. (Watzke and German 2009: 160)

The discussion of these matters in the literature among food scientists inside and outside the industry makes it clear that the very nature of processed foods may be an important, overlooked contributor to both overconsumption of food and diet-related ill health.

Conclusion

Agricultural developments have led to changes in the food supply, with implications for food processing, retailing and eating habits. While the growth in bodyweight among the population overall, and the widespread experience of health consequences of overconsumption, are unique in history, there is a dimension of historical continuity in the globalisation and processing of food. This chapter has cited early examples of the reliance of lower classes on unhealthy processed foods. Food suppliers in the nineteenth and early twentieth centuries altered foods and lowered their quality and safety until regulations challenged these practices.

Advances in food production technologies encompassing both agriculture and processing, and the globalised nature of their structure and financing, have combined with food product development to enable dramatic changes in the food supply to suit the tastes of groups identified as likely consumers for a given product. Current trends in diets and bodyweights are rooted in dramatic changes to food production, and this linkage has been traced in this chapter.

Marketers and food scientists engaged with what is recognisable as a commercial version of Bourdieu's habitus and industry's awareness of the need to interact with it as it designs and markets its products. Food industry texts acknowledge the lifelong influence of flavour and dietary preferences established in childhood, the reinforcing nature of purchasing behaviour, and the limits to conscious thought in these processes.

Food industry science and marketing naturally encompass and study all these phenomena in their continuing desire to design appealing products and understand and shape consumption behaviour. Thus the psychological dimensions of food choice, socially shaped as they are acknowledged to be even by the food industry, are not a separate category from industry activities or the nature of processed foods – they are intimately connected. Food product developers and marketers aim to cue and reinforce food behaviours, interacting with and shaping consumer psychology where food choice is concerned. The habitus can most easily absorb new products modelled on existing ones which are already part of food consumption patterns, but can also be expanded to include *new* foods; it is a matter of engaging with the habitus of a target group and positioning the food as something that, despite being new, is appropriate for people like them (and may well build on products they already consume). The lifestyle in which it is contextualised in marketing and advertising campaigns is recognisable to target purchasers. The portrayal of others like them (or as they may see themselves) eating the product allows them to assimilate it into their habitus without resistance.[3]

Some marketers acknowledged consumer confusion regarding the health implications of functional food and drink products, and advised working with that confusion so that 'energy drinks', for example, are promoted to and apparently understood by consumers as healthy, even though they are not. Low fat products may not originally have been seen as a prompt for overconsumption, but that evidence is now well established. Yet the language and imagery of such products continues to construct a 'health halo' effect around it, adding to consumer confusion and potentially increasing consumption.

Observations regarding the nature of choice and habit prompted industry scientists' concerns about the health implications of diets based on processed foods; they identified low income groups as particularly at risk. Their own surveillance of developments in the field led them to identify emulsifiers as a potentially significant factor in overconsumption; research into emulsifiers and the biology of digestion by scientists outside industry proposed lessons to be learned in a public health context. The focus on foods high in salt, fat and sugar is important in understanding how health is put at risk by overconsumption of these foods. But there are additional potential problems for health stemming from the chemical structures of processed foods and their influence on digestion.

The following chapter focuses on marketing, placing it in its historical and political economy context. It further explores the role of psychology and consciousness research in illuminating food consumption and the particular use made of it by food marketers. Chapter 7 additionally investigates the applications and expertise of market research, its capacity to track consumption in terms of place, rank and, given digital platforms, even time, and how all of this informs marketing interventions which reinforce class-differentiated consumption.

Notes

1 In 2013, sales grew again after four years of decline (Soil Association 2014).
2 Adipocyte hyperplasia: increased production of fat cells, found in some types of obesity (Naaz *et al.* 2004).
3 This does not always succeed – marketing failures are discussed in Chapter 7.

7 Critical perspectives on marketing and market research

Introduction

The pervasiveness of food marketing and the consumption of snack and convenience food is often commented upon by researchers in social sciences, nutrition and epidemiology. In addition, advertising to children has been the target of much debate, and some regulation. But the detailed activities of food product development and food marketing have not been studied by social scientists in terms of their role in shaping the relationship between diet, class and health. In this chapter, all these activities are put in context, beginning with a historical overview of how marketing emerged alongside the growth of consumer industries, and how it has flourished in a neoliberal age.

A key dimension of neoliberalism is the discourse of personal choice and individual responsibility for one's choices (Chapter 1). This discourse has suited the food industry well in its defence of its own practices, and has been backed by public health promotion campaigns and commentary which emphasise personal responsibility, often in a positive and encouraging way, for a healthy diet. But the powerful role of the industry in transforming the food supply and shaping our diets and, indirectly and unintentionally, our health – by social class – is too often missed.

In this chapter, I focus on the growth and flourishing of marketing, analysing both critiques of its power and marketing's claims of its own weaknesses and limitations, alongside its capacity to mobilise the insights of psychology and the complex algorithmic techniques of market research and consumer purchase data in support of corporate goals. A critique of marketing by marketing scholars assesses the claims and discourse of applied marketing and insists that marketing must be understood – and should be taught – in the wider context of corporate power in a neoliberal age.

Hackley, for example, decries marketing's lack of acknowledgement of its activities as emblematic of a neoliberal society and business model (2001, 2009, 2010). Skalen et al. (2008) challenge marketing's claims to be consumer focused, pointing instead to the larger goal of increasing capital accumulation. They explore the internal contradictions and self-referentiality of marketing discourse, supplying what is essentially a critical discourse analysis, as urged by Fairclough (though they do not call it that). From food marketing practitioners cited in this chapter, analysis of industry activities tends to be instrumental in nature, as one might expect: they are naturally interested in how companies can operate most effectively to increase or sustain product sales, though the language of engaging with customers and satisfying consumer needs is also regularly invoked. But in this chapter practitioners also supply valuable insights into how the industry operates.

In Chapter 6, corporate food scientists discussed their concerns about the health implications of a diet based on processed foods. In this chapter, marketing practitioners recommend research methods that social scientists – and indeed some marketers – might consider invasive or manipulative. Chapter 8 discusses in greater detail the debate among marketing academics and practitioners about the ethics of marketing, but marketers air some of their disquiet in the diet-related examples given in the present chapter.

Having set out a critical framework for evaluating the contribution of marketing to consumption, this chapter then provides an overview of how the industry sustains and reinforces both larger socio-economic structures as well as individual business goals. Examples from food industry texts illustrate how the industry interacts with an array of cultural, technological and social forces to shape our diets and, ultimately, if not intentionally, influence our health. A detailed examination of market research, and especially geodemographics, is included, because this is the (ongoing) stage in the marketing process when consumers are closely and continually tracked, and data is amassed for the purpose of targeting and segmenting consumer groups. The leading firms which carry out this research are very large-scale and global in nature; they are major players in the consumer economy and increasingly influential in a public policy context as there is a growing public sector demand for their services in researching social and health problems.

Marketing in a historical context

> Marketing in all its forms is a cultural force of extraordinary proportions.
> (Hackley 2001: 22)

Lang and colleagues (Lang *et al.* 2009: 224; Lang 2009: 328) refer to marketing and advertising as consciousness industries, with a vastly increased penetration throughout the twentieth and twenty-first centuries. Marketing is key to the development and retailing of food products, and to mobilising class distinctions while doing so (while almost never using the language of class); this has been understudied by social scientists. In seeking to understand its role and significance in a food–health context, a look at the origins and development of marketing offers valuable insights.

While the marketing techniques of today might rely on highly sophisticated tracking technologies, marketing a product or service to its most likely buyers is 'as old as commerce' (Egan 2008: 4). Georgian pottery entrepreneurs Boulton and Wedgwood used 'market segmentation, product differentiation, [and] prestige pricing ... [to create] interest in their innovative ware' (Hackley 2009: 37). Advertisements and promotions using persuasive slogans and images can be traced back hundreds of years (McFall 2004 cited in Hackley 2009: 37).

In the nineteenth century, many new foods arrived in the UK and were advertised by their purveyors. Additives and adulterations were common (Wilson 2009), often aiming to make food appear more palatable. Marketing was sometimes very aggressive, with purveyors and advertisements making outrageous claims about their products (Blythe 2006: 58).

By the early twentieth century, it became clear that mass production would require mass consumption. What might be viewed as a crisis of accumulation – more was being produced than there was a demand for – required the nurturing of desire in the consumer. Crucially, this desire needed to be 'increased and manipulated by factors ... other than the mere existence of supply' (Egan 2008: 4). One early marketer wrote that 'the more progressive businessman is searching out the unconscious needs of the consumer, and is then producing the goods to gratify them' (Shaw 1912 cited in Egan 2008: 5). Marketers today continue to speak plainly on this point, alluding to more than just passive tracking of consumer 'need'. Instead, companies must try to 'discover what consumers either cannot find, or do not know yet that they need' (Cox and Delaney 2009: 286). The latency of need, the nature of free choice, and implications for marketing ethics are subjects of longstanding debate in marketing.

Demographic profiling arose after World War Two, with an increasingly statistical orientation beginning in the 1950s (Cox and Delaney 2009: 286). Claims of a scientific basis to marketing and the development of theoretical frameworks also started around that time, and continue today (Egan 2008: 6; Hackley 2001; Blythe 2006).

Market segmentation as we might recognise it nowadays arose in the 1950s, and what is still called the marketing mix was defined in 1960 as the 'four Ps': price, product, promotion and place (McCarthy 1960 cited in Egan 2008: 8). Marketing was increasingly seen as the way to ensure that 'consumption kept up with output' (Packard 1957 cited in Egan 2008: 8). Kotler, a leading marketing educator in the later twentieth century, began writing textbooks in the 1960s and shaped marketing research by combining statistical techniques with behavioural sciences (Wilkie and Moore 2003 cited in Egan 2008: 9). Academic marketing thrived, and is itself today a huge market for textbooks, journals, universities, research funding and marketing education and training (Hackley 2001, 2009; Skalen *et al.* 2008).

In the 1950s in America, Dichter applied Freudian psychology, an interest in the unconscious and psychoanalytic methods, to introduce motivation research, which 'tapped into the consumer's subconscious to discover feelings about products' (Stern 2004: 165). A trained psychoanalyst himself, Dichter found that 'Freud's notions of subconscious urges and socialised inhibitions seemed to make intuitive sense' (*Economist* 2011). This thinking contributed to a growing understanding, even in Dichter's time and acknowledged more recently in 'nudge' theory, of the limited consciousness underlying some consumption behaviours.

As competitive pressures intensified, the new goal for marketing became to secure 'competitive advantage', with market share 'its primary indicator' (Ambler 2004 cited in Egan 2008: 10). But in the past decade, marketing has been articulated as a process in which 'value is defined by and co-created with the consumer' (Egan 2008: 14). The strategic realities of corporate goals and the mission of marketing in a neoliberal era do not generally enter this discourse of a partnership with consumers, which features strongly in the way marketers understand and speak about their work and role (regularly, for example, in *Marketing Magazine*). Certainly much effort is devoted to finding out what consumers want and 'need', not only by tracking their activities and purchases in ways in which consumers remain unaware; but also by engaging with them creatively online and in product launches, campaigns and public events. There is often an element of entertainment and fun in these activities, and marketers find that they can learn a great deal about their consumers while promoting a given product or brand. But ultimately – naturally – the aim is to increase sales, and in a larger sense, in many cases, to provide sufficient returns to shareholders. Consumers may not always be aware (and if they are aware, they may not mind) that they are being both studied and marketed *to*.

Marketing increasingly permeates our lifeworlds, to use Habermas's term. According to one marketing textbook, 25–33 per cent of civilian workers in Europe and the US carry out marketing activities (Dibb and Simkin 2009: 14). Globally, market and opinion research is worth about £10 billion annually, with a few international agencies dominating the field (ibid.: 206). Put another way, of the 70 per cent of a British family budget (before taxes) spent on goods and services, half that amount finances marketing activities (ibid.: 16).

The power – and weaknesses – of marketing: a critique

> Marketing communication: 'a technique for analysing, planning, intervening in and ultimately controlling the consuming behaviour of people from the vantage point of a commercial organisation'. (Hackley 2001: 135)

> ... marketing doesn't work. (Blythe 2006: 112)

The above quotes, the first from a marketing academic and the second, expressed ironically, from a marketing practitioner turned academic, reflect the debate within marketing about its role and power. These authors acknowledge criticisms of marketing, as well as marketing's defence (i.e. the insistence that it often fails, so cannot be accused of successfully manipulating consumers; or that marketers are only focused on meeting consumer needs). Marketing undergraduates are told in one textbook that:

> although marketers try to understand and influence consumer buying behaviour, they cannot control it. Some critics credit them with the ability to manipulate buyers, but marketers have neither the power nor the knowledge to do so. Their knowledge of behaviour comes from what psychologists, social psychologists and sociologists know about human behaviour in general. (Dibb and Simkin 2009: 106)

While acknowledging that it is the instrumental use of such knowledge that informs marketing activities, making this claim to knowledge 'borrowed' from other, more established disciplines is problematic, and the subject of some critique (discussed later in this section).

So there is some discussion within the discipline over whether it can 'control' consumers, but the desire to *influence* buyer behaviour is acknowledged – and entirely logical, in line with overall business goals. The textbook recommends close study of personal, demographic, psychological, family and social influences on buying decisions (Dibb and Simkin 2009: 110), describing these in what amounts to a retail-oriented understanding of Bourdieuan habitus. They note that demographic factors can affect a consumer's decision-making process as well as their use of a given product (ibid.: 115).

In an example of how these influences are mined, 'marketers often capitalise on the tendency towards impulse buying – for example, by placing magazines and confectionary next to supermarket checkout counters' (Dibb and Simkin 2009: 109, in an example of marketing's instinctive use of 'nudging' techniques). They also acknowledge the importance of children's influence on buying 'breakfast cereals, ice cream and soft drinks' and note that 'this influence is increasingly reflected in the way such products are designed and marketed' (ibid.: 115).

One of Kessler's anonymous food industry consultants describes his industry as 'the manipulator of the consumers' minds and desires' (Kessler 2009: 21). These observations challenge marketing's invocation of co-creation of value with consumers, and its description of a collegial process between equal partners. When marketers speak to each other, or speak as anonymous informants, the discussion is sometimes more frank.

Yet there are limits to marketing power, and examples of marketing misjudgements and product failures abound. There are also problems with product longevity in the FMCG (fast moving consumer goods) sector, but food manufacturers make this tendency work for them, deliberately using 'limited edition variants' and pulling them as soon as profitability declines – ideally with something similar to replace it (*Marketing Magazine* 18/02/09a).

Product longevity, while achieved by many brands in different sectors, including food, is not the only indication of marketing success. Continual developments in processing, packaging and logistics, alongside new merchandising techniques and formats, make it possible to produce new products or new product variants in a range of styles, sizes and amounts. Fast food companies are advised that they should constantly review and adjust their target market segmentation, ensuring that the right products are aimed at the correct consumer segment (Michman and Mazze 1998: 34). In order to prosper, businesses must innovate, exploring the potential for expanding production and sales in new directions. So it may be that marketing discourse regarding the failure to achieve longevity, at least where food products are concerned, is something of a diversion. Food companies need to be able to bring new foods on stream quickly, replacing them regularly. The frequent appearance of new products is apparently normal practice in this sector; not an indication of failure per se.

But sometimes, marketing does fail. *Marketing Magazine* (03/08/11) ran a feature discussing ten cases of in which a marketing turnaround was required to address problems with product positioning/branding. Elsewhere the magazine estimates that there are three times as many marketing failures as successes, and that large budgets are no guarantee of the latter (*Marketing Magazine* 18/02/09a). A BBC programme, *Business Nightmares with Evan Davis: Marketing Mess-ups*, highlighted such failures (BBC 2011a). Scammel-Katz's (2012) book *The Art of Shopping: How We Shop and Why We Buy* found that some products fail because they are inappropriately sited and signposted in stores. Marketing failures are the subject of an entire book by one marketer, who maintains that asking people to explain their consumption choices is pointless: 'the unconscious mind is the real driver of consumer behaviour … what matters is not what consumers say but what they do' (Graves 2010: 10). This author recommends close study of consumer psychology, particularly the power of the unconscious (ibid.: 18–19). Market research which tracks consumer purchases is another effective way of learning what consumers *do*, bypassing what they might *say*. Its sheer scale and insight makes it increasingly effective, according to both supporters and critics, as the subsequent discussion of geodemographics and digital tracking will reveal.

Marketing is most likely to succeed when it is 'designed to appeal to a well-defined market' (Dibb and Simkin 2009: 123). Drucker, a leading twentieth century management consultant and writer, describes this process: 'The aim of marketing is to know and understand the customer so well that the product or service fits him and sells itself' (cited in French *et al.* 2010: 100). The successful product or service is conveyed with the appropriate images and language, and in the location – from street, to shop, to shelf, to home computers and smartphones – which will reach and be noticed and purchased by the target customer. When products or formats are truly novel, marketing efforts can normalise them, easing this process.

Kessler's interviews with food industry executives provide numerous examples of normalisation of new kinds of consumption. A former Coca-Cola executive, Mike McCloud, discussed his company's efforts to shift the norm regarding soft drink sizes from 8 to 12 ounces. Consisting only of carbonated water and syrups, these drinks allow the company to make a large profit margin on sales, and retailers did not resist this enlargement strategy. Coke also 'discouraged water giveaways'. Thus, '"When the beverage companies throw their weight behind a change in norms, they're often successful", McCloud noted. "Coke and Pepsi are so big and strong, they have the horsepower to change people's habits"' (Kessler 2009: 130). (It is worth noting here that whereas marketing enters the supply chain at a relatively late stage, the reformulation of soft drinks and its larger sizes came about in part because of farm subsidies on corn, which made high fructose corn syrup so much cheaper than sugar that even major increases in the *size* of soft drinks like Coke and Pepsi necessitated no more than small increases in *price* (Hawkes *et al.* 2012: 348)).

The normalisation of frequent snack consumption and meal deals consisting of a sugary drink, sandwich and packet of crisps, was achieved by marketing. This is an illustration of the habitus being diverted by outside forces and external actors; no one was drinking such large containers of sugary drinks or eating crisps daily with lunch until these formats and combinations were presented to consumers and marketed as normal behaviours for the target group. The normalisation of them is key to mass market sales. However unintentionally, the sheer normality of a lunch of crisps, sugary drink and sandwich diverts attention from any health consequences. Thus these products are more overtly associated with palatability and low cost than with risk of, say, the longer term prospect of chronic illness. Lifeworlds have been both disrupted and colonised by these practices, as health is put at risk among those for whom such foods constitute a routine, disproportionate amount of their diet – that is, those whose habitus led them to assimilate these new products and meal combinations without conscious thought or challenge.

This phenomenon is encapsulated in the comment by a working class woman in a 2005 BBC TV programme, who serves her family only prepared foods heated up at home. Her refrigerator and freezer are full of pizzas, chips and ready meals. She is filmed picking up a vegetable (which she is unable to identify) given to her by the producers and saying, 'This is completely alien to me. I don't cook from fresh' (BBC 2005). Cooking, then, has become for her a matter of reheating prepared foods; fresh foods are not a part of her dietary habitus, or, by extension, that of her family.

Some marketers have reservations about the role of marketing in this process. One marketer expressed the view that pack sizes have become too big and that low status consumers are more likely to consume large quantities of them: 'If the knock-on effects of that trend are seen to hit the most vulnerable hardest, even marketers of relatively healthy food and drink brands will find themselves on the back foot. Too much of anything is still too much' (*Marketing Magazine* 02/05/12b). There is some uneasiness about the effect of package and product sizing and the targeting of these items at low status people (Chapter 8 has a longer discussion of ethical concerns among marketers).

It is arguable that the power of marketing to engage with culture and society (and to influence eating behaviour) has been underestimated or at least under-analysed, with marketing often dismissed as lightweight: 'Marketing is seen as a popular and safe, if relatively undemanding, elective choice at university' and even that 'you need no marketing knowledge to be good at marketing' (Hackley 2001: 22). Hackley's own critique finds much marketing scholarship 'epistemologically disjointed, temporally discon-nected, epistemically nebulous and thematically kaleidoscopic' (ibid.: 136). Fuller concludes that despite advances in marketing expertise, marketing remains 'looked down upon by true scientists' (Fuller 2005: 111).

Nevertheless, the 'managerial discourse' which has emerged in marketing has 'a power based on truth claims that are legitimated by its position in the academy' (Hackley 2003 and Marion 2006, cited in Skalen *et al.* 2008: 3). Marketing is highly successful at marketing itself in academic, business and public policy contexts, and academic marketing research is well supported by funding bodies (ibid.). Some university marketing and psychology studies are funded by consumer firms; in this way, academic disciplines can themselves be colonised, their research useful to industry but possibly uncritical in a broader context.

Some marketers stake their claim to academic legitimacy by emphasising their multi-disciplinary approach, bringing 'many perspectives (e.g. consumer research, sociology, psychology, anthropology, grounded theory, phenomenology) to the study of the consumer experience as told by the consumers themselves' (Beckley and Ramsey 2009: 235).

But Hackley finds fault with marketing precisely for this 'borrowing' of concepts from more established disciplines, without acknowledging their 'drawbacks, controversies, history, contradictions and theory' (Hackley 2001: 130–3, 136). This is said to be true of marketing's plundering of sociology and psychology (Gronhaug 2000 and Foxall 2000 cited in Hackley 2001: 131); these authors feel that the ideas of such disciplines are not used by marketing with 'the intellectual integrity of their use in their original habitat' (Hackley 2001: 131). Blythe acknowledges marketing's borrowings from sociology, anthropology and psychology, supplying the concepts of 'motivation, perception and attitude formation and change', but finds that despite a tendency to 'pinch' concepts from other disciplines, there is little ongoing study or reference to them (Blythe 2006: 28–31).

Hackley criticises marketing academics and practitioners alike for using theories such as Maslow's hierarchy of needs to explain consumption behaviour: 'For Maslow, the highest state of self-actualisation occurred when humans rejected selfish (including material) values and instead gave back to their fellow humans in some way. One could hardly think of a less appropriate model for advertising or marketing' (Hackley 2010: 147). Blythe, concurring that Maslow's theory is widely taught in marketing, also finds it inadequate to the task, but for more practical reasons: it fails to portray the myriad ways in which people experience and define their needs, which constantly change (Blythe 2006: 97–9). Or as another marketing writer phrases it, customers are 'moving targets', so it is vital to track their changing needs and social experiences (Schmidt 2009: 225).

Mainstream marketing texts rely on basic descriptions of consumer attitudes, beliefs and desires, with the assumption that such things are 'largely under the volition of the thinker, except, of course, when subject to a carefully planned marketing intervention' (Hackley 2001: 134). The marketing techniques openly described in campaign literature, the growing encroachment of fast/snack food into public spaces, the resources devoted to advertising and marketing, and the way such campaigns are promoted and evaluated indicate that the industry hopes at the very least to influence the 'volition of the thinker'. Indeed, this is entirely and logically in line with larger commercial goals.

To achieve this influence, commercial messages are increasingly found in ambient media, tracking consumers as they move through their day, looking for what marketers term 'dwell time': 'for example, on the morning commute, in the hair salon, in the back of a taxi, during a coffee break, filling up with petrol … in the Post Office queue, at the GP's surgery. Brands should look to engage consumers within these rare moments' (*Marketing Magazine* 22/09/10).

But, of course, these moments are not rare – they permeate and punctuate our days and our lives. In reaching consumers in this context, one fast food company has found outdoor media effective: 'We want to drive that impulse to eat … when people are thinking about food and are hungry, a poster is there, making us top-of-mind' (*Marketing Magazine* 25/01/12).

Another problem with marketing is that it has resisted grappling with language in social, historical, biographical and political contexts (Hackley 2001: 134). Thus it uncritically accepts notions such as lifestyle choices and attitudes, rather than seeing them as social constructions – indeed, discourses – within market limitations (ibid.). As a discipline, marketing does not reflect critically on its own rhetoric (ibid.: 22). Hackley takes aim at 'fatuous' statements, made repeatedly in marketing texts, that marketers are operating in an increasingly turbulent and complex world (ibid.: 140). After all, 'the world's marketing managers have the benefit of more market data, a greater degree of transference of technology and information and, in the largest companies, more monopolistic market power than they have ever had before' (ibid.) – powers belied by the complexity rhetoric. As if conceding the point that even in a complex world, products can easily succeed, one marketer wittily describes his company's successful marketing of drinks products to different countries and cultures as simply a matter of 'moving shit that works from one place to another' (*Marketing Magazine* 23/02/11d). Nevertheless, it is a process which must be facilitated by market information and market research techniques.

But his comment reveals an intriguing insight into the workings of the habitus, seemingly contradicting the idea of cultural specificity of food practices. While not arguing that cultures are not significant influences on food/drink consumption, the marketer quoted above reflects the undeniable success of many western food and drink products in utterly different non-western cultures. So a habitus can be disrupted with new notions of what is good to eat or drink; the very foreignness of some products, and the aspirational lifestyle with which they are associated, is actually instrumental in their success, not an obstacle to it.

Hackley decries much business and marketing education for its tendency to omit rigorous, theoretical, original marketing research (as he insists the best of it truly is; several such studies are cited in this book) from its syllabus (Hackley 2001: 177). Marketing's quantitative capabilities can produce impressive statistical research, garnering lucrative consulting opportunities, but such research 'deflects critical attention and offers a spurious legitimacy' to the discipline (ibid.: 132). He particularly opposes the use of consulting frameworks in undergraduate courses: 'Young people deserve an education. Grown-up marketing executives can look out for themselves' (ibid.).

Thus marketing discourse conceals its inherent power – a power which 'legitimizes and reproduces the market economy' – and should therefore be evaluated in the context of a critique of market economics (Skalen *et al.* 2008: 166). Instead, much academic marketing concentrates on 'prescribing how to do marketing' instead of studying the process and effects of marketing (ibid.).

These are serious faults, since marketing 'forms our world in telling ways through discursive mechanisms which are often invisible to us ... it is precisely because these mechanisms are largely invisible that they are so powerful' (Hackley 2001: 22). Marketing not only influences consumer behaviour but also underpins capitalist economies; this needs to be acknowledged and investigated.

Marketers are encouraged to get close to consumers via a range of market research techniques which have the potential not only to track but also to shape human behaviour; this merits detailed analysis in a social science context. Psychological insights have long been used by marketers in understanding consumer behaviour. The use of psychological testing and analysis in marketing is explored below.

Psychology and marketing

In marketing literature, much is made of a technique known as psychographics, in which participants are tested for attitudes and character traits. In a food context, psychographic testing measures variety-seeking, food neophobia (unwillingness to try new foods), restraint (flexible intake control, food guilt, bodyweight concerns), and food involvement (how important food is to participants) (Meiselman 2009: 346–53). Psychographic tests have been widely used in research on food consumption, though little has been published concerning how test results are applied to food product development (ibid.: 346).

But Hackley dismisses psychographics as a pseudo-science developed by advertising agencies for the purpose of persuading clients that 'in spite of the breakdown of traditional mass audience characteristics, they still understood the motivations and behaviour of discrete consumer groups' (also Hackley 2010: 147). Marketing textbook writers Dibb and Simkin find that testing buying decisions on the basis of personality characteristics is inconclusive, but believe more reliable measuring techniques will be developed to reveal the relationship between personality and consumption (Dibb and Simkin 2009: 124, 182).

In a more intrusive technique known as neuromarketing, 'functional magnetic resonance imaging [reveals] activity regions within the brain ... people's reactions to products, services and advertising can thus be studied, enabling researchers to locate the preference center of that participant's brain' (Lovell 2002 cited in Fuller 2005: 119). One marketing agency describes neuromarketing as exploring 'the science behind emotional engagement with a brand'; they advise that 'marketing with a greater emotional uplift is likely to increase sales' (Mail Media Centre 2009). This technique is big business: the advertising company Nielsen recently paid $5 billion for NeuroFocus, a neuromarketing research firm which measures brain impulses against the emotions aimed for by advertisers (*Guardian* 15/01/12). The neuromarketing firm Neurosense, founded by a neurologist, tests food textures and aromas to predict consumer behaviour (ibid.). One marketing author has called for industry standards 'that banned ... efforts to find the brain's "buy buttons" in this manner' (Lindstrom cited in Houpt 2011).

Psychographics and neuromarketing are just two manifestations of marketing's longstanding association with psychology. Consumer behaviour and marketing constitute 'one of the traditional areas of cooperation between economics and psychology' which can be traced as far back as Bentham's 'hedonic calculus' (Lea 1978: 441–3; hedonic calculus is 'a method of working out the sum total of pleasure and pain produced by an act, and thus the total value of its consequences' (Bentham 1789)).

An expert understanding of consumers emerged in the psychological research at the Tavistock Institute of Human Relations (TIHR) from 1950 to 1970, and their work with advertising agencies in that period (Skalen *et al.* 2008: 14). The TIHR studies questioned contemporary marketing approaches, finding that 'people did not know what they wanted; people did not tell the truth about their wants and dislikes even when they knew them; and one could not assume that individuals would behave in a rational way when selecting one commodity rather than another' (Miller and Rose 1997 cited in

Skalen *et al.* 2008: 14). These findings anticipated 'nudge' theory, which accepts the non-rational, not completely conscious behaviours in some areas of human life. Psychological insights could thus help retailers to know customers 'better than they know themselves' (Skalen *et al.* 2008: 14).

The TIHR work is noteworthy for its observations of consumers unaware of their true desires, and the potential for this to be exploited by businesses. It is an insight repeated by marketing texts since, in the language of anticipating consumer needs, and then making these needs felt via product development and marketing and advertising campaigns. In a business context, this practice has an undeniable logic. It can also be helpful to consumers. Many of us would consider the convenience and variety now available in many product categories an improvement over the past 20 or 30 years. Hackley acknowledges that 'there does seem to be a large amount of marketing activity which makes consumer life better and is really quite fun and which, furthermore, is conducted by decent people working in good faith' (Hackley 2001: 141). The point is not to condemn all marketing activities and strategies, but to trace the ways in which effective marketing, in influencing consumer desires and consumption, can also shape diets and – unintentionally – health, and along class lines.

Psychology and food consumption

Human beings are thought to have a natural (evolutionary) preference for energy-dense, fatty foods, which are appealing and pleasurable (Kessler 2009). These generate weak satiety and increased tolerance for heightened consumption, resulting in weight gain along with a natural resistance to weight loss (Canoy and Buchan 2007: 3). As sociology frames it:

> pleasure and desire, as libidinal forces, may be regarded as pre- or non-discursive; they are innately undisciplined and undisciplinable. Pleasure and pleasure seeking is thus conceived as the weak link in the chain of command from authoritarian discourses of health governance to docile compliance for body maintenance. (Lupton 1995 cited in Coveney and Bunton 2003: 166)

When we eat pleasurable foods, we experience weak satiety and a greater capacity for consumption, resulting in weight gain, along with a natural (biological) resistance to weight loss (Canoy and Buchan 2007: 3). This is a major focus for psychology research, which has been instrumental in public policy. The evidence review on lifestyle change for the UK's 2007 Foresight report on obesity was undertaken by (social) psychologists, who observed that:

> People know that rich foods are bad for them and that moderate exercise is beneficial. But people get positive sensations from eating foods

that are laden with calories or excess salt, while, on the other hand, finding the time to exercise is difficult. No one escapes this psychological conflict. (Maio *et al.* 2007: 1)

Indeed, obesity is present in all social groups. But energy-dense, nutrient-poor diets are more likely to be consumed by those of lower socio-economic status (Darmon and Drewnowski 2008 cited in Chapter 5). Most such foods are not developed *for* or marketed equally *to* all social groups and there may be differing susceptibility to palatability and a consequently weakened sense of satiety, despite instinctive, biologically based responses. The habitus might include, for example, an awareness of the health effects of such foods. If one has been instructed in the family setting to eat a healthy, balanced diet, and to be sceptical of food industry strategies and claims, this can become as much a part of one's make-up and habitus as the actual foods and combinations of foods eaten. The awareness of the benefits of eating a balanced diet, and indeed a status-based notion of the kinds of foods people like us are meant to eat, could override the biological impulse and attraction to (over) eating flavourful but unhealthy foods. Thus palatability and even hyperpalatability might have a weaker hold on some individuals and social groups than others. The role of habitus is present for all, but one type of habitus might have as a priority healthy and balanced eating; another might prize taste; another might focus on affordability above all.

But the specifics of 'the role of habit and limited volitional control' over health behaviour are not well understood, and campaigns to encourage behavioural change will not suit all socio-economic groups (Maio *et al.* 2007: 2–3). One problem is that, as indicated above, 'readiness to change may fluctuate according to social and environmental contexts and in relation to other goals and demands that impinge on self-regulatory processes' (ibid.: 16). In addition,

> despite the current Government's emphasis on 'choosing responsibly', it is clear that many of these behaviours do not arise from conscious choices. There is a need to understand the social factors and internal variables that predict habitual, counter-intentional behaviours. (ibid.: 27)

If the use of marketing data and techniques used to influence behaviour are added to the list of 'social factors' referred to here, then the process described in the Foresight report is recognisable from the social theories of Bourdieu and Habermas and their analysis of how habits are formed, and how they are altered and permeated by external forces.

Coveney and Bunton note the potential for studies of 'food, pleasure and the problems posed for health promotion intervention' (Coveney and Bunton 2003: 175). Such studies would benefit from investigating the food industry's understanding of the experience of palatability, which has been mobilised to stretch our capacity for consumption by appealing to our pleasure response. Effective health promotion interventions would also acknowledge the differing status of food products, how they are targeted at social groups of different status, and the insights of psychology which challenge the notion of conscious choice where food is concerned.

One food industry psychologist, discussing the role of psychology in enhancing the appeal of food products to consumers, lists food behaviour fallacies, including that of conscious choice (Koster 2009: 73). He describes seminal research between the 1970s and 1980s which found that 'intuitive thinking and decision-making ... is characterised by operations that are "fast, parallel, automatic, effortless, associative, implicit (not available to introspection) and often emotionally charged; they are also governed by habit and therefore difficult to control or modify"' (Kahnemann[1] 2003 cited in Koster 2009: 76). This characterised Kahnemann's system 1 in his dual process model; system 2 was 'slower, rule-governed, deliberate and effortful' (Kahnemann 2010). System 1 is prone to generating error; system 2, when activated, may spot and correct these errors. There is an interplay between intuitive and reflective systems which 'sometimes allows biased judgments and sometimes overrides or corrects them' (ibid.). Kahnemann's work lies at the heart of 'nudge' thinking, and the growing acceptance that some behaviours are largely intuitive. Thus, from a sociological perspective, varying degrees of reflexivity are mobilised to incorporating health considerations to food consumption. There can be a social class dimension to this process, and food marketing engages with the intuitive, class-differentiated nature of food consumption. The food industry more broadly addresses health matters only when subgroups of consumers cite health as a concern in their food purchases, or when it is pressed to do so by regulatory requirements or public policies.

Consciousness-based methods are inadequate for sensory consumer research, and especially hedonic research, which investigates the pleasure and reward experiences of food (Koster 2009: 80). Koster's interest is a very instrumental one – improving the appeal of food industry products to consumers – but it is possible to apply these observations to a public health understanding of why people eat the way they do. For example, policies which focus on advising people to 'choose' to eat a healthier diet and exercise fails to acknowledge gaps in consciousness where such choice is concerned, as well as the powerful hedonic appeal of some foods.

Koster's and Kahnemann's ideas substantiate the Foresight psychologists' conclusions, who refer to a high degree of implicitness and automaticity leading to unreflective behaviours, and observe that health promotion campaigns which encourage people to think about what they are eating, rather than telling them what to eat, might be more effective (Maio *et al.* 2007: 31).

This observation was tested by a team of psychologists who found that when people who ate little fruit were instructed to imagine themselves eating fruit, their fruit intake increased (Knauper *et al.* 2011: 614).[2] This study provides a healthy eating version of a marketing technique which aims to embed images of products in target consumers' minds. For example, packaging is designed to appeal to a given consumer group; the design and marketing/advertising messages lead them to imagine people like them eating the food. Some people eat little fruit or vegetables (perhaps for reasons other than cost), relying largely on ready meals. Could 'targeted mental imagery' overcome the imaginative gap which they are not even aware exists (i.e. 'people like me don't eat fresh fruit and vegetables')? The study illustrated a dimension of what happens subconsciously with food consumption: we eat what we can picture ourselves eating. We imagine eating foods that we see reflected in marketing campaigns and advertisements which are targeted at people like ourselves.

Once the patterns of our diets are established, we experience an impulse to eat when visual cues with sufficient 'incentive salience' are triggered (Kessler 2009: 52–3). This may include seeing the food itself, or the restaurant where we've eaten it, or an advertisement for the restaurant (ibid.). Food is omnipresent now; we are rarely far from a food retailer, restaurant, vending machine, or snack foods and drinks even in non-food stores. A weight management scientist tells Kessler that 'the number of cues, the number of opportunities to eat have increased while the barriers to consumption have fallen … the environmental stimulus has changed' (ibid.: 128). Additional cues include TV advertisements or a pop-up ads on the internet, food-product 'advergames' promoted via social network sites, or smartphone alerts from fast food retailers. The use of images is crucial:

> The food industry understands exactly what it's doing when it markets foods with such compelling imagery, said my source [an industry consultant]. In the face of the pleasure that pizza promises, consumers 'suspend more rational thought and are drawn to the indulgence of it' … 'Indulgence is the primary driver in premium products', he says. 'Generally they're higher in flavour and often higher in fat, and a lot of imagery goes with them. It's a very profitable place for the food and beverage industry'. (Kessler 2009: 79)

But these cues do not operate on all of us uniformly. As consumers we are targeted with those products which will appeal to the consumer segment of which we are a part. The market research techniques which track consumption patterns, in order that they may be fully understood and reinforced, are discussed below.

Market research: investigating (and reinforcing) consumption behaviour

> Here at MegaFood Corp, you're more than just a customer … you're a completely predictable compilation of spending habits and product data. (PC and Pixel cartoon by Thach Bui and Geoff Johnson depicts

sign at a supermarket entrance; text but no illustration cited by Fuller
2005: 120)

Even marketing pioneers could describe 'customer characteristics that
enabled the abstract market to become comprehensible from a company
point of view' (Skalen *et al.* 2008: 131), but since the late twentieth century,
technological advances have enabled marketing to track, segment and
target consumers to a highly sophisticated degree; the cartoon cutline cited
above makes the point with humour. Many texts written by and for those
working in the food/market research industries describe the centrality of
consumer market research:

> A conscientious agency will … want to understand the lifestyle prefer-
> ences, consumption habits, media consumption, patterns, values, atti-
> tudes, drives, aspirations, income, priorities and influential peer groups
> of its target segment. Qualitative research in the form of discussion or
> focus groups, or surveys, can be of assistance … Secondary data
> sources detailing demographic and other information important to
> segmentation and targeting can also be invaluable. (Hackley 2010: 85)

In assembling focus groups, 'market research companies keep lists of
consumers whose backgrounds are well documented. With little effort they
can enlist consumers with any desired profile that the client wishes' (Fuller
2005: 115).

Schmidt describes a range of market research techniques: 'one-on-one
interviews, ethnographic-style interviewing (on-site observations and
interview – in-home, in-car, in-office, etc.); shopalong interviews; online –
bulletin boards, live chat groups or interviews, online video diaries' (Schmidt
2009: 225). When doing ethnographic research in people's homes, researchers should look inside kitchen cupboards and refrigerators since, she notes,
the consumer doesn't always tell the truth about what they eat (ibid.).

If this recalls Habermas's observation of the colonisation of the lifeworld,
the process continues as product developers are urged to

> become a regular part of your target consumer's day to day life.
> Consider how you can fit in to her wake up, breakfast, daily nutrition,
> energy, workout, snacks, lunch at work, away from work … health
> practices … relaxation time, on the go, kids … hunger pangs, dinner-
> time, dessert and when entertaining friends. (Schmidt 2009: 232)

Targeted consumer research should aim to understand people's lives so as
to anticipate the kinds of needs they might have. Thus researchers should
ask, 'What makes them "tick"? What are their values? What or who influences their lives? When and how might my product fit into their consumption patterns?' (Schmidt 2009: 219). One market research firm researching

attitudes to frozen foods recruited a sample of adults representing different demographic groups:

> They had to videotape themselves planning meals, be interviewed evaluating a new product concept, and were questioned extensively about their lifestyles, satisfaction levels with current products, and talk about the role of frozen foods in their lives. (Schmidt 2009: 225)

The result was several 'distinct consumer profiles' which were still used by the company's product development teams (Schmidt 2009: 225). This could be one illustration of how marketers work with consumers to 'co-create' value. Marketers are genuinely interested in consumer experiences so as to improve products and increase sales. They are, in a sense, learning about the habitus of the target group so that they can understand not just what products might appeal, but how these products would be used and absorbed into their purchasers' lives. However, one food industry consultant acknowledged that the increasing success of market research techniques has come at the cost of public objections to invasive approaches and breaches of privacy; he describes 'a rebellion against consumer researchers' hunt for information about people's habits and a growing feeling on the part of some consumer groups that customers/consumers are being manipulated' (Fuller 2001: 77).

One consumer product company has used video diaries to observe how customers use their products. Company researchers 'hope this direct observation approach will help them identify and address problems *that consumers do not even know they have*' (Dibb and Simkin 2009: 204, emphasis added). Excerpts are then made available to staff on a secure website (ibid.).

Others affirm the importance of observing consumers in the right context during the product development phase:

> Whether in a staged context ... or in the consumers' environment, we find that a more familiar and comforting situation for the research allows the subject to feel more at ease and tends to stimulate ... less guarded discussions. (Beckley and Ramsey 2009: 234)

In these circumstances, their habitus, in sociological terms, is more completely revealed to marketers. Participatory action research is also recommended as a way of identifying problems and solutions for specific marketing scenarios (ibid.: 239). An extraordinary degree of empathy with research participants is encouraged:

> walk gently with the person ... To value them as people and to create a comfortable and engaging situation that allows them to be close to who they are *while* we are with them, as they were before we came into their lives, and the way they become when they leave. (Beckley and Ramsey 2009: 244, authors' emphasis)

In commercial-ethnographic research, marketers are urged to engage with participants to learn about their tastes in food, their skills, time and space for food preparation and consumption, and which products might suit these circumstances. This will enable products to be presented and packaged so that they are absorbed seamlessly into consumers' lives, and indeed habitus; they will, for example, be relevant in terms of convenience and time-saving features as well as sensory appeal. Products and brands can be designed to appeal to particular groups and marketing strategies appropriate for reaching those groups can be developed (Dibb and Simkin 2009: 169).

In supermarkets, researchers may position hidden cameras to follow shoppers, tracking the aisles they visit, how their eyes move and how long they view a product: 'areas where they are attracted ... or sections that they bypass entirely or visit less frequently are carefully noted' (Fuller 2001: 53–4). Food retailers also need to know 'what items are purchased together, so that customer flow can be laid out strategically within the store' (ibid.: 55).

The UK marketer who piloted eye-tracking technology in stores, now used worldwide, claims that without it, many products failed. Eye-tracking allows retailers to go beyond what shoppers *say* to looking at what they *do*, understanding why they bought or passed by products: 'shoppers obey the law of entropy: understanding that they conserve momentum is the key to designing spaces that help them shop more effectively' (Scammel-Katz 2012: 28).

Long before eye-tracking technology, telemarketing services were developed for fuller consumer profiling. As long ago as 2001, US companies could subscribe to a service which gave them the phone numbers of callers to a 1-800 service – caller and address could be identified from this which allowed the food company to identify the person's socio-economic status as well as that of their neighbourhood. With this information, 'Food manufacturers can then develop products that fit the demographic niche' (Fuller 2001: 56). Clearly, consumer tracking technologies have advanced considerably since then. Yet in Christakis and Fowler's influential research as late as 2009 (discussed in Chapter 5), the 'amazing' power of social networks, as they described it, was not linked to this capacity to differentiate the food supply by neighbourhood and socio-economic status.

Marketers are advised to develop 'consumer personas' for each target segment: this ensures that the 'entire marketing mix (product development, promotions, packaging, communications and pricing strategies) reflects the needs and wants of the target consumer' (Schmidt 2009: 225). This is what large marketing firms do in their constant updating of consumer profiles based on a vast array of data. This aims to build a complete picture of types of consumers, how they live, their tastes, family type, neighbourhood, ethnicity, etc. – it is a marketing version of the habitus. Then each step of the marketing chain can be tailored as much as possible to the nature of each type of consumer.

Word of mouth is a vital marketing tool among all consumers, including children: 'we learn by seeing people we know/respect try something and we think we will, too' (Urbick 2009: 258). This reflects how social networks operate in a food context. Word of mouth regarding foods in a given neighbourhood or among a group of friends is likely to have a class dimension, reflecting the class status of the area or group.

Other dimensions of the consumer are also central to marketing efforts. Many 'brands have a natural gender fit', though it is possible to target men while still reaching female consumers by addressing women through witty advertisements during TV programmes women are known to watch (they cite *Dancing on Ice*), as well as more traditionally male ad spots (football matches) (*Marketing Magazine* 02/03/11a). An advertising campaign for chocolate bars featured the slogan 'Yorkie: it's NOT for girls!' which, used and interpreted in an ironic way, resulted in increased sales among both sexes (ibid.).

McCain's Rustic Oven Chips brand was aimed at young women interested in healthy eating (*Marketing Magazine* 02/02/11); whereas Ginsters' new filled, breaded snack products targeted men and students (*Marketing Magazine* 08/06/11d). Women may eat these products as students, then, but grow out of them, while men apparently do not; social class may (re)assert itself in food consumption for educated women in a way that it does not to the same degree among educated men. Obesity statistics show a clear social gradient among women, but it is less clear among men; here we may have food industry evidence of these diverging trends in early adulthood. It has long been the case that 'men are more likely to purchase impulse items, to spend more on food shopping, and to purchase certain types of food, especially snacks and convenience products' (Michman and Mazze 1998: 5).

Subway has traditionally targeted young men working in offices and students but they have also begun marketing to women, aiming to appeal to those interested in healthy eating by including calorie information on menu boards (*Marketing Magazine* 25/01/12). But there is no plan to stop catering for traditional customers with indulgent products (ibid.). As Hawkes *et al.* (2012: 350) concluded, 'food consuming industries' are unlikely to change their emphasis on 'energy-dense, nutrient-poor foods' without the 'incentive' provided by health standards aimed at the entire supply chain (see Chapter 6).

The market research methods described here are aimed at assessing customer 'needs', whether consciously expressed or latent; meeting consumer need is a dominant feature of marketing discourse. But the accompanying assumption is that although commercial decisions to develop and market a given set of products results in consumption of those products, consumption itself – and its effects – is the responsibility of the consumer. An ethical role for the firm, or its marketers, is not always central to the discussion, though the concerns of many marketers are cited in this book.

The focus on serving customer needs can also divert attention from larger business goals. One brand marketer describes commercial-economic pressures:

We don't get given this money [marketing budgets] to entertain the public. We get given it to build strong businesses that make bigger returns to shareholders and pensions and bigger tax for governments – and more secure employment for people who work for it. (*Marketing Magazine* 23/02/11d)

In other words, it is obviously essential to bring the ability to meet customer 'needs' together with corporate – and even, for this marketer – societal goals.

The discourse of meeting customer needs and co-creating value with consumers must be understood in this highly instrumentalised context: 'marketing texts … deploy the rhetoric of consumer orientation to promote a sense of connection between the little consumer and the big corporation' (Hackley 2010: 225). But this does not dent the 'rhetorical production of dominance and control which underlies so much research in the field' (Hackley 2001: 21).

Marketing discourse acts ideologically 'in framing the conditions for social relations on a huge scale' (Morgan 1992 cited in Hackley 2001: 22), while never admitting to doing so. Yet 'the pervasive effects of mediated marketing activity constitute cultural and psychological life in developed economies to an extent which it is hard to appreciate' (Hackley 2001: 22). One technique which has enabled marketing to reach, study and segment consumers with a high degree of accuracy is geodemographics.

Tracking consumption by neighbourhood: geodemographics

One's residence is a crucial, possibly the crucial, identifier of who you are. (Savage *et al.* 2005 cited in Burrows and Gane 2006: 808)

The discourse of geodemographic information systems is an apotheosis of instrumental reason. It promises to measure, represent, and classify consumer identity with the explicit intent to predict and manipulate behaviour. (Goss 1995: 161)

Commercial geodemographics is a consumer profiling technique which combines the output of geographic information systems (GIS), census and purchase data, and some qualitative styling of resulting groupings (Longley and Goodchild 2008: 183) – but its power is more starkly conveyed by the citations above. It has its origins in the nineteenth century, when Charles Booth documented poverty in Victorian cities – probably the first systematic measurement of neighbourhood population characteristics. Further conceptual work was undertaken from 1916 in Chicago, with a burgeoning academic analysis of 'social area analysis' by the 1950s/1960s.

UK national classifications were developed in 1971 to guide local government policy, and this model was developed into commercial applications (such as ACORN – A Classification of Residential Neighbourhoods – and Mosaic).

By 1993, 85 per cent of business information had 'geographic attributes' (Baker and Baker 1993 cited in Goss 1995: 144). Public sector geodemographic approaches have been developed along commercial lines to enhance their effectiveness (Longley and Goodchild 2008: 181).

For Harvey, the amassing of data of this nature is part of the neoliberal project. Given neoliberalism's identification of the social good with

> the reach and frequency of market transactions ... it seeks to bring all human action into the domain of the market. This requires technologies of information creation and capacities to accumulate, store, transfer, analyse, and use massive databases to guide decisions in the global marketplace. Hence neoliberalism's intense interest in and pursuit of information technologies. (Harvey 2005: 3)

Such data is also used in the marketing of foods, one of the last stages in food production and the one which must help to foster consumption of a continually developing food supply.

An emphasis on lifestyle choices and personal responsibility for dietary health was a natural outgrowth of neoliberalism (Guthman 2011). To recap this discussion from Chapter 1, a free market (however imperfectly designed or functioning) needs to be populated with freely choosing individuals who are encouraged to be less reliant on the state. Ideally, then, they will avoid making choices which will result in problems like ill health. While data gathering of the scope of market research tracks 'choices', these choices are a response to a food supply constituted by the agricultural–financial–retail forces discussed in Chapter 6, and one which is marketed according to consumer type (including social status). The data is then used to further refine consumer profiles which will be used, in turn, to further shape future choices. While Murcott (2000: 122, see Chapter 1) observed that it is difficult for academics to get access to commercial market research data, we *can* learn about techniques like geodemographics, and what they mean for consumption and health.

Clustering is a key geodemographic concept. Socio-residential patterning is repetitive – similar social groups live in similar types of neighbourhoods in different cities. People tend to live among other people like themselves, and separate themselves from those who are different (Phillips and Curry 2003: 143). However, there are exceptions. One commentator observed that the consumer profile for his postcode did not describe his purchasing patterns accurately (Lawson 2009). A similar finding was reported by a group of sociologists when they gave residents in four streets in different parts of the UK their consumer profiles: many said the classification did not describe them but it did describe their neighbours (Parker *et al.* 2007: 913). Ethnographic observation led the researchers to conclude the classifications *do* give some socio-economic and cultural understanding of who lived in the four areas (ibid.: 913): 'In general, we and the residents thought they were frighteningly accurate' (Burrows, who worked on the study, cited in *Guardian* 11/09/07). This comment was considered to be of interest to marketers and reprinted in *Marketing Magazine* (02/10/07).

In fact, the characteristics of any given household can differ from the neighbourhood average or consumer profile for a given neighbourhood (Longley and Goodchild 2008: 178). Mosaic descriptions of consumer groups are 'pure examples to which individual cases approximate only with various degrees of exactness' (Mosaic cited in Burrows and Gane 2006: 800). A neighbourhood may be assigned to a category 'because it is the most similar of the available options ... [but] within each class [category] there is substantial variation around any mean or median value' (Longley and Goodchild 2008: 180).

Nevertheless, geodemographic profiles provide useful guidance for retailers and service providers: 'improvements in targeting of goods and service offerings [using geodemographics] improve measured profitability' (Longley and Goodchild 2008: 190). However accurate the original profiles are to begin with, the more they are used, the more 'true' they become:

> the fact that the final geodemographic classifications are meaningful and useful is ... a deliberate part and aim of the method. It is a circular argument. They are both meaningful and useful because they are useful; and they are increasingly meaningful because they are increasingly used. (Parker *et al.* 2007: 914)

The use of these classifications is thus a 'deeply political and ethical' matter (Parker *et al.* 2007: 914). In developing and applying them, the 'classifications interact with the classified' in a kind of 'dynamic nominalism' (Hacking 2002 cited in Parker *et al.* 2007: 915–16).

Geodemographics and the academy

Geographers Phillips and Curry critique those who developed these systems for having 'abjured the use of related academic work in geography, sociology and political science' (2003: 137), which probably accounts for the suspicion with which they are regarded within the academy. This critique parallels that aimed at marketing and its relationship with other disciplines. But academic inattention to geodemographics means that its social importance has remained insufficiently explored, except for critiques of consumer surveillance (ibid.: 145–6). In the process, structural effects such as 'the management of taste, increased inequity in market knowledge, and the creation of a society fractured into increasingly precise and exclusive market segments' have been ignored (ibid.: 147). The image in Figure 7.1 encapsulates this phenomenon as these young people eat food products designed for and targeted at them, in a place they are normally to be found.

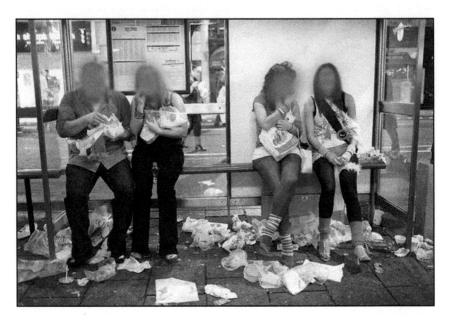

Figure 7.1 Young people eating fast food in a UK city centre at night. Maciej Dakowicz ©. Photograph reproduced with kind permission from the photographer.

Sociologists Savage and Burrows speculate on reasons for academic resistance to geodemographic approaches:

> we can emphasize our superior reflexivity, theoretical sophistication, or critical edge ... yet the danger is that this response involves taking refuge in the reassurance of our own internal world, our own assumed abilities to be more 'sophisticated' ... [But] from their perspective, the research they [market research firms] do ... is productive and is 'effective' in its own terms. (Savage and Burrows 2007: 887–8)

The academy's neglect of geodemographics has left it ignorant of 'the empirical knowledge that has been built up by marketers on the relationship between purchasing patterns and the patterns of neighbourhood segregation which characterize modern societies' (Webber 2004 cited in Burrows and Gane 2006: 794).

The detail of this constantly updated market research dwarfs anything academics have access to by way of public sector research. But 'key agents in the research apparatus of contemporary capitalist organisations now simply don't need the empirical expertise of quantitative social scientists' (Burrows and Gane 2006: 891). Their survey tools are more powerful in terms of quantity, reach and instantaneousness, as 'data on whole populations are routinely gathered as a by-product of institutional transactions' (ibid.).

Some social scientists have, quite separately from the commercial world, taken a 'spatial turn' (Parker *et al.* 2007: 905). They conclude that 'class places people into different types of places … [and] the application and impact of geodemographic classifications recursively reinforces this spatialization of class' (ibid.: 917). Lyon argues that the proliferation of organisational classifications – which are not free of stereotypes – have played an increasing role in determining life-chances (Lyon 2003: 21–2).

As Burrows and Gane observe, 'The success of such classification systems lies in their ability to map out and structure patterns of consumption that in turn aid both the enhancement and regulation of the capitalist market' (Burrows and Gane 2006: 807). If what we consume increasingly defines us – both our health, in the case of food, and our status – then geodemographic classifications are themselves influential in this process. Yet most of us, invisibly networked to a range of retailers and purchasing patterns, embedded in the consumption of a given set of goods and services aimed at other people like us, are unaware of this process, given that the classifications are the result of 'complex algorithms that remain hidden from the user's eye' (ibid.: 809; Goss 1995: 140).

Savage and Burrows conclude that only commercial transactional research technologies are able to provide nuanced explanations of diverse population groups (Savage and Burrows 2007: 894). Nevertheless, academic research should try to link 'narrative, numbers and images in ways that engage with, and critique, the kinds of routine transactional analyses that now proliferate'. There is a need to investigate the 'social construction of the classifications that have come to dominate our social world' (Bowker and Starr 1999 cited in Parker *et al.* 2007: 903) with vital new centres and systems of power. But if we are to engage with these commercial data sources, we will need to campaign for greater access to them (Savage and Burrows 2007: 894).

However, Webber, who developed geodemographic techniques in the commercial world several decades ago, finds it difficult to see how neighbourhood classifications could be 'translated into forms which can contribute to academic discourse' (Webber 2007: 185). Academic awareness of these classifications is 'fragmentary' and access to the classifications themselves is limited (ibid.), presumably for commercial reasons. Nevertheless, Webber sees some similarities between Mosaic classifications and sociological discourse (on globalisation and neighbourhood gentrification, for example) (ibid.). One health classification service has noted that its public sector team includes academic specialists (CACI 2014).

Geodemographics and health market research

Commercial marketing data houses have also developed neighbourhood classifications for non-commercial clients such as health authorities and policymakers – another reason for academics to pay attention to them, as commercial market research firms are increasingly consulted in developing public policies. CACI's HealthACORN profiles, for example, offer insights into local health, fitness and dietary profiles, including in their data even those who do not regularly attend GP surgeries (CACI 2011).

One ACORN profile of families on very low incomes living in council housing notes that they eat more fast food and takeaways than the population average (CACI 2009). HealthACORN profiles describe the poor diets of a disadvantaged, low status group: such diets include very little fruit or vegetables, and rely on snack and convenience foods high in fat. This group is also described as having higher than average levels of illness (especially circulatory) and obesity (CACI 2012).

These profiles, which amount to a description of diet and health habitus, have been used by the government's Central Office of Information and a range of public health bodies and helped develop the Change4Life health promotion campaign. HealthACORN can provide data-rich insights into local use of and future need for health facilities and services, including social marketing/behaviour change campaigns, and it can do so by local area.

Using the same types of data for both commercial and health behaviour classifications, there is a consistent logic running through both. Thus, while information is gathered on food consumption patterns by neighbourhood alongside emerging health needs by neighbourhood, the latter must result at least in some measure from the foods routinely purchased from local food stores and outlets, particularly over time, as these foods form dietary patterns.

Here is an illustration of how this process seems to work: health profile classifications assess and predict health problems such as diabetes or heart disease by neighbourhood. One group, which is to be found in public housing, takes little exercise and has a poor diet, with almost no fruit or vegetables, but much snack and prepared foods (CACI 2011). Such information, provided on a neighbourhood by neighbourhood basis if desired, could usefully alert health services to the kinds of health problems that might result from such diets; but it also reflects the local food supply and, in a presentation to food retailers, could provide relevant information for those seeking new locations or wishing to learn about local food preferences. Those who sell the above foods will apparently be well advised to site similar businesses in these areas.

Mosaic classifications include one which specialises in grocery purchases by neighbourhood using its own demographic data and lifestyle surveys as well as government Expenditure and Food survey data (Experian 2011). Its public sector service includes health studies analysing location, demography, lifestyle and behaviour. This service enables policymakers/service providers to 'understand the needs of customers and local areas to optimise the allocation of resources ... develop personalised messaging and communication that changes behaviours and improves service adoption, and accurately measure the risk and value of customers' (Experian 2011).

The use of geodemographic data for both marketing foods and planning for health needs which might be the result of poor diets characteristic of some areas, poses the question: could this kind of research about a neighbourhood's food consumption patterns and health consequences have the unintended side effect of reinforcing the siting and availability of such foods, and the patterns of consumption themselves? The following cases illustrate the interaction between low status, illness and food retail type.

A social marketing initiative to raise awareness of diabetes combined commercial geodemographics with a database listing hospital admissions in England since 1996. Each patient's health and demographic details are compiled along with their postcode (Farr *et al.* 2008: 458). There are an estimated 850,000 undiagnosed cases of diabetes in the UK; overall diagnoses number 400,000 (Type 1) and 3.4 million (Type 2) (Hex *et al.* 2012). In the study by Farr *et al.*, those most at risk of untreated diabetes were segmented into four groups: 'South Asian Industry, Families on Benefits, Low Horizons and Ex-Industrial Legacy' (Farr *et al.* 2008: 459).

All four groups were considered 'economically stressed', so local discount retailers were targeted by the awareness campaign. The study reported anecdotal evidence of increased screenings, but an independent evaluation found no significant change in diagnoses of diabetes in adults over 50 (Farr *et al.* 2008: 460). The benefits of social marketing campaigns may only be measurable in the longer term, but this type of initiative is downstream by its very nature. The problem originates at least partly in local food supplies and dietary patterns; both are linked to the social class status of the groups identified above.

The power of geodemographics: the perfect panopticon?

Even by 1995, geodemographic systems were growing rapidly, and the companies which had pioneered them were merging into IT conglomerates (Goss 1995: 131). Public datasets could be integrated with finance/insurance and health company data, consumer surveys and other consumer data, and finally, each client's customer data (ibid.: 150). Already the quantity and depth of the resulting data was remarkable (ibid.). Goss believes the industry flourished because of the capacity 'to monitor, model and control consumer behaviour, and ultimately because they promise the capability to manipulate the market and consumer identity to enhance profitability' (ibid.: 131). Lyon observes geodemographic surveillance technologies capturing personalised data and argues that these 'abstractions' are then used 'to place people in new social classes of income, attributes, preferences, or offences, in order to influence, manage or control them' (Lyon 2002 cited in Burrows and Gane 2006: 802).

Thus we should be concerned not just with privacy issues stemming from increased commercial surveillance, but also with the use of this knowledge to categorise and characterise groups of people, areas and even social relations, 'and to reify those models' (Phillips and Curry 2003: 148). If geodemographic insights lead to the siting of food options according to our home and work neighbourhoods and the routes we take between them, for example, then this structures an individual's 'foodscape' and food consumption. In managing the consumer's environment, 'desires are predicted (or manufactured) and sated before they have fully entered the consumer's consciousness' (Williamson 2000 cited in Phillips and Curry 2003: 148). This recalls the conclusions of behavioural economics regarding the automaticity of some types of consumption behaviour, and illustrates how the habitus can be subtly steered by industry strategies and activities in twenty-first century foodscapes.

Geodemographic research produces customer profiles that reflect a rational, predictable social world which is appealing to commercial clients (Phillips and Curry 2003: 132). When consumers purchase the goods marketed at them – and as they use and make meaning from them – they are in the process of constructing 'appropriate' identities (ibid.: 156, 162). So those who control market information influence 'the means of production of social identity' (ibid.: 162). While this does not render consumers 'dupes facilely manipulated by capital and the state ... geodemographics does at least promise that ... systematic manipulation of consumers is possible' (Goss 1995: 141).

The conceptual order inherent in this process would also hold powerful appeal for public bodies, to whom it is marketed in a public policy context. Market research and analysis is one mechanism for increasing 'governmentality by both capital and the state' (Phillips and Curry 2003: 148). It offers a kind of 'geostrategic technical control over the everyday life of the consumer, through the collection, consolidation and circulation of information necessary to predict behaviour' (ibid.: 162).

We as consumers assist efforts to track our movements, for example, when we participate in surveys or focus groups, complete applications for a variety of goods and services, navigate the internet, or use smartphones or bank or loyalty cards. Even 20 years ago, Goss concluded that this created 'the perfect panopticon' (Goss 1995: 146) – a highly accurate yet invisible surveillance system, constantly updated and increasingly able to track and rank individuals accurately in time and space. The confidentiality of company profiles and any resulting marketing strategies offer a powerful draw for prospective clients, and enhance the effectiveness of the 'panopticon' (ibid.: 143).

The permeation of the public domain enabled by geodemographics marketises it in a sense, such that 'the character of lived regions becomes the product of the goals and strategies of ever fewer, more interlinked, well-capitalized, and private corporate interests' (Phillips and Curry 2003: 149). At the level of the individual, his or her lifeworld, to use Habermas's term, is changed, moulded – colonised.

Tracking consumers digitally

Facebook is at the centre of the gold rush of marketing spend. (*Guardian* 05/03/12)

The practice of segmenting potential consumers by tracking evidence of their existing preferences is being further transformed by access to patterns of internet/digital usage (Pariser 2011[3]), as the comment above illustrates. Since December 2009, Google has used a range of signals – 'everything from where you were logging in from to what browser you were using to what you had searched for before – to make guesses about who you were and what kinds of sites you'd like' (ibid.). Each Google user has a personalised profile, making computers 'a kind of one-way mirror, reflecting your own interests while algorithmic observers watch what you click' (ibid.). Google says it will not sell this data, but other personal data firms or 'behaviour market vendors' will (ibid.). Personalisation will thus shape what we purchase and even the news we consume. Social networking sites are already a prime source of 'personalised news feeds' for 36 per cent of those under 30 in the US. Internet filters extrapolate from things we like to predicting future behaviour: 'they are ... constantly creating and refining a theory of who you are and what you'll do and want next' (ibid.). This places each of us in an invisible filter bubble which we are not aware of and which we have not chosen to enter. It is a form of 'informational determinism' which 'can affect your ability to choose how you want to live ... you can get stuck in a static, ever-narrowing version of yourself' (ibid.).

For example, Facebook knows its users' real names, gender, who their friends are, what they are doing online at any given moment, interests, and educational background. While there have been assurances that personal identities will not be sold to advertisers, they will have enough information to target users with a high degree of precision (*Observer* 21/11/10). One marketing commentator concludes that 'Facebook is positioning itself as a formidable advertising platform. With its wealth of personal information – helpfully supplied by users – Facebook enables advertisers to target consumers according to demographics, their locations and even their interests' (*Marketing Magazine* 'Revolution' supplement 09/10a).

Online advertising accounts for 25 per cent of marketing budgets; advertisers spent £4.1 billion on online advertising in 2010 (*Marketing Magazine* 30/03/11; the figure for the first half of 2013 was £3 billion (IAB 2013)). One business commentator emphasised that the challenge was to figure out how to use social media to generate sales (*Marketing Magazine* Conference supplement July 2011a). Social networks, tracked via social media, are a rich source of demographic and behavioural data, continually updated by users (ibid.). A customer relations consultant noted that among the many things people talk about on social media was their food preferences (*Marketing Magazine* Conference supplement July 2011b). With continual input from users, digital technologies will enable better targeting of advertisements at relevant individuals, with content that will appeal to them (*Marketing Magazine* 25/05/11).

Mobile handheld devices, with their 'ecosystems of apps, tags, geo-coding, augmented reality, micro-blogging, synching, avatars and the like ... will proliferate as personal informatics and the internet of objects wirelessly interconnect the sensors that will soon be embedded in everything in order to capture and act upon real-time information' (*Marketing Magazine* 12/01/11). This phenomenon will typify the 'demographic hand-off from the generation over 50 to the generation under 30' already under way (ibid.).

One restaurant chain described the benefits of smart phone technologies:

> in the first three months of launching our iPhone ordering app, we took more than £1m, purely through natural adoption ... the opportunity to target and home in on our potential customers through demographic and behavioural targeting, as well as using time and new location propositions, is exciting. (*Marketing Magazine* 19/01/11)

A UK market research firm used an app to recruit consumers as field researchers – photographing merchandise, counting products displayed, checking point-of-sale material. Participants (7,600 as of June 2011) are paid a small fee (*Marketing Magazine* 08/06/11a). The resulting data was considered to be of a high standard (ibid.).

Even before Google had introduced its new filter monitors, one marketer questioned whether too much filtering, with the reinforcement of existing interests this implies, gives consumers less scope for stepping outside their existing preferences to try new products (*Marketing Magazine* 04/03/09, also cited in Chapter 8). As this technology develops, Google's executive chairman observes that 'it will be very hard for people to watch or consume something that has not in some sense been tailored for them' (Schmidt cited in Pariser 2011).

Analysing where the most likely customers are to be found, tracking what they already buy, then tailoring products via the use of images, language, packaging and product placement/siting have long been central to marketing. But should there be limits on the technologies, both online and offline, now used to do this? One marketer comments that 'today's dark arts are practised with the aid of MRI scanners, facial EMG electrodes and ... eye-tracking and video surveillance techniques'; gleaning 'veracity from respondents [is] deemed to be too unreliable to be taken at face value' (*Marketing Magazine* 13/04/11). Describing these high-tech methods as 'creepy', this commentator recommends a more openly co-operative approach. In such a scenario, 'active subjects, fully aware of the objectives of the research, [would be] fully participating in the exploration of their own behaviour and the extrapolation of meaningful conclusions' (ibid.).

Another commentator notes that the intensive degree of tracking of online behaviour would be unacceptable on an actual shopping excursion (*Marketing Magazine* 26/01/11). In online retail, 'the techniques we can apply are growing in sophistication, and some of them cross the line' (ibid.). As another marketer subsequently wrote, 'Will consumers be happy with a future of ubiquitous, pervasive surveillance and stalking, where every place they go and every online conversation they have is monitored and fed to back-room real-time ad servers?' (*Marketing Magazine* 23/02/11a). He feels this takes marketing's previous information-gathering on customers a step too far. It is one dimension of an emerging critique of marketing ethics by and among marketers (discussed further in Chapter 8).

Still developing is marketing's use of Twitter, with the launch of branded pages in February 2012 (*Marketing Magazine* 15/02/12b). By that time Cadbury already had 1 million fans on Facebook, and planned to use Twitter to bolster interest in its newest chocolate campaign (ibid.). Social media 'conversations' between customers and brands can be entertaining for participants, but they are also meant to foster brand loyalty and promote products, and may be opportunities for data-gathering. At the same time they are an example of the systematically (if co-operatively) distorted communication Habermas warned of long before the advent of social media.

Conclusion

This chapter has revealed the role of marketing in selling products and services, but also, having mined the insights of psychology, in nurturing desire itself. Hackley's critique noted the power of marketing not only in driving consumer purchases but beyond that, in laying the foundation for capitalist economies, even as it underestimates its own role and influence. Marketing shapes dietary patterns but is not usually observed by those whose lifeworlds are permeated and altered by it – that is, all of us.

I have cited examples of marketing strategies which normalised the consumption of HFSS foods – in meal deals; foods targeted at low status people; and the language of marketing discourse, which masks the ways in which foods are designed for and targeted at differing population segments. Yet higher status people are also tempted by 'indulgent' (HFSS) foods, despite an expressed interest in healthy eating. Marketers grasp this contradiction and, in co-operation with food product developers and retailers, cater to it. As discussed in Chapter 5, many higher status people are overweight or obese. Marketers will not be surprised by this phenomenon. They describe the persistently health-seeking eater as only a subset of higher status consumers, recalling Skeggs's notion of the subset of middle class people characterised by a reflexive approach to social life.

By tracking and classifying consumers by social group, market research has a role in reinforcing those groupings and the consumer identities and purchasing patterns that flow from them. Geodemographic research reveals neighbourhood consumption but also – separately, for different clients – neighbourhood health profiles, even when medical records are lacking (among those who have little contact with health services), partly by assessing things like food purchases and dietary patterns by household. These distinct yet complementary types of market research may contain a contradiction, as the unhealthy foods which blanket some neighbourhoods and dominate the diets of residents also generate diet-related illness over time. In this case, the market, broadly conceived, leverages both the food supply and the health policy solutions to problems flowing from it.

Social scientists who research food consumption should be aware of commercially oriented research engaged in the same task. This research and the influence it has on consumption is, in critical realist language, a generative mechanism shaping diet, yet people are mostly unaware of the degree to which they are tracked and supplied based on consumption identities that are continually updated through purchase data and geographic and online roaming. Nor is this research all quantitative; in this chapter, examples of qualitative, ethnographic research were described, amid the stated aim of marketers to identify 'needs' consumers are not yet aware they have.

Doubtless many of those who carry out market research and analysis are trained in social sciences. Those who practise these disciplines within the academy are well placed to research the researchers who inhabit the commercial world and the techniques they use. Their research is used not only to market products and influence consumption practices but also to market health analysis and health policy advice to government. The material presented here has highlighted the pervasiveness, quality, resources and reach of commercial marketing research.

Such research perhaps unintentionally strengthens the argument for looking at consumption in class terms. The marketing classifications sampled in this chapter depicted the inhabitants of deprived neighbourhoods in terms which did not try to imply that these people were all making free choices; indeed, the types of housing and amenities they experience, their education, family structure and employment profiles, are all listed as part and parcel of their classification. Patterns of food consumption, characterised by poor nutritional quality, are described alongside the health risks arising from them. Though it is not the stated aim of these classifications, they illustrate in a Bourdieuan way the package of life experiences and environments in which such behaviours arise.

The following chapter focuses in greater detail on one of the key tasks of marketing: segmentation. The discussion will reveal how marketing targets consumers and how consumer segments relate to concepts of social class; how supermarkets and food products are ranked and distinguished both by consumers and producers of food, and how consumers identify and interact with their segmentation profiles in their shopping and eating habits. The chapter concludes with a review of an ethical debate among marketers regarding the role of their discipline in altering norms and contributing to problematic consumption.

Notes

1 Daniel Kahnemann's work on prospect theory formed the basis for 'nudge' theory (discussed in Chapter 1), uniting psychological insight with economic behaviour. Unusually for a psychologist, he won the 2002 Nobel prize for economics for this work.
2 I accessed this study after reading about it in a 'Bad Science' column by Ben Goldacre, a medical doctor, in *The Guardian* (09/07/11). Though small-scale, the study was good science, he concluded.
3 Citations are from an excerpt of Pariser's book in *The Observer* (12/06/11), so page numbers are not given.

8 Social class in food retailing and marketing and reflections on marketing ethics

Introduction

> The homogenizing and illusory notions of the consumer and of the consumer interest will tend to come up against differences of income, gender, race, region, nationality, class, etc. (Fine 2006: 306)

> Any substantial group of people develops shared beliefs and behaviours. (Blythe 2006: 44)

These statements, the first by a critic of consumer discourse, the second by a marketing academic, approach the notion of consumption from different angles. For marketers, noticing how people develop and share beliefs and behaviours is an important step in effective consumer marketing. For critics of the way consumption is portrayed, it is important to go further than that, and to acknowledge that structural matters over which people have little control can also shape their activities as a consumer – and the consequences that flow from that consumption.

Marketing uses the term 'segmentation' to describe 'the process of classifying people into groups that have some set of similar characteristics, resulting in the ability to be studied and targeted', in the words of one marketing agency (Xtreme Impact 2011). It is informed by the qualitative and quantitative market research techniques and data described in the previous chapter, and lies at the heart of how social class is *reflected* in food consumption, even if it is not openly acknowledged by the industry.

Marketing's engagement with social class as a way of understanding and serving consumers will be discussed in this chapter, showing how shoppers, supermarkets and even food products are 'classed'. Consumers are shown participating in this process; as discussed previously, successful marketing engages in a highly interactive way with consumers. The chapter concludes with an analysis of the ethics of food marketing, with marketers themselves expressing reservations about aspects of marketing and the ethical limits which practitioners must continually negotiate.

The role of segmentation in marketing

In segmentation, existing and potential consumers are

> profiled, categorized and sorted into groups in order to 'target' them with marketing initiatives ... Marketing segments have to be viable in the sense that they must have the necessary disposable income, the segment must be large enough to sustain the required level of sales, and it must be accessible. (Hackley 2009: 90)

Segmentation has been instrumental in Tesco's success:

> It developed a clear marketing strategy based on a desire to fully satisfy a carefully targeted set of market segments. Tesco is continuously upgrading its stores, adding new services and product lines, and innovating with channels of distribution ... with the aim of addressing its targeted-segment customer needs ... Tesco has [also] led the way in creating over 400 'ethnic stores'. (Dibb and Simkin 2009: 48, 128)

There is nothing wrong with this practice; indeed it might well be experienced as good customer service. Tesco has been alert to the changing ethnic make-up of populations local to its stores, for example.

But Tesco and other supermarkets also serve distinct social class groups. For one business commentator, Tesco 'has succeeded in making itself largely classless, with price ranges designed to cater across the board' (*Observer* 25/04/10). In fact, it appeals to several different social groupings with products of varying quality and status; this is not the same as being classless. An ad agency executive describes the appeal of Tesco products for different groups of shoppers: 'The middle classes buy their wine, petrol and insurance from Tesco. The working classes buy their food, clothes and everything else from Tesco' (*Marketing Magazine* 09/03/11b).[1]

Tesco tracks customers via its Clubcard and its own market research group, with customer demographics, location and preferences being gleaned from its consumer data (*Marketing Magazine* 09/03/11a). Detailed tracking of shopper behaviour is also carried out by market research firms. In the 67 household types and 15 groups listed in Experian's Mosaic publicly available profiling tool, descriptions of typical food consumption feature in most categories. The same is true for CACI's ACORN segmentations, which also describe how each profile would be educated, employed, and housed, without referring to social class per se.

One problem with using segmentation to target consumers is that it can have the effect of 'cocooning' them – potentially stultifying broader consumption by offering people the kinds of products that only reaffirm the kinds of consumers they already are, as one marketing commentator observed (*Marketing Magazine* 04/03/09). Marketing does seem to have some capacity to reinforce both personal identities and consumption patterns.

Edwards, a sociologist of consumption, queries the 'tendency of contemporary patterns of consumption to individualize every activity into a lifestyle miscellany' and finds that 'the creation of a plethora of mutually exclusive lifestyle categories seems paradoxically to reinforce the economic inequalities it seems to undermine' (Edwards 2000: 186). There are many ways in which consumer groups can be segmented, but the social ranking of potential customers is fundamental for product developers, marketers and retailers. This chapter examines how marketing academics, marketing practitioners and retailers engage with concepts of social class via segmentation, and the role it plays in food consumption.

Marketing and social class

> Primary socialization within a consumer culture creates a mass of 'good' consumers, behaving in consonance with the aims of corporate capitalism. Since the ... [consumption] code prescribes meanings in advance, individuals are channeled into certain forms of class and consumer behaviour. (Cherrier and Murray 2004: 517–18, describing a Baudrillardan analysis)

> Social class is based on a very old-fashioned view of economic structure. (Market research executive, Interviewee A, 2011)

These quotations illustrate the differing stances of consumption theorists and marketers working in the field; the former links consumption with class and behaviour, the latter finds class a dated concept altogether. Yet marketing has long classified populations as consumers into six broad groups: A, B, C1, C2, D and E. Each is associated with a 'class' label and occupational status, based on official national statistics, ranging from higher managerial/ professional to pensioners/unemployed (Dibb and Simkin 2009: 126). In Figure 8.1, an artwork which appeared in a 2009 exhibition on social class in British history, the artists have brought together these marketing classifications with images of cutlery representing different social classes as they are segmented and labelled in marketing practice. The lists in the caption link marketing designation with professional status and type of occupation.

These marketing categorisations are referred to constantly in marketing discourse. Dibb and Simkin mention the innovations of the official NS-SEC categorisation in 2001 but do not cross-reference it with the A–E marketing classification, though they comment that the NS-SEC 'aims to more closely reflect consumers' purchasing power on the basis of their position in the labour market' (Dibb and Simkin 2009: 127). This may not have been the

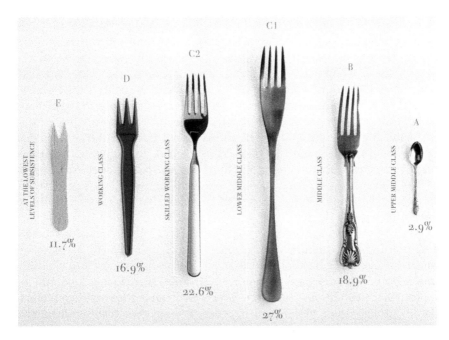

Figure 8.1 A rendering of social class and marketing classifications using differing styles of cutlery to represent each group. Image by Ben Branagan and Gareth Holt (originally appeared in *RANK: Picturing the Social Order 1516–2009*, Northern Gallery for Contemporary Art, Sunderland). National Readership Survey/Ipsos Mori.

Alphabetical socio-professional classification, updated 2008. Social class: A, upper-middle class (higher managerial/professional; doctor, director); B, middle class (intermediate managerial; teacher, engineer); C1, lower-middle class (supervisor, clerical or junior; salesman, artist). C2 skilled working class (skilled manual worker; bricklayer, electrician). D, working class (semi-skilled and unskilled manual; operative, machinist). E, subsistence levels (state pensioner/no other income; casual labourer).

intention of the originators of the NS-SEC, but it is undoubtedly one of its outcomes. The NS-SEC categories and even marketing's adaptation of them leave us a fragment of Marx's original idea of class relations in their labour market context.

Social class in consumer research has had a trajectory broadly paralleling that of class in sociology, with a strong focus from the 1940s to 1960s, but fading since the 1970s (Henry and Caldwell 2008: 388). In the 1990s, Bourdieu's ideas began to circulate among marketing theorists, who saw class-based behaviours in daily life as habitual rather than deliberate. Holt's (1998) research showed how class influenced the consumption of food and other household items in the US. Class had *not* faded, as many had concluded, but the class structure had changed 'in terms of the overt markers that identified each social class group' (Holt 1998 cited in Henry and Caldwell 2008: 398).

But class is a relatively arcane idea for marketing practitioners today. A market research executive I spoke to said, 'We rarely if ever talk about social class with clients. It's a kind of concept that's irrelevant to the conversation we're having. They're more interested in: what are they [customers] spending, what are their lifestyle characteristics?' (Interviewee A, 2011). Nevertheless, he likened the ABCDE classifications to social class: simplifications of more complex segmentations which can only be assessed by detailed geodemographic research. As he put it, retail clients just want to be able to understand that a given segment is, for example, 'predominantly educated urbanites – but in old money, in social class terms, they're AB'. Geodemographics and focus group data can provide a more specific picture which links numbers and types of potential customers according to where they live.

The rise of the 'quantitative project' of multivariate statistical marketing research indirectly admits the influence of social class, with its measurements of income, education and occupational status (Henry and Caldwell 2008: 400). Marketing as a discipline understands that 'a set of co-occurring holistic lived conditions tends to follow a predictable trajectory from childhood through adult maturation that creates outcomes such as distinctive dispositional tendencies, and a range of wellbeing outcomes such as health, wealth and consumption practices' (ibid.: 402). This recalls not only Bourdieu's concept of habitus but also Weber's description of class in which 'a specific market position accrues a similar mix of living conditions and life chances that in turn shape members' outlooks' (ibid.: 395).

When asked if brands illustrate class distinctions, a retail marketing lecturer described how vodka is marketed to different social groups:

> Diageo spends more than £1bn a year on advertising ... to create the 'right' image for the drinkers of its brands ... Red Label Smirnoff is the market-leading brand ... Glen's Vodka is targeted at less affluent members of society, whereas Grey Goose is positioned to attract the more discerning and affluent customers. (Ellis-Chadwick interviewed in *Sesame* 2010: 41–2)

In this way, she says, there is a link between the vodka people drink and their social class (ibid.). But class is rarely addressed overtly within marketing discourse. Consumer marketing literature, marketing profiles, and the media more broadly use a range of alternatives when referring to different social groups: terms such as premium, discerning, educated, affluent (and less affluent), upmarket, high end, good taste, ABs (highest status marketing category), DEs (lowest marketing category), low income, disadvantaged, deprived and vulnerable denote the social and economic status of consumers. These terms are arguably proxies for social class, including socio-economic status, and link questions of taste and dietary type with status, housing type and geographic location.

The way class is approached in marketing education is worth examining, since it is not often referred to in marketing practice itself. The undergraduate marketing textbook cited below describes it in quite instrumental and simplistic terms:

> Within all societies, people rank others into higher or lower positions of respect. This ranking results in social classes. A social class is an open group of individuals who have similar social rank. A class is referred to as 'open' because people can move into and out of it ... In the UK, many factors are taken into account, including occupation, education, income, wealth, race, ethnic group and possessions ... To some degree, people within social classes develop and assume common patterns of behaviour ... Social class influences many aspects of people's lives ... whom they marry, their likelihood of having children and the children's chances of surviving infancy ... Social class affects the type, quality and quantity of products that a person buys and uses. Social class also affects an individual's shopping patterns. (Dibb and Simkin 2009: 126)

Historical contextualisation and the potential obstacles to social class mobility are not alluded to, nor is any link between the reinforcement of 'an individual's shopping patterns' and the way that individual is marketed *to* over time. Nevertheless, students are learning about the link between status/rank and behaviour/consumer choices, and segmentation by class is clearly acknowledged, even without any further exploration of social inequality or social structure. This textbook is broadly comparable to other undergraduate marketing textbooks in its treatment of social class in marketing education.

Between September 2010 and September 2011, two articles in *Marketing Magazine* cited the same study on social class. These were the only references to social class in this industry magazine during that time. One article was entitled 'Defining the new middle class: a new study gives fresh insight into the growing proportion of consumers who describe themselves as middle class. Its findings are critical to brands' (*Marketing Magazine* 23/03/11). The article describes the study's conclusions about self-defined social class, political orientation and brand preferences among both middle and working classes by political and consumer research firm BritainThinks (2011). Ten focus groups and an online survey of adults in 2003, weighted to represent the UK population, were asked to self-assess their social class and select their preferred brands. Some 71 per cent of participants considered themselves middle class (7 per cent upper middle; 43 per cent middle, 21 per cent lower middle) and 24 per cent working class. No one self-identified as upper class.

The report presented six subgroups: 'Bargain Hunters, Daily Mail Disciplinarians, Comfortable Greens, Urban Networkers, Deserving Downtimers and Squeezed Strugglers' (*Marketing Magazine* 23/03/11). A subsequent report on the working class found it to be more homogeneous, despite north–south differences (*Marketing Magazine* 06/07/11). Food brands favoured among this group included Iceland, McDonald's, KFC and Asda.

One marketer interviewed talked about the importance of remembering to serve the self-identified working class group, as they can be forgotten (*Marketing Magazine* 06/07/11). But all consumer groups are tracked, with products developed, marketed and sited to suit each group. Sometimes the only marketing tool that is used is simply siting ('place'): at the lowest end of the market, there may be little or no advertising, but people know which products and outlets are meant for them. In the case of independent fried chicken shops in low income areas, their target consumers – mostly young men with low incomes – know it instinctively (this case is discussed later in this chapter).

One critique finds that as consumers meet their 'socially sanctioned "needs"',

> they reproduce the conditions for their own domination. Here, the consumer is determined, controlled, and even alienated by marketing practices. Ultimately, consumers do not choose their consumption life-styles; it is the system of marketing practices that chooses for them. (Studies cited in Cherrier and Murray 2004: 520–1)

Cherrier and Murray reference this perspective but find it one-dimensional. Marketing is not always insightful or effective: sometimes it fails (see Chapter 7). Sometimes it does allow for ambiguity in consumer identities; and it is possible to find one's life improved by consumer products appropriately marketed so that we find out about them, use them and benefit from them. But food consumption *is* often shaped by industry trends and forces: 'Many food businesses historically arose to find markets for agricultural products – not to find products which matched consumer needs' (Wennstrom and Mellentin 2002: 28). It was marketing's role to make those needs felt. Engaging with consumers as members of social classes is part of that process, even if the language of class is not used.

The classing of food

An academic marketing study references Bourdieu's linkage of cultural capital with taste to show that 'social class position and consumption patterns remain intertwined', whether that position is high or low (Henry 2005: 766). Among lower status groups, he observes a 'disempowered tendency to self-restrict' (ibid.: 767). Disempowerment is, for Henry, 'a primary shaper of habitus' and even of class reproduction (ibid.: 767, 776). His notion of self-restriction could be applied to food consumption in the context of the poor quality of products consumed by (some of) those of lower social class, as confirmed by epidemiological research (Chapter 5) and observed – with concern – by food industry scientists in Chapter 6.

Henry's insights are also reflected in a research study presented at the 2011 British Sociology Association conference (Thompson 2011). Accompanying low income shoppers (individually) from a deprived area around a supermarket, the researcher asked one shopper why she picked up a particular product:

RESEARCHER: You seem quite excited about this ... what is it?
SHOPPER: [Dairylea] Dunkers. You never had a Dunker? ... I like these. They're called Jumbo Tubes. (She puts 4 packs in her basket and walks off). They're quite weird. They're not particularly nice. I have this weird obsession with them. They taste nice but they taste weird ... I can't eat this cheese (pointing to a block of cheese) ... In this form I don't like it. (Thompson 2011)

Dairylea Dunkers would not be marketed to high status, health-conscious consumers, who may not even have heard of this product; they are not, for example, sold at Waitrose. The salient feature about this shopper's description of them is that she is not sure why she buys them. She says she likes them, but also that they taste weird and are not particularly nice. Yet she is comfortable buying them. She knows how to eat them. She subsequently says she can't eat cheese in a block of cheddar; perhaps she doesn't know what to do with it, or the taste may be too strong. But Dairylea Dunkers have been designed for someone like her; they are, in sociological terms, consistent with her habitus, even though she has had to work at liking them. For her, the concept of cheese has been 'colonised' (to use Habermas's phrase) by the marketing of this product to people like her.

A nutritional analysis of food advertisements used readership rankings according to marketing categories. In 30 UK magazines, only magazines read by affluent readers advertised diet drinks and sweeteners; as on television, fruit and vegetables were rarely advertised, and again only for affluent readers; magazines with lower status readers had more advertisements for foods higher in saturated fat, sugar, sodium, protein and carbohydrate; higher status magazines had fewer advertisements for prepared meals and sauces, perhaps reflecting a higher degree of food preparation skills among readers (Adams and White 2009: 144–8).

A study on the effect of sugar information on food labels found that where this information was provided and consulted, sugar consumption was lower (Weaver and Finke 2003). But the study also found that it was those already aware of the health problems associated with a high sugar intake who were more likely to seek out these labels and make consumption decisions accordingly. This is a classic case of reflexivity – but one limited to a certain sector of the population trained via their habitus in this kind of reflexive thinking, as Skeggs has described in non-food contexts. Dietary information might be aimed at improving people's capability to make healthy choices, using capability in Sen's sense of the term (Sen 2004). But Sen argued that such measures are not always sufficient: 'the informational basis of justice cannot consist only of capability information, since [other] processes too are important' (Sen 2004: 24) and these processes are not always fair (ibid.: 31).

Moran, a cultural historian, traces the linkages between food and class which became apparent with the rise of convenience foods in the UK. By the 1960s, frozen foods and especially fish fingers were popular but of low status. It wasn't until the 1980s that frozen food transcended its previous class restrictions: by then, 'the ready meal was no longer for sad singletons or lower-class layabouts' (Moran 2007: 156). Later, M&S produced refrigerated ready meals which were considered posh; other supermarkets soon followed, targeting 'the young, middle-class professional' using language such as 'fresh', 'slow-cooked' and 'home-grown' (ibid.: 157). Frozen meals are still available, targeted mostly at low income shoppers (Moran 2007: 157). Lower priced refrigerated dishes are often presented, in primary colours, simply as value (or even 'valu') meals.

As ubiquitous as chilled ready meals are, the most commonly consumed prepared food in the UK is sandwiches (constituting 41 per cent of fast food consumption; the next is burgers, at 18 per cent (Burch and Lawrence 2005: 7)). In 2013, 1.69 billion sandwiches were sold in the UK (Sandwich News website 2014).

Both ready meals and sandwiches are highly diversified product categories, produced in a range of prices and quality, and with different consumer groups in mind. Greencore, which makes sandwiches for a range of British supermarkets, reported an 8.4 per cent increase in sales in late 2010 to early 2011, which it attributed to 'stronger demand for its higher end sandwich and alternative lunchtime options such as sushi, wraps and salad' among office workers who are considered affluent enough to purchase such products (*Guardian* 25/05/11).

Supermarkets contract out much food preparation to manufacturers, who manufacture different versions of their products for different customers. Hazlewood Foods produces chilled lasagne for many UK supermarkets (Harvey *et al.* 2003 cited in Burch and Lawrence 2005: 8). Companies like these are characterised by a high degree of innovation and flexibility, allowing them to meet demand for products ranging from pizzas to Thai meals to organic soups. Yet even within basic food categories, there are gradations of quality. The case of pizza illustrates the different 'classes' of food produced within one product line:

There is a definite pizza hierarchy – a top of the range product (hand crafted, low volume); there is a middle range or mainstream product (thin and crusty, or deep pan); and there is a bottom of the range economy product (made with basic ingredients) ... The new food manufacturing companies which necessarily produce large numbers and varieties of pizza for niche markets on the same 'assembly line' are required to adopt highly flexible systems of production. (Burch and Lawrence 2005: 8)

This 'classing' of foods happens in many product types. Henley (2010) traces the classing of crisps to the arrival of Kettle Chips in the UK in 1987. In addition to their irregular shape and flavourings, Kettle Chips came in large bags for sharing, and were more expensive. Sales of Kettle Chips rose 16.8 per cent during 2009, suggesting a thriving market for upmarket crisps (*Marketing Magazine* 03/03/10). But upmarket crisps are not necessarily healthier, though crisp manufacturers overall have been reducing salt, sugar and fat (Savoury Snack Information Bureau dietician cited in Henley 2010). A 2006 British Heart Foundation (BHF) study found that 69 per cent of lunchboxes contained a packet of crisps, with half of British children eating the equivalent of five litres of cooking oil per year in crisp consumption (cited in Henley 2010). In 2011, a third of British children were eating crisps and sweets three or more times a day and were more likely to have crisps with lunch than fruit (BHF 2011). Given the normalisation of a packet of crisps as a part of lunch, it is unlikely that most people realise the quantity of fat being consumed as part of this 'normal' practice. The British Heart Foundation created an image of a child drinking from a bottle of oil to make the point (Figure 8.2).

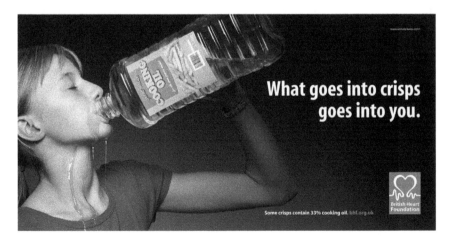

Figure 8.2 'What goes into crisps goes into you.' Image from 2006 BHF campaign, supplied by BHF for use in this book.

Sales of crisps overall in the UK rose by 27 per cent between 2006 and 2011, reaching £3.16 billion (*Marketing Magazine* 04/04/12); two-thirds of purchasers look for price promotions (ibid.). The trajectory for upmarket crisps was flatter; but 'the premium segment has performed well ... so it would seem that consumers are paying little heed to the government's healthier-eating messages where crisps are concerned' (*Marketing Magazine* 16/03/11). As sales figures indicate, crisps are big business. In recent years Kellogg bought the crisp brand Pringles for $2.7 billion from Procter & Gamble (*Marketing Magazine* 30/05/12).

The biggest buyers of crisps are families with children aged 5–15. Because of restrictions on selling such foods in schools, consumption outside the school environment has increased, with sales of crisps expected to increase another 21 per cent by 2015 (*Marketing Magazine* 30/05/12).

In further examples of how marketing links food consumption and social group, 'women, over-35s and the D socio-economic group are the most ardent sweet biscuit eaters ... [while] women, the over-55s and the lowest (E) socio-economic group' buy more savoury biscuits (*Marketing Magazine* 15/06/11a). Nuts, seeds and dried fruit 'are more popular with the affluent and the over-45s', although 'retailers have launched "value" ranges of mixed nuts and fruit to cater for more cash-strapped consumers' (*Marketing Magazine* 10/11/10). In the magazine this comment is illustrated with pictures of a packet of Red Hot Chilli Big Nuts and the contrasting dried fruit and raw nuts; the juxtaposition of these images represents in graphic terms their differing consumer categories. The Big Nuts packaging is a fun image in strong colours, in sharp contrast to the austere simplicity of the unadorned fruit and nuts.

One less visible category of consumption is the food produced by independent food restaurants/fast food providers, especially those supplying fried chicken, burgers, kebabs and curries. These businesses are very localised, often set up by people who know the area and customer base well, although they may make use of a discounted neighbourhood profiling service offered by market research firms (Interviewee A, 2011).

The salt and health research charity CASH found high salt concentrations in a study of 784 curry products from both grocery stores and independent restaurants (CASH 2010). An Iceland curry meal contained 7.2g of salt; a takeaway curry from a London restaurant had 6.81g (6g is the recommended daily maximum salt intake); at the other end of the spectrum, Sainsbury's Be Good to Yourself range included a curry meal with .91g of salt. While the government's discussions about health with food manufacturers and retailers have focused on chain stores and restaurants, independent providers are not so easily reached. Nor are they visible in lists of voluntary participants in the government's Public Health Responsibility Deal. However, the Department of Health notes that it 'has produced guidance for SMEs and is seeking to engage with them through relevant representative bodies. We are also exploring how action might be taken at a more local level to broaden the scope of participation' (DoH 2011a).

The case of fried chicken

A councillor in Oldham who objected to another fried chicken outlet opening in an area that already had 16 fast food businesses commented, 'We literally have streets that consist of nothing but kebab shops, chippies, curry houses, pizza, chicken and burger outlets' (*Guardian* 18/02/11). The class dimension of such foodscapes does not escape one north London fried chicken purveyor: 'Fried chicken won't work in Chelsea, Kensington or Hampstead, or anywhere like that. It's only places for the lower middle class or working class. That's the only place you can do it' (ibid.). Notably, he cites both class and place – targeting neighbourhood and class are crucial to the success of these businesses. Fried chicken sales grew by 36 per cent between 2003 and 2008, faster than the 22 per cent growth in fast food overall. In London's most deprived borough, Tower Hamlets, there are 42 fast food retailers per school compared to a national average of 25. One 20-year-old man said he ate fried chicken 'a lot. Probably daily. It's, like, addictive or something' (ibid.).

The case of fried chicken outlets underlines a dimension of marketing, and one of the four Ps – 'place': the importance of locating where your customers will find you easily, and recognise that you are selling food for people like them. Advertising doesn't always come into this type of food provision, though price promotion (on storefronts and leaflets) may be part of efforts to attract customers.

Larger global trends underlie the increase in fried chicken consumption. Chicken prices have remained stable in comparison to other meats; production is less affected by adverse weather and consumers rate it highly in terms of versatility, taste and nutrition (Gatfield 2006: 34). Also, 'value added segments are growing in line with changes in consumer tastes and preferences'; much less chicken is produced and sold as raw (ibid.: 35). A major development is that chickens eat 'less than half the amount of feed compared to 25 years ago ... feed represents 50–60 per cent of production costs' (ibid.: 39). Developments in soya processing allowed its fat and lecithin to be removed and used in food processing, while the remaining soya meal is fed to intensively reared chickens (Lawrence 2008a).

Prompted by these global agro-scientific developments, fried chicken has become popular even in areas where it has no previous cultural resonance. Bagwell (2011) explores this paradox in Tower Hamlets in London, a predominantly low income, Bangladeshi area, with already high rates of obesity, which has easily absorbed fried chicken into its dietary routines. Although it is a novel item, it has been adapted and is culturally sanctioned because of its compliance with halal requirements and the addition of spices to the crumb mixture (Bagwell 2011: 2225).

The halal status of independent fried chicken outlets there is even a marketing tool, and the novelty of the dish, which is not prepared in people's homes, is seen as a positive feature, in that it provides a treat (ibid.: 2226). The broader socio-economic needs of this consumer group are met via the low pricing of fried chicken and an accessible, welcoming social space for patrons. Many are young people looking for a more youthful atmosphere than that provided by more traditional curry restaurants in the area – but one which is still culturally sanctioned, as no alcohol is served (ibid.: 2226–8). A strong element of trust has entered the relationship between halal fast food outlets and their customers, which is leading to the replacement of 'more mainstream retail outlets' where less trust is experienced (ibid.).

This is another example of how a distinctive habitus is permeated, adapted and changed by a combination of interacting global, cultural and local forces. Cultural norms are respected while being slightly extended to include an unfamiliar food, which in turn is slightly adapted to preexisting tastes and is priced in line with limited local incomes. This is possible because of changes in global chicken production, feeding and processing technologies. The habitus is not consciously disturbed, but the food lifeworld has been colonised. Culturally, this development is not necessarily problematic, but the health effects of frequent fried chicken consumption are unlikely to have been considered by a primarily young clientele.

The government's policy announcement on obesity in October 2011 acknowledged that 'a number of local areas have also taken steps to use existing planning levers to limit the growth of fast food takeaways, for example by developing supplementary planning policies' (DoH 2011b: 28). But Bagwell's study found that some areas were already saturated with such businesses (Bagwell 2011). Fast food does not have to be unhealthy; promoting healthier fast foods could be one strategy, but deeper structural inequalities should also be addressed (ibid.: 2232).

Food quality and the classing of supermarkets – and shoppers

What are the health implications of a diet reliant on 'budget' or 'value' meals, and is the quality of ingredients appreciably better in health terms in 'premium' meals? How can supermarkets be assessed on these measures?

A report on supermarkets, diets and health by the National Consumer Council (NCC) in 2006[2] found that lower status supermarkets produced some poorer quality items in terms of fat, sugar and salt content, as well as labelling and price promotions, most of which were for highly processed foods rather than fruit and vegetables. However, the salt research charity CASH found that 'despite a nine-fold difference in the price of sausages (per 100g), there was no notable difference in the salt content of economy versus standard or premium supermarket ranges', with many sausages higher in salt than a packet of crisps (CASH 2011b).

Budget or value products are in some cases significantly less healthy than standard versions of processed products. By 2008, the next NCC report found that at Tesco, six out of ten products did not meet FSA health targets, while 'a third of economy range products still fail to meet the targets, despite retailers saying they are giving special attention to these products' (NCC 2008). The inspectors commended Tesco for 'some prominent and eye-catching promotions in fruit and vegetable sections but these messages are overwhelmed by promotions for fatty, sugary and salty products throughout the store' (ibid.).

There is evidence for increased consumption of supermarket products purchased in promotions (Ailawadi and Neslin 1998 and Chandon and Wansink 2002, both cited in Hawkes 2008: 279). Some 42 per cent of grocery products were sold on promotion in the year to June 2011, an all-time high (*Marketing Magazine* 14/09/11b). One marketer described the strategy as good for customers: 'The economic conditions are tough, and price promotion is the way customers cope with that' (*Marketing Magazine* 14/09/11b). Kantar Worldpanel data showed that 'Saturated fat is the most promoted nutrient: 40 per cent of saturates in the shopping basket are bought on promotion' (Kantar 2011).

Promotions for fatty/sugary foods increased at Tesco from 26 per cent in 2006 to 56 per cent of total promotions in 2008; at Morrisons the figures went from 39 per cent to 63 per cent. Morrisons' three economy range versions of a standard product had higher salt content than the standard one (NCC 2008). Sustain's Children's Food Campaign report in 2012 found that Asda, Morrisons and Iceland were the 'worst offenders' in displaying unhealthy snacks at tills, but all supermarkets were criticised on this point, as were non-food retailers now displaying snack foods at tills (Sustain 2012). The increasing appearance of snack foods, large displays of chocolate and drinks machines in UK newsagent/bookshop and discount general store chains was notable by 2012.

This is one example of Mikkelson's and Winson's ideas regarding the expanding foodscape, but also, more broadly, Habermas's description of how lifeworlds are colonised. One goes into this kind of shop for a newspaper or a greeting card or a book, but is then faced with the visual cues of food product displays. Additionally customers can be asked by staff if any of the food items displayed are desired; these techniques reflect commercial 'nudging' (discussed in Chapter 1).

At higher status supermarkets, consumers are thought to be more health aware, and inclined to purchase more costly, high quality foods. Yet a survey of 526 pie, mash and gravy processed foods by CASH, sampled from supermarkets, chain restaurants, cafes and takeaways showed that two Waitrose steak pies had the highest amount of salt per serving among supermarket pies. At 1g of salt per 100g, both were three times that found in an Asda chicken pie (CASH 2011a; and the Waitrose portions were almost twice as large). But supermarket pies were lower in salt than their restaurant counterparts – the highest salt content was a chicken pie with chips and gravy from JD Wetherspoon, with 7.5g of salt (ibid.).

By 2008, Waitrose had doubled its promotions of fatty/sugary foods since 2006 and lowered its fruit and vegetables promotions from 26 per cent to 13 per cent of all promotions (NCC 2008). Marks & Spencer pizza and sausages had not met FSA criteria for salt content, though healthier options did; labelling was inconsistent and M&S had almost doubled its promotions of fatty/sugary foods in the previous two years. It also continued to offer fatty/sugary snacks at child height at checkouts. But M&S did have the highest proportion of promotions of fruit and vegetables, at 25 per cent of the total (NCC 2008).

In a *Marketing Magazine* article about Marks & Spencer, one source said the company was

> shifting away from its premium positioning, particularly where its foods are concerned … when 'Your M&S' was launched, the food ads were all about the premium and quality, but now they seem much more populist in their approach … Perhaps 'Only at M&S' [a recent campaign] and its renewed focus on premium will bring some of that quality feel back to the food offer. (*Marketing Magazine* 17/11/10)

M&S has also announced a refit of its stores according to local demographics and preferences, based on insights from focus groups and online purchases, and a demographic analysis (*Marketing Magazine* 08/06/11b). M&S's marketing director, commenting on the value of segmenting, said, 'Segmenting based on [people's] lives, attitudes and actions at least gives a credible way to maximise relevancy of the message' (Sharp cited in *Marketing Magazine* 23/03/11). Meanwhile, some less upmarket retailers have also embraced segmentation (ibid.). Morrisons is assessed by an anonymous marketing director as 'a little downmarket'; as it considers stocking clothing merchandise, it is urged 'not to try to push too far upmarket' (*Marketing Magazine* 16/02/11).

Marketers are essentially observing here that grocery stores are themselves 'classed'; nor is this a recent phenomenon. The grocery company advertised in the Figure 8.3 describes itself as 'high class'. The image is a reminder that the association between class, status and food retail operations is not new. The woman pictured and the house and neighbourhood she occupies represent the desired (prosperous) clientele.

What is different today is that high status grocery stores such as Waitrose or Marks & Spencer do not describe themselves in the language of class; it is instead implied. Marketers comment more directly on the matter: Waitrose has 'an upmarket image and attracts middle-class customers' with

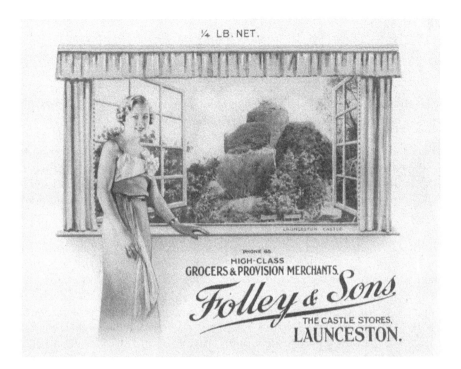

Figure 8.3 The women pictured and the house and neighbourhood she occupies represent the desired (prosperous) clientele © Wellcome Images.

good design, high standards of customer service and 'intelligent signage' (*Marketing Magazine* 29/06/11).

The class boundaries still observed regarding grocery stores by consumers themselves were revealed in an exchange of comments by *Guardian* readers, following a letter by one reader asking if others had tried discount food chains and asking for recommendations (*Guardian* 02/07/11).

In response, one reader listed various products which were acceptable to her at Lidl, but added, 'in spite of discovering the joy of Lidl, I still usually shop at Waitrose'. Another advised: 'what we now tend to do is buy our staples at Aldi and "treats" like quality breads, cheeses and wines from a so-called higher-end supermarket'. Another shopped regularly at Lidl: 'it is noticeable in the last two years or so that there are more middle-class shoppers. Suddenly, it has become acceptable to shop at Lidl'. A reader who had 'tentatively entered a Lidl store about five years ago' concurred. Class barriers as signified by vehicle status were observed by a subsequent respondent to the letter: 'I knew my local Lidl had definitely arrived when after shopping there for about a year, I noticed all the BMWs, Mercedes and Porsche cars that were starting to fill up the car park' (*Guardian* 24/06/11).

The debate continued, with one reader approving of Lidl but drawing the line at Asda:

> Lidl opened in quite a posh road and met with strong opposition from local residents ... [Admittedly] the layout's weird, e.g. there were crates of ring binder folders and plug extensions plonked amongst the fruit and veg. But ... the snobbery surrounding these kinds of places isn't justified. I'd go to Lidl before Asda. (*Guardian* 24/06/11)

This and other comments showed that it was important for the participants in this discussion to shop in a place in which their sense of their own social status does not clash too strongly with the social status of the store itself.

Challenging the association and image of working class people and poor quality foods, a group of organic companies placed an advertisement in a grocery store magazine (*Real Food*, Spring 2011, back cover). The man is shown at work as a painter and decorator; he acknowledges that he might not look like the sort of person who eats organic food, but that it is important to him and his wife to buy it, even if they have to pay a little more for it, for the good of their children. The image and message of the advertisement is aimed at people not normally associated with eating organic food. It also reflects the notion that in order to get people to change their eating/shopping patterns to adopt new foods, they need to see other people like them doing so, even if only in advertisements.

One geodemographic profile for a low income group describes them shopping mainly at Asda, Somerfield or Co-op. This reflects the usually unspoken classing of supermarkets and their shoppers; certainly the middle class *Guardian*-reading, Waitrose-accustomed shopper in the excerpt above felt that Asda and its shoppers were of a different (lower) social dimension.

Supermarket advertisements naturally do not discuss their social or class differences in such terms, but shoppers know which stores they feel most comfortable in. As the shoppers' comments above indicate, it is not just a matter of choosing the store which supplies the foods suitable for us; it is also important that other people like us will be there – people of a similar social status, who dress and behave more or less as we do. Some middle class people are prepared to endure discount store environments for certain items at lower prices, but only up to a point. In the *Guardian* example, foods recommended for purchase at discount stores are those which are purchased more frequently by higher status groups, such as fruit, vegetables, olive oil and smoked salmon; readers are advised to shun the discounters' meat for both quality and animal welfare reasons.

But overall, a switch from Waitrose to Lidl is made more reassuring by the observation that other people like themselves have also made this switch. The habitus has been expanded to take on unfamiliar, slightly uncomfortable surroundings, but the lifeworld is not disrupted – the foods purchased are not of a different order or quality, they are merely presented in more basic surroundings and at lower prices. But a healthy and varied diet is still being consumed by such consumers. Their purchases did not vary widely even when they crossed a class divide to shop at a discount store; healthy foods can be purchased there, too, and they could return to higher status retailers when delicate matters such as meat quality were at stake. While higher status people may make some purchases at lower status supermarkets, they are unlikely to switch to what they would consider a lower status diet, with inferior foods which people like them simply would not eat.

Yet a commitment to healthy eating is not always demonstrated by this group. Some consumers who might prefer organic chicken will not usually find organic meats in ready meals, which they nevertheless buy. As one food industry analyst noted, 'Consumers want healthy but buy convenience' (Fuller 2005, citing industry newsletter). Another comments on consumer interest in healthy eating: 'upscale and sophisticated buyers prefer fresh vegetables', for example, but where fast food is concerned, they may 'say one thing and do another' (Michman and Mazze 1998: 34). These authors identify 'a small health-conscious segment' but 'the overriding majority of consumers indulge themselves' (ibid.: 184). Similarly, in food industry tasting panels, participants might say they avoid fat, but in blind tastings, they tend to prefer foods with a higher fat content (Kessler 2009: 101). In a marketing survey, only 20 per cent of those buying pizza look for low calorie options and fewer still check fat content, yet 43 per cent said they would buy a pizza with a wholegrain crust and 39 per cent would like lower salt content (*Marketing Magazine* 14/09/11c). There seems to be interest in healthier options, but there is an apparent contradiction between an articulated preference for such foods which purchasing behaviour does not always bear out.

Advising readers on food and drink innovations, a Business Insights report (2011) describes what motivates affluent consumers: health concerns, convenience and indulgence. A market research firm spots the inconsistency: 'the desire for health and indulgence represents a trend clash ... consumers looking to satisfy seemingly contradictory desires represent an important market opening' (Datamonitor cited in Kessler 2009: 130). They may be describing the significant proportion of people of higher social status who are obese or overweight.

In any case, food retailers know their customers well through purchasing data. Loyalty cards have 'vastly increased the capability of supermarket operators to target promotions more closely at consumers' (Euromonitor 2004e cited in Hawkes 2008: 679): each supermarket transaction can be analysed 'to determine which products are likely to attract their attention, which promotions could find appeal, and then the consumer receives promotional information particularly targeted at him/herself or their family' (Euromonitor 2004e cited in Hawkes 2008: 679).

In UK supermarkets, such sales promotions may increase sales by 200–300 per cent (Cooper 2003 and Competition Commission 2000, both cited in Hawkes 2008: 679). This may be one way in which supermarkets are contributing to weight gain – promotions aim to increase consumption, so with this technique supermarkets 'counter the health promotion message to eat in moderation' (Hawkes 2008: 684).

With a team of researchers, Winson quantified the dietary quality of the foodscape, measuring the amount of shelf space in Canadian grocery store chains stocked with what he terms 'pseudo foods' – products high in sugar and fat but low in nutrients (Winson 2004). Results ranged between 26 per cent and 37 per cent of total shelf space stocking edible products; 70 per cent of shelf space was occupied by 'pseudo foods' in convenience stores, which are more commonly found in poorer neighbourhoods (ibid.: 306–7).

The UK foodscape is one in which petrol stations, book/stationery shops, public transport networks from large city centre stations to commuter station platforms, universities, fitness/leisure centres, offices and even hospitals – and routes to and from these spaces – are sites of an ever increasing array of snack foods. This is a further illustration of the visual cues provided by such installations, and in unlikely places (see Figures 8.4, 8.5, 8.6, 8.7 and 8.8).

Habermas's notion of the lifeworld being colonised is evidenced by this phenomenon, as with the snack displays which appeared in previously non-food shops and spaces. People's instinctive reaction to visual cues, as marketers themselves described in the commercial version of 'nudging' in Chapter 1, can be tapped into to expand food merchandising opportunities, increasing sales and consumption of snack/convenience foods.

Apart from simply placing products before consumers wherever possible, there are marketing techniques to address consumer 'extremeness aversion' (tendency to avoid large or small sizes and consequent increase in mid-range sizes/volumes) and 'bundling', which offers processed foods in combination with each other (i.e. meal deals, which also increase consumption) (Sharpe *et al.* 2008: 420).

In addressing problematic societal eating patterns, less attention has been focused on structural factors such as an omnipresent, targeted foodscape than on individual behaviours, as even marketing academics have observed (Hoek and Gendall 2006: 415). Indeed, marketers themselves are conducting a robust debate on marketing ethics, which is discussed below.

The ethics of marketing: a debate among marketers

> Marketers are now more overtly conscious of the need to create meaning and identity, or literally to colonize the lifeworld. (Habermas 1970 cited in Goss 1995: 160)

The industry literature on food science discussed in Chapter 6 revealed concerns regarding the health consequences of a diet overly reliant on

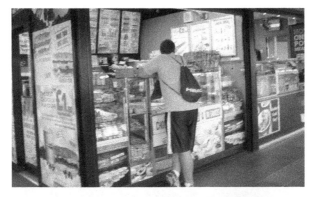

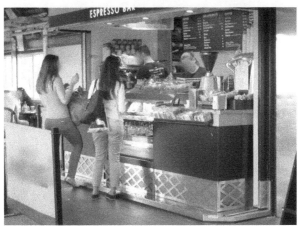

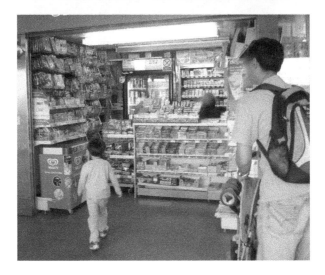

Figures 8.4, 8.5 and 8.6 The increasing supply of fast food for commuters. These hutch-style fast food/snack installations arrived in a UK city centre train station in 2013 in a previously empty corridor used by passengers changing trains. Photographs by Melanie Jervis.

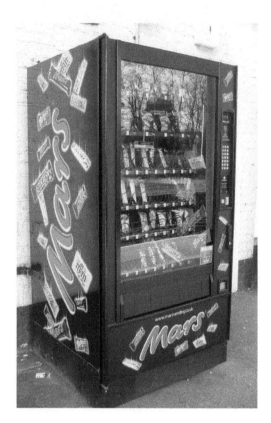

Figure 8.7 Vending machine in a UK suburban commuter station. This machine, new in 2013, is on a train platform. Photograph by Melanie Jervis.

processed foods. Food product development literature emphasised the importance of tracking consumer ideas of healthy eating with a range of products – some of which, like energy drinks, are not necessarily healthy. Both these issues raise questions about the influence of the food industry on dietary health. Given the conclusions made by psychologists and economists, now accepted by government, via 'nudge' theory, that some behaviours, including eating, are automatic, and by epidemiologists and sociologists that there is a link between poor diet, social class and poor health, there are ethical questions to be addressed about the nature of the food supply, strategies used to target-market it, and the language sometimes misleadingly used to describe it.

Even by the 1920s, some of the 'dangers' of consumerism had begun to be voiced in moral terms (Egan 2008: 6). This debate continues today among marketers (Mick 2007; Hackley 2001; Skalen *et al.* 2008), with marketing ethics discussed regularly in the *Journal of Business Ethics*.

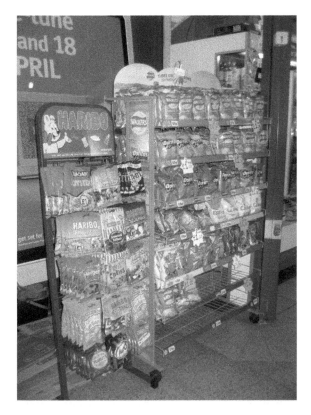

Figure 8.8 Snack food displays in a UK suburban commuter station. The candy and crisps racks are downstairs in the same station as the image in Figure 8.7, having arrived in recent years in a previously empty space. Photograph by Melanie Jervis.

Some marketing educators acknowledge the pitfalls of marketing, warning students that

> society becomes concerned about marketers' activities when those activities have questionable or negative consequences. For example, in recent times, well publicised incidents of unethical behaviour by marketers and others have perturbed and even angered consumers. (Dibb and Simkin 2009: 83)

Fuller's food industry text repeatedly acknowledges the ethical issues surrounding market research and marketing:

> Retailers can wield considerable power by … manipulating, or being a major influence through selling techniques, on what customers

can/will purchase. Can this power of the retailer be abused or will it be abused? Some consumer groups believe both questions can be answered, 'Yes'. (Fuller 2001: 261)

There is a consistent strand of marketing research and marketing industry comment on the ethics of marketing. Simon Houpt, the author of *Buyology: Truth and Lies About What We Buy* (2009) and *Brandwashed: Tricks Companies Use to Manipulate Our Minds and Persuade Us to Buy* (2011) is a marketer who reveals what he believes are unethical marketing ploys to consumers, in the hope that his revelations will pressure companies to change (Houpt 2011). In Chapter 7, there was evidence of ethical concerns among marketers over internet surveillance for marketing purposes. One marketer described 'stalketing, the creepy and tactless use of retargeting and other data techniques', though this critique is also made as a warning of a consumer backlash – so it is a commercially self-defeating practice, apart from an ethically dubious one (*Marketing Magazine* 07/12/11). Another commentator describes the 'self-serving norms, nod-and-a-wink deceits and illusions that conspire to put [the product's] own interests ahead of those of paying customers. These are usually so accepted and universal that even consumers can fail to notice them; but you [i.e. marketers] must' (*Marketing Magazine* 27/10/10). One example is when 'supermarkets put the milk and eggs at the back of the store, to force customers to walk past tempting goodies and encourage them to buy things they never came in for' (ibid.).

A subsequent marketing commentary pointed to studies showing that lower status people are more likely to 'overconsume' and become obese; people consume more when they purchase larger pack sizes though they may not be conscious of this (*Marketing Magazine* 02/05/12b). Therefore 'marketers have a moral incentive to reduce pack size'. There may also be a commercial advantage here: US researchers showed that 'even people with perceived low status opt for smaller sizes when primed to believe that this is the choice influential people would make' (ibid.). Conceivably, then, supersizing could be portrayed as unappealingly lower status and in health terms, constitute a marketing achievement (ibid.). This example reflects concepts of social class, status comparisons, marketing strategies and nutritional intake.

Ethical issues surrounding unhealthy snack and fast foods are addressed by marketers in a special issue of the *Journal of Public Policy and Marketing* examining food marketing in a public policy context. The editor notes that 'much of the existing empirical research in this area has focused on advertising, with little attention given to questions regarding food composition and availability' (Moore 2007: 3).

Activities described under the rubric of corporate social responsibility (CSR) are one effort to address criticisms of food industry ethics. Alongside efforts to convince us to consume more food products and to make it easy to do so by blanket siting of foods, from snacks to meals, some food companies have also adopted a pro-exercise discourse. These strategies arguably fall under the marketing rubric, bolstering 'brand value', reinforcing healthy eating/personal responsibility discourse in a very general way, shifting responsibility for health and bodyweight outcomes onto individuals and their food choices, and diverting attention from the industry's own role in influencing food consumption patterns (Herrick 2009: 57). For Sklair and Miller (2010: 492), 'CSR ... prioritizes private profits, market share, stock market valuation and regulatory capture'. CSR strategies may also compete with public health promotion efforts; if they promote food industry products with dubious health claims, this can undermine 'the legitimacy and authority of public health' (Herrick 2009: 54–5, 60). This recalls Fairclough's warning of 'the colonisation of institutions in the public domain by types of discourse which emanate from the private domain' (Fairclough 2010: 135), in an echo of Habermas. The larger problem is that quite apart from healthy food promotion, 'commercial interests dominate food messaging space', drowning out healthy eating messages, which are funded to a lesser degree than commercial food marketing (Lang 2009: 327).

Marketing to children

> All consumers base their interpretation on what is familiar, on knowledge already stored in memory. (Dibb and Simkin 2009: 118)

> Like it or not, children are susceptible to marketing. (*Marketing Magazine* 24/08/11b)

In a 2011 leaflet publicising a conference on marketing to children, organisers described the importance of understanding children's behaviour and communicating with them via social media in order to market products successfully to them, while abiding by regulatory guidelines (*Marketing Magazine* 22/06/11). To succeed in this growing market, marketers must appeal to child audiences, but they also need to engage with parents, since they are the ones who do the purchasing; and parents should be consulted on how they want brands to communicate with their children (ibid.).

The leaflet also spoke of ethical campaigns in marketing to children (ibid.). In fact there is a growing critique among commercial marketers of some of the strategies and activities employed to appeal to children, and concern regarding the quality of some food products developed for children.

An editorial in *Marketing Magazine* comments that, 'for the increasingly regulated UK market, it is no longer enough simply to reduce the level of fat, salt and sugar in their products ... for the likes of, say, PepsiCo, a more radical response is required' (23/02/11c). A separate article cites the example of Innocent Kids Smoothies, which have increased sales by 30 per cent;

but 'there's a way to go before NPD [New Product Development] of healthy kids' products is considered the norm. The number of fruit and vegetables products launched in the past year? One' (*Marketing Magazine* 23/02/11b). The top brand in the Kids Brand Index for 2011 is Walkers Crisps (*Marketing Magazine* 24/08/11b).[3]

There was also criticism of Coke, which had concluded that 'mothers do not consider its products when planning family meals' and so developed a campaign with the slogan 'Meals taste better with Coca-Cola' (*Marketing Magazine* 11/05/11). One marketer wrote in to query the ethics of this approach: 'there are just too many things wrong to list out about targeting mothers [with Coke] when planning family meals ... offsetting against social responsibility campaigns just doesn't make it taste any better' (*Marketing Magazine* 18/05/11b).

The focus on regulating TV advertising to children has obscured the rise of other marketing techniques for children such as food website 'advergames', in which brand messages are embedded. The British Heart Foundation's Food4Thought 'Lardbar' campaign produced a series of mock advergame designs on their website alerting parents to the way some of these are put together, engaging children's attention in an entertaining way while marketing products to them (BHF 2014).

Given that 90 per cent of the foods promoted on these websites were assessed in a study as unhealthy because of high levels of fat, sugar and or salt, and that children were encouraged to email their friends about the brand-promoting game, the authors of the study concluded that some protections should be considered (Moore and Rideout 2007). Along these lines, in 2011 Consumers International launched a toolkit for governments and consumer/health interest groups wishing to monitor the marketing of unhealthy foods to children, with the aim of supplying a database of evidence to be used in developing policies to tackle such activities (CI 2011). It was developed for both developed and developing countries in response to a World Health Organisation call to member states to 'reduce the impact of marketing of foods high in saturated fats, trans-fatty acids, free sugars or salt to children' (CI 2011: 6).

Marketing fast foods to parents in deprived communities and ethnicities can be a pathway to childhood obesity; there is evidence that it influences their food preferences (Grier *et al.* 2007: 223). They cite nutritional research showing that parents who ate fruit and vegetables also fed them to their children (Nicklas *et al.* 2001 cited in Grier *et al.* 2007: 223). The same pattern occurs if parents eat large quantities of fast food. Both may constitute lifelong dietary patterns:

> Parents' brand preferences create comfort in children and set the stage for compliance with their children's request for a brand (McNeal 1999). The formation of children's attitudes and beliefs about fast food in the context of family life may imbue the attitudes and beliefs with

sustaining characteristics over time (Moore, Wilkie, and Lutz 2002). Accordingly, the fast-food industry focuses on children because childhood memories of fast-food products may translate into adult visits. (McNeal 1999, Schlosser 2001, cited in Grier *et al.* 2007: 224)

This recalls the theories of Marx and Bourdieu in terms of family food provision, but also the conclusions of food industry scientists regarding the powerful, lifelong role of early years food consumption.

Fast food marketing aims not simply to sell more fast food, but also tries to shape perceptions so that eating fast food is normalised among target consumers:

> fast-food marketers aim for their activities to create positive attitudes and to influence social norms such that they increase the consumption of their products ... Fast-food marketing contributes to consumers' beliefs through the persuasiveness with which strategies communicate specific benefits and reinforce existing behavioral patterns ... more positive fast-food attitudes and the degree to which parents perceive fast-food consumption as socially normative are associated with children's greater fast-food consumption. (Grier *et al.* 2007: 224)

So even if marketing does not *create* an interest in fast food, these authors are concerned that it can *reproduce* it (ibid.: 230). Thus consumption of a given food or meal becomes embedded in a target consumer's way of life and dietary routines – and those of their children.

This process requires repetition. An article about marketing food to children emphasises the importance of repeating exposures and behaviours: 'it can take between 8–13 positive exposures for kids to be strongly familiar with a food or beverage' (Urbick 2009: 257). This could be conceived in terms of the habitus – that is how long it takes for the habitus to be expanded to assimilate a new product and for it to be considered a normal dietary practice. Once this familiarity has been achieved, food companies can build on it by modifying products: this technique 'seems to be highly successful in developing new food trends with kids' (ibid.). Furthermore, marketing should target boys separately from girls: 'when you must target both, always skew the positioning to boys. Girls are more accepting of "boy" products, yet boys are more likely to reject something that is "too girly"' (ibid.: 258). An example of this same strategy in adulthood was the overt (but ironic) marketing of a chocolate bar brand to men, with the intention (and achievement) of increasing sales among both men and women (Chapter 7).

The advertising of food products for children has been limited by regulation in recent years. An Ofcom ban on television advertising of HFSS foods to children under 16 came into effect in 2008. The text of the ruling refers to the psychological content of advertising and engages with ethical matters, describing the need 'to reduce children's emotional engagement with HFSS advertisements, and reduce the risk that children and parents may misinterpret product claims, and to reduce the potential for pester power' (Ofcom 2007: 3). As a consequence, 'manufacturers have boosted their marketing presence across other media, such as outdoor and online' (*Marketing Magazine* 19/10/11). A subsequent study, not suggesting any influence from the food industry but exploring food cues presented to children, has also observed a high degree of consumption of unhealthy (unbranded) foods portrayed in children's television in both Ireland and the UK, reflecting a similar pattern previously observed in the US (Scully *et al.* 2014).

While 305 dairy, confectionery and ready meal products for children were introduced in 2008 in the UK, there were just 220 in 2010, a fall of 32 per cent, raising concerns among marketers about the potential for UK regulation to block innovative products (*Marketing Magazine* 23/02/11b). However, some brands are still increasing sales by introducing adaptations of existing products such as individualised serving sizes or film character licensing (ibid.). Kellogg's was unable to promote Coco Pops to children, so introduced Coco Pops Choc'n'Roll, with reduced quantities of sugar, salt and saturated fat (ibid.). It also developed Krave, a chocolate cereal (*Marketing Magazine* 19/10/11) aimed at young adults who had eaten chocolate cereals as children but who do not want to eat cereals aimed at older age groups (*Marketing Magazine* 'Revolution' supplement 09/10b) and to whom advertising is not restricted. Alongside TV ads for the product, an accompanying Facebook campaign invited consumers to bid for various prizes (ibid.). This campaign was later criticised by the British Heart Foundation (2014) in a report which critiqued internet marketing of such products to children in general.

When the children's drink Fruit Shoot was battling an unhealthy image, its producer, Britvic Soft Drinks, developed a website offering interactive games for children, aimed at developing skills, and a link to a parents' website (*Marketing Magazine* 08/06/11c). A back-up TV ad also directed children to the site. Sales increased.

Marketing analysis of the power of advertising: academic and applied approaches

Marketing Magazine (15/06/11b) is clear about the value of advertising: 'The direct link between advertising and sales is proven, not least courtesy of the IPA's[4] databank case study service.' Marketing academics challenge the argument that advertising does not affect 'primary' demand for food products, and that there is, therefore, no need for further regulation (Hoek and Gendall 2006: 409–10). They cite a systematic review of research which provides evidence for advertising affecting primary demand; it found 'only weak evidence of brand switching and much stronger evidence of category switching' (Hastings *et al.* 2003 cited in

Hoek and Gendall 2006: 412). One reason for this might be the rise of 'category management' in which products are grouped together according to consumer perceptions (King and Phumpiu 1996 cited in Hawkes 2008: 670). These categories are then managed to '"maximize the effectiveness of the demand creation process" through optimum product variety, new product introductions, product promotions and efficient assortment' (Bhulai 2007 cited in Hawkes 2008: 670).

It is also argued that, given the acceptance of advertising's influence on smoking rates, which justified its banning, removing advertising for fatty/sugary foods would have a similar effect (Hoek and Gendall 2006: 413). Consumption of such foods is normalised for target consumers by the reinforcement of advertising (ibid.). Marketing strategies include bundling, in which food products are grouped together in 'meal deals'.

'Up-sizing' also presents consumers with the notion of quantity and good value, normalising the consumption of HFSS foods. A sandwich, a soft drink, often in large sizes, and a packet of crisps are now widely available as a normal lunch combination. One crisps brand succeeded in their campaign to increase the crisp/sandwich combination by encouraging stores to place displays of crisp packets alongside sandwich displays (*Marketing Magazine* 08/06/11e).

Given the resources and insights that go into targeting relevant consumer segments, it is unsurprising that 'food advertising reflects, and may reinforce, socio-economic and gender variations in food choice and adiposity' (Adams and White 2009: 1), or that more is spent advertising highly processed, packaged, sweet, high fat food products than on other foods (Winson 2004: 301).

Ehrenberg's 'weak' theory of advertising (1974, cited in Hoek and Gendall 2006) viewed it as a form of 'operant conditioning' rather than a 'persuasive force' capable of prompting new consumer behaviours. Advertising thus merely 'maintains' behaviour, according to Ehrenberg. But this does not mean it is irrelevant for health: 'by supporting the continuation of unhealthy behaviour patterns, advertising reduces the likelihood that individuals will either recognise the behaviours as unhealthy or seek to change these' (Hoek and Gendall 2006: 414). This is because advertising normalises the eating of whatever food is being presented. It is portrayed being eaten by people the target audience feel comfortable emulating; people like themselves. This effect is intensified by increasingly personalised advertising online.

And there may be a flaw in Ehrenberg's argument: trials of a new product are often proposed by food companies, which may bring about the kind of category switching earlier described by Hastings *et al.* (2003, cited in Hoek and Gendall 2006). Other strategies such as discounts and loyalty programmes then foster increased consumption (Hoek and Gendall 2006: 414).

Given the capacity of marketing and advertising to alter norms regarding food consumption, Grier *et al.* note attempts by social marketing to bring these norms back to a more critical attitude towards fast food (Grier *et al.* 2007: 230). Thus one social marketer writes that

> the marketing of fast food ... can and should be reined in. And this means much more than curtailing advertising. The entire marketing effort has to be scrutinised: product design, distribution, pricing strategies and packaging – as well as communications – have to be put under the public health microscope. (Hastings 2006: 5)

Another (commercial) marketer, commenting on obesity, concludes that 'marketing plays a key role in moulding the future shape of people and the health service alike', and suggests that unhealthy brands should subsidise healthy foods (*Marketing Magazine* 07/09/11).

Public health campaigns themselves have not been successful in altering eating behaviour at a population level; commercial marketing and the omnipresent retailing of palatable foods may be powerful and dominant enough simply to overwhelm health promotion efforts (Grier *et al.* 2007: 232). This further undermines arguments that advertising does not cause people to change their behaviour (Hoek and Gendall 2006: 415). But it also raises questions about why the food industry supports healthy eating and exercise campaigns; if advertising doesn't work, why bother (ibid.)? Perhaps it bolsters the industry's efforts at managing its image; promoting physical fitness is uncontroversial, and where obesity is concerned, it helpfully (for the industry) shifts the focus onto exercise and individual initiative.

There is a key distinction here: consumer marketing is aimed at needs as experienced by *consumers* (whether conscious or latent, but detected through market research), whereas social marketing takes aim at health needs as identified by *experts* (Donovan and Henly 2003 cited in French *et al.* 2010: 100). This may be why one approach works, while the other is less effective. Social marketing might only work among those who have already identified a need to change their eating habits or begin exercising. Meanwhile, obesity is a 'normal response to an abnormal environment' in which palatable food is omnipresent (Eggers and Swinburn 1997 cited in Hoek and Gendall 2006: 416). The conclusion of these marketing academics is that changes to the food environment via regulation and public policy, altering food manufacturing, must 'logically precede' health promotion campaigns (Hoek and Gendall 2006: 417, 420).

Moore concludes that 'Marketing's role as both a contributor to the problem and a force in its alleviation is complex, and many significant questions are yet to be addressed' (Moore 2007: 4). A stronger challenge comes from Mick (2007), who argues that it is time to 'elevate the focus and scope of marketing to a higher ground for which the public, marketing professionals, and marketing students are yearning' (Mick 2007: 289). Like Hackley, he takes aim at the ambiguous language of marketing (ibid.: 290).

Terms like 'value meals', for example, may divert attention from poor quality nutrition in some such products.

Mick interprets an American Marketing Association definition of marketing which speaks of the need to manage relationships with consumers as manipulative and controlling; these are sometimes criticisms of marketing and the association's ethical code (Mick 2007: 290). Where it does encourage members to market 'for a better world', this is only in the context of non-profit organisations (ibid.). Well-being, he argues, should motivate all marketers in all organisations, including profit-making businesses (ibid.: 291). He hopes that corporate social responsibility activities will be sincere, yet even 'among the most ardent defenders of market capitalism, the new commitment to corporate social responsibility has been called "harmful" and a "sham"' (*Economist* 2001 cited in Mick 2007: 291). He recommends an ethical 'macromarketing' perspective, in which the long-term effects of marketing are routinely considered (ibid.).

Conclusion

This chapter has revealed evidence for class-based food consumption and illustrated some of the contradictions of marketing highlighted in an ethical debate among marketing academics and practitioners. Together with the preceding two chapters, it aimed to substantiate the earlier theoretical, exploratory context-setting work of the book.

To summarise the narrative of the argument thus far: the introductory chapter outlined the dominant power of healthy eating/personal responsibility discourse driving both public understanding and public policy, and highlighted its weakness in addressing problematic consumption–health trends. The second chapter established the analytical framework, identifying discourse as an object of analysis, and outlining the guidance provided by critical realism and critical discourse analysis in tracing mechanisms which are often unobservable (or at least unobserved) in the formation of diets and their health consequences.

The third and fourth chapters challenged a powerful yet misleading healthy eating discourse via an exploration of social theories, analysing the role of social class in consumption for which marketing literature later provided much evidence. In providing a social context for behaviour – and behavioural economics – and explaining how communication about public issues can mask deeper truths, these theories illustrated how the activities of the food industry could play a major role in shaping our class-differentiated diet, and the health that flows from it, even if we are not normally aware of this. The very notion of reflexivity, a cornerstone of sociology in recent decades, was called into question.

Chapter 5 discussed epidemiological and other evidence for the link between food consumption, health, class and political and market ideologies. Chapter 6 revealed how the food industry interacts with consumer interest in health and the emerging health concerns of food scientists regarding the consumption of industrialised food, particularly among lower status groups, who consume more of it. It also traced the origins of this phenomenon in the changing nature of the food supply, relating agricultural developments to food product changes, food marketing techniques, changing dietary patterns, and public health. Chapter 7 investigated the growing technological power and psychological insights of market research in tracking and ranking populations, learning where and how we live, how we move about our cities and towns and what we eat, alongside a theoretical critique of marketing by academic marketers.

This chapter revealed marketing's 'proxies' for the language of class and linked these proxies to the quality of food and even the supermarket experience for shoppers and how this interacts with their ideas of their own social rank. The ranking of consumers, products and food retail outlets is an essential part of positioning products successfully in the marketplace.

But what is important in public policy and population terms is the effect of diet on health. This book has discussed the strong links between poor diet and poor health and has traced growing bodyweights alongside an omnipresent supply and normalised consumption of snack and convenience foods. The earlier epidemiological evidence for social class as a factor in diet quality and health was reflected in this chapter's discussion of the marketing of foods by consumer segment in stores and outlets that themselves are socially ranked.

Limits to the marketing of HFSS foods to children have been set, but this chapter traced the activities of some companies in seeking to find other ways to sell their products: marketing to parents; developing creative content to engage children online; and targeting slightly older groups of young people with products traditionally aimed at children.

The concluding chapter which follows brings together the insights of the varied perspectives and disciplines explored throughout this research regarding the problems of food consumption and diet-related ill health in order to distil the lessons of this investigation and suggest how it might be carried forward.

Notes

1 In 2014 Britain's traditional food retailers are being seriously challenged by discount food stores such as Lidl and Aldi. Tesco's profits have been falling for three years and Sainsbury is working with the Danish discount retailer Netto. Lidl has just announced a major UK expansion (*Guardian* 28/06/14a, 28/06/14b). See below in this chapter, 'Food quality and the classing of supermarkets – and shoppers', for a further discussion of social class and grocery retailers.

2 There had been a previous report and a subsequent one in 2008. The NCC merged with other organisations to become Consumer Focus in 2007 and after 2008 the

reports were not continued. The merger had resulted in food being dropped as a policy focus because food policy was thought to be sufficiently studied by other organisations and the new Consumer Focus needed a smaller list of priorities. This was a missed opportunity to continue the work and achievements of the NCC investigations. Consumer Focus later became renamed Consumer Futures and was closed in April 2014. Its functions were transferred to Citizens Advice (Consumer Futures 2014).

3 With parental approval, 4,000 children were interviewed online, ranking 166 household brands: 'Children enjoy participating in surveys online, they spend a great deal of time online and feel at home in front of a PC' (*Marketing Magazine* 24/08/11b).

4 Institute of Practitioners in Advertising.

9 Conclusion

> Critical sociologists looking at issues of health and healing, locally, regionally and nationally as well as globally, need to 'do it big'.
> (Scambler 2002: 157)

In this book, in order to reveal gaps in the way we as a society understand and address food consumption problems, it was necessary to 'do it big', as Scambler advises. The surface-level explanation of obesity and diet-related illness as resulting from poor dietary choices ignores a complex relational context structuring both the production and consumption of food. The longstanding ineffectiveness of individual choice discourse in explaining consumption trends has been made more obvious by the rise of 'nudge' theory and the acceptance by behavioural economics – and the UK's Coalition government – that some behaviours, at least, are not fully conscious, shaped instead by deep and enduring social and cultural forces. These forces are in turn permeated by food production trends and practices, and are not easily amenable to conscious change.

Uniting theory and practice

The discourse of personal responsibility for diet and health, broadly corresponding to Marx's theorisation of the power of a ruling idea, is pervasive, and on an individual level, commonsensical – this is how it is mobilised in a neoliberal era, as discussed in Chapter 1. The freedom of the market has been coupled with the freedom of consumer choice, and an accompanying responsibility of individuals for their own lifestyles (Harvey 2005: 42), as well as 'bodily practices' and 'self-control' (Guthman 2011: 53). In challenging this individual responsibility discourse, a range of social theories helped to illuminate food consumption patterns in the context of an increasingly industrialised, pervasive and targeted food supply. There were striking continuities between sociological theorisations of choice, social change and the structuring role of class on the one hand, and epidemiology, psychology and marketing understandings of these matters on the other. In the way social class is assessed and described by official national statistics lie the roots of marketing classifications, which were themselves explored in later chapters.

For a time, even sociology was distracted by notions of consumption allowing individuals to construct their identities and free themselves of structured notions of class. Yet Bourdieu and others, including many British sociologists, who have continued to study social and health inequalities, never wavered in their attention to class, seeing within consumption another arena for embedding and enacting class identities and practices. By tracing the persistent role for social class in shaping identities and consumption patterns, and generating habits ('acquired dispositions', as Bourdieu described them), a clear picture emerged of how this process could be manifested in the domain of diet; how these habits could become a matter of routine, and less than fully conscious, as psychology would similarly explore. Marx and Bourdieu both described the role of childhood learning and experience in shaping later life, observations which psychologists, food scientists and food product developers would similarly make regarding diet. Food systems analysts focused on the agricultural dimension of the food chain, the financial interests driving it, and its role in altering the food supply and consumption patterns.

The theoretical analysis in Chapters 3 and 4 laid the groundwork for understanding the emergence of consumerism and marketing, their role in shaping food consumption, and the resulting challenge for governance and democracy itself in balancing the sometimes conflicting needs of commerce and public health. The relationship between social theory and the empirical world is not always clear, but the case of diet presented a unique opportunity to draw some linkages between the two. The objective was always to enhance understanding of the structural influence on human action in this domain, given the limitations to conscious choice observed by social theorists, psychologists and food industry practitioners, and hence the often unobservable impact and experience of being marketed *to*. This theoretical exploration also enabled a move beyond social science's more characteristic focus on food consumption to consider the activities of food *production* and how industry interacts with and reinforces a food-classed society (though Hawkes and others have done groundbreaking work on global food systems and their implications for health). In the context of the food industry's goals and requirements in a neoliberal era, the logic of the industry's approach is unassailable. This highlights the importance of public monitoring of their activities – the way food is produced, sited and marketed – given the centrality of the food supply for human well-being.

Methodologically, the research described in this book aimed to move beyond the traditional qualitative–quantitative binary which characterises social research, though both play a role in this investigation. This study of powerful forces in industry could not rely heavily on personal, qualitative access to the world of food producers and processors, and use of quantitative information had to be limited to studying production, consumption and health outcomes. Instead, researching the role of industry in structuring diet and influencing health required a critical, textual approach, locating industry commentary and challenging discourse which focuses on consumption while diverting attention from food production. It required an investigation of a range of perspectives and disciplines, but it needed to begin with social theory – the story of how different theories and disciplines simultaneously missed and traced what was happening with class and consumption, and the consistent strand of research which focused on structure, the formation of habit and behaviour, and class.

Habermas revealed the disembedding capacity of science, technology and capital to distort discourse and meanings when unattended to by public monitoring and policy. The case in Chapter 6 of the food industry researchers who noted consumer confusion over the health benefits or risks of caffeinated 'sports' drinks, and pointed out the advantage to industry of working *with* that confusion through the careful use of descriptive language, was one example of this.

Habermas's concept of the way in which systems can be manipulated to alter and even distort the experience of our own lifeworlds is resonant here, particularly given a general lack of awareness of these shifts taking place. Indeed, the habitus can remain outwardly unchanged, even as dietary patterns assimilate more processed foods high in fat, salt and sugar, and fewer fresh foods. Several examples of this were highlighted. The useful distinction between Bourdieu's habitus and Habermas's lifeworld shows how a habitus which seems such a powerful influence on human action, emerging from strong social and familial conditioning, can nevertheless permit ultimately dramatic changes in the domain of food consumption. The countervailing power of industry, with its technologies to produce and site new and palatable foods alongside its market research techniques enabling effective targeting of new products, explains the paradox. By understanding consumers' lives – understanding, in essence, their habitus – new products and meal combinations can be portrayed in ways which fit that habitus. The images and language used in designing and marketing such foods, and the palatability which characterises them, explain their overall success. Several industry experts also recommended building on existing products and consumer preferences in introducing modified 'new' products – this is obviously an easier sell than a completely new product. Nevertheless, the normalisation of some products and meal combinations alongside large portion sizes are new in human experience. Marketing insight and ongoing data analysis has managed to access and reveal the human habitus in its varied types, enabling it to be permeated by new practices and products, ultimately altering the character and routines of the habitus dramatically. In this process, the lifeworld of those who assimilate new convenience foods to the virtual exclusion of more nutritious ones, has been colonised and distorted, whether they are aware of it or not.

But at a certain point, should this dietary pattern continue over time, the health lifeworld can overtly disintegrate. In the context of diet-related health, for example, the diagnosis of diabetes or circulatory disease could shatter one's previous idea of health, well-being and diet, and radically alter many of the routines of the lifeworld. By this stage, the healthcare system has entered the lifeworld and neither the patient's social class nor the way his or her diet developed is the focus of either patient or clinician; it is anyway too late for the individual concerned to *avoid* diet-related illness (though diet has a role to play in managing some chronic illness). But epidemiology picks up this thread; Chapter 5 traced the comprehensive analysis of the relationship between diet and health, and between socio-economic status and quality of diet.

In 2012, the UK's King's Fund published a study showing that over time, while higher status people were reducing behaviours considered unhealthy, those of lower status were increasing them (Buck and Frosini 2012; a similar pattern was reflected in a study of US adolescents by Frederick *et al.* 2014). The King's Fund study recommends a holistic, integrated public health approach uniting interventions addressing smoking, excessive alcohol consumption, poor diet and sedentariness, and the targeting of such interventions at those most likely to experience them – people with the least education and the lowest incomes (ibid). But even these valuable insights are unlikely to yield decisive dietary change if the deeply structuring role of the food industry and the nature of the food supply are not taken into account. This book has investigated why food consumption varies by social class in ways which might usefully apply to the recommendations flowing from the King's Fund study.

Food industry activities and health outcomes

The language, style and techniques of food marketing and food product development are key to understanding broad consumption trends and indeed food industry influence on population diet. The discussion of industry texts not normally aired in public health or social science discussions of food consumption aimed to get beyond traditional industry responses to the problems of overconsumption of food and associated health effects – namely, industry's attempt to turn the focus back to individual choice and responsibility for healthy eating and exercise, and the insistence that no food is bad or good.

Yet some industry scientists revealed concerns about the altered nature of processed food as a possible contributor to obesity, and the particular problems associated with extensive consumption of processed foods, especially by people on low incomes. In tracing the habitual nature of such consumption, they laid bare the weakness in the argument that it is diets, not individual foods, which are the problem. The industry itself combines foods into meal deals, consumed daily by some, and has normalised the eating of crisps and fizzy drinks with sandwiches, for example. A regular feature of food marketing is the bundling together of items in promotions, normalising combinations and frequent consumption of palatable but often unhealthy foods and drinks. Some product categories designed for and marketed to lower status social groups feature a preponderance of items which, industry scientists acknowledged, cannot be the basis for good health.

A more plentiful food supply since the 1970s and lower food prices in relation to incomes were probably likely to increase consumption and population bodyweights over time, regardless of the types of foods produced and consumed. But strategic decisions made at every step, beginning with agriculture, subsidy programmes, crop science, and then advances in processing, food product development, siting and marketing, resulted in a food supply which came to emphasise frequent eating of highly processed, ever present snack and convenience foods. As Habermas warned, when the scientific and technical progress that characterises these complementary phases of production takes place 'without being reflected upon ... new technical capacities erupt without preparation into existing forms of life-activity and conduct' (Habermas 1987: 60). The dramatic changes in population bodyweight and metabolic health have, therefore, 'the accidental character of uncomprehended events' (Habermas [1981]1996: 312). Their origin in a changed, unbalanced, omnipresent food supply, and in the tracking, segmenting and targeting of consumers, has been obscured, and a focus on individual behaviour was summoned as the explanation – though the behaviour was a clear response to unprecedented change in the quantity, style and accessibility of the food supply. Meanwhile, the food supply continues to expand into previously non-food spaces. This is still not well understood or tracked, at least by public research, and the consequences are likely to remain uncomprehended, if they are observed at all.

Class and health

Although most of us are now considered overweight in clinical terms, this book traced an evident ranking in the quality of foods designed for different social groups, and a social gradient in diet quality, diet-related illness, and, among women and young people, in bodyweights. Different decisions dating back decades could have produced a global food supply that addressed food security as well as dietary health. But most of the foods which constitute a healthy diet are not those which require a high degree of processing, or the kind of 'value added' which results from product design and marketing expertise. Technology made possible and capital made necessary the engineering of a highly processed, highly palatable diet, and the spreading of this diet among different cultures and countries, while allowing for a higher quality of food for those who could both discern and afford it.

Yet the dramatic public health consequences of these food industry innovations were not anticipated and could not have been desired by any actor in this process. As Johnson's (2010) model of the 'adjacent possible' proposed in Chapter 4 and 6, this is what results when technological developments and cultural change combine to produce initially incremental but ultimately decisive change. Without the consistent, anchoring presence in this process of a disinterested, Habermasian, monitoring, balancing, public health and governance perspective, the combined power of science, technology and capital were able to bring about unexpected change in patterns of food consumption, with some startlingly negative results. For Habermas, good governance would have detected this process, revealed the underlying interests at work, illuminated technological progress with political consciousness, and ensured public awareness, debate and action regarding developments which might threaten the public good. Bourdieu, too, called for the restoration of politics in the context of a depoliticised public realm. Political engagement with public health problems enables them to be addressed; but historically, there has been strong resistance to political engagement in a regulatory context, and this struggle is under way now in food regulation. Links between politicians and industry, the phenomenon of regulatory capture, and the return of many politicians to industry after their political careers, complicates the policymaking process in many different domains.

Marketing: relations with consumers

This book has traced the enormous technological, statistical and financial resources marketers have at their disposal. Marketing firms track and engage with consumers in a variety of ways, observing trends and behaviours, and marketers often speak of co-creating value with consumers. Engaging and interacting with consumers aims to reveal useful data and insights for firms, and strengthens claims for marketing's effectiveness. This helps marketers and the consumer firms they advise to develop and target products and services appropriately. A marketing category termed 'experiential' allows for personal interaction with consumers 'allowing for instant data capture as well as the flexibility to make changes' (*Marketing Magazine* 18/02/09b). Nor is this interaction and engagement with consumers an inherently negative phenomenon; marketing strategies are developed for most product and service categories, many of which are helpful to consumers and add to the public good.

But the central task of this book was to reveal the development of problematic dietary patterns and practices which have been normalised by marketing strategies, while carrying significant risks to population health. Several rigorous academic marketing studies cited in this book challenge food industry claims on this point, and even commercial market research has studied dietary health problems in support of public health.

It is a rare occupational category which defends itself with arguments of its lack of effectiveness, as marketers sometimes do; it is a peculiarly modest, disingenuous and one-sided view of what they do. This underlined the need to analyse how marketers talk *to each other* about what they are doing, in their own literatures; track successful strategies reflected in sales figures, examples of which appeared in Chapters 6–8; examine the financial resources and data mobilised in market research; and trace the normalisation of constant snacking and large portion sizes, the dominant promotions of unhealthy foods, and critiques of these activities by fellow marketers, both in the academy and in the field.

The way forward

The social gradient in dietary quality and associated health problems, the growing acceptance by economists, psychologists, marketers, public policy and the food industry of the unconscious nature of food consumption, and the acknowledgement by industry of the techniques it employs in shaping and growing that consumption, can provide policymakers and public health specialists with a way forward. The more the activities of the food industry and its marketers are analysed in the context of population health, the less effective personal responsibility discourse will be in deflecting attention from the role of the industry in structuring an ever expanding class-differentiated foodscape. The government's policy of requesting voluntary reductions of unhealthy content by the food industry may be a useful approach, alongside industry reformulations of HFSS foods, but these measures need to be seen in the context of a distorted food supply which is continually permeating new areas of public space, both in the physical world and in social media.

This point was assessed in a US context by Moore *et al.* (2009), who found associations between neighbourhood exposure to fast food and poor diet. The study provided evidence which earlier studies had lacked, and the authors noted the importance of defining and measuring neighbourhood food exposure and the quality of diets in nuanced ways. In the UK, the expansion of fast food outlets and the role of vending machines in public transport, non-food shops and fitness centres in fuelling snack food consumption is something which researchers and policymakers should monitor, as the Oldham councillors did when they found too many fried chicken outlets in one deprived neighbourhood (Chapter 8). The NCC inspections of supermarkets described, also in Chapter 8, consistently revealed marketing practices and convenience food formulations which could not support public health goals; the cessation of these inspections, with the discontinuation of the NCC itself, reduces the opportunity to contribute to public awareness and understanding. A new set of regular third-party inspections could redress this loss.

Several other ways forward emerge from this research. The UCL Institute of Health Equity (2012) has been consulting widely on the education of healthcare staff regarding the social determinants of health and health inequalities, as is being piloted in some universities. This would deepen medical understandings of the social experience of illness, and would enable clinicians to help patients to deal with or even avoid some illnesses. A report issued by the institute in 2013 reflects the contributions of a wide range of health and social care professionals and the commitments by 20 professional associations to training staff in the social determinants of health, alleviating inequalities and advocating for change (UCL 2013). Specifically, those training in health and social care work should be taught 'the graded distribution of health outcomes, and how social and economic conditions can help to explain these unequal outcomes' (ibid.: 7). The way in which neighbourhoods are supplied with foods according to social status, industry understandings of the psychology of cueing consumption behaviour, the segmentation and tracking of individuals' consumption, and the promotion of foods and constant snacking via a range of media and platforms are all important elements in the social and economic background to diet-related health – and its unequal outcomes.

The King's Fund study cited previously calls for a segmentation approach to public health interventions so that they reach the poorest and least educated, who are now known to be increasing risk behaviours, even as higher status people decrease them (Buck and Frosini 2012). They also call for special training for NHS staff in guiding behaviour change in this new context. Recent obesity guidelines from NICE echoed this call and noted the particular needs of vulnerable groups (NICE 2014a).

But this heightened awareness of the role of social class in bodyweight and states of diet-related health should be accompanied by an awareness of how people are targeted differently by the food industry and the power of these strategies. If healthcare professionals remain unaware of the permeation of our social life and our public spaces – even our psyches – by the food industry, and along class lines, they will miss a key opportunity for understanding the obstacles to dietary health among their patients. This lacuna could be addressed in clinical curricula, within the context of a critical public health. It seems equally important for students of food marketing, food science and food product development to be trained in critical thinking regarding the social factors, including class, which influence food consumption and health.

Additionally, informing young people in formal education (and perhaps patients with diet-related health problems of all ages) how they are being tracked by market research and targeted by food companies might allow them the capacity to reflect on this dimension of food production and consumption, and their own experience of how they are targeted. Seeing how their dietary lifeworlds have been colonised, as Habermas would describe it, could spur a conscious 'process of unlearning' (Habermas [1981]1996: 331). This recalls Fairclough's exhortation to educate young people in the distorting effects of discourse: 'a critical awareness of language and discursive practices is ... becoming a prerequisite for democratic citizenship, and an urgent priority for language education' (Fairclough 1993: 142). The insistence by Hackley, a marketing academic, that university students studying marketing should be taught critical thinking, not simply the consulting frameworks used in the field is also resonant ('Young people deserve an education. Grown-up marketing executives can look out for themselves' (Hackley 2001: 132)).

A future for academic/market research co-operation?

Burrows and colleagues in various papers cited in this book urged social scientists to try to access industry data to better understand consumption patterns. We have seen the extent and depth of market research resources which bolster industry's understanding of consumer food behaviours. Market research incorporates official statistics and other public data, but much knowledge is derived from commercially sensitive transactional data. A pioneering example of academic–commercial co-operation in data sharing to study salt consumption and health suggests that more might be possible (Ni Mhurchu *et al.* 2011). One area which may be worth exploring is the type and amount of fats consumed by different social groups as recorded by tens of thousands of consumers purchasing food products over time, both in and out of home; data only the market research sector possesses. The academic–commercial sodium study discussed overall consumer purchases of foods containing salt, but did not analyse consumption by different classes of consumers. However, the market research firm involved in the study confirmed that such analysis would be possible (Interview B, 2012). Even without it, the study was able to reveal which product categories contain the most salt and sell the most, and therefore those which could be most usefully reformulated in a public health context (Ni Mhurchu *et al.* 2011). Commercial data is a new area for diet–health research, and it has its limitations; naturally, specific brands cannot be revealed, nor can grocery store identities or data. The academic researchers in the sodium study stressed that commercial data may be a useful supplement to, but not a replacement for, public nutrition datasets.

Summing up

> ... the task is to deepen collective understandings ... (Harvey 2005: 198)

This book has revealed several areas for further research and future policy development. In food science, the structures and constituents of processed foods can be studied and altered to lessen the damage to public health, as food industry scientists are urging. In local areas, licensing of fast food businesses and snack installations can be more closely monitored and restricted in the interests of public health. In schools and universities, young people can learn about nutrition and develop an awareness of how they are targeted as consumers. In medical and other healthcare training institutions, healthcare professionals can be taught to think critically about the role of the food industry in structuring the problematic diets of prospective patients, and the social class, body-weight and health effects of food targeting and siting. Health and social researchers can ensure that the activities of the food industry are central to diet and health research.

But will this address the deep inequities in food consumption in the UK? The limitations of personal resources and capabilities, combined with the power of habitus, studied and catered to by an alert food industry in its many manifestations, cannot easily be tackled, though more attention could be given to a sufficient wage to allow those on low incomes to eat a nutritious diet. Nor can the influence of the industry on public policy be easily traced or challenged. A significant employer and a sophisticated lobbyist, its power will remain formidable. There is a long tradition of industry resisting public intervention on the grounds of health, as the history of both pharmaceutical development and food provision describes. Eventually, accounts of the health consequences of flawed industrial products, growing ethical concerns and the leadership of key individuals combined to bring about change, as happened in the nineteenth century.

A more recent example of this was the ban on transfats in 2006 in New York City, which prompted subsequent reductions even by UK food producers (*Guardian* 01/06/12). But a subsequent New York City ban on the sale of soft drinks larger than 16oz/500ml by restaurants and cinemas was overturned by a state judge following lobbying by soft drink companies (Reuters 2013). The city's Board of Health appealed, but in June 2014 the Court of Appeal upheld the earlier decision (BBC 2014).

The argument against the ban was that it limits free choice. In this book I wanted to challenge arguments like that. There is something un-free about the way we eat, based on the nature of the food supply and the class-differentiated way in which diets are formed and health influenced, as discussed in the research from a range of disciplines cited here. Not only is it connected subconsciously to the way we are raised to eat, and the social class of which we are a part; but it is also true that new foods are normalised by tapping into this same subconscious nature of the way we consume food and make our food 'choices'. There was nothing normal about bucket-sized soft drinks until recent decades. But now it is normal to drink them, at least among those at whom they are targeted. Technical agricultural developments lowered production costs, and marketing's achievement was to make it seem normal to drink such large sizes. Coffee and other food and drink items have also increased dramatically in size. The ever spreading siting of snack foods and drinks is another growing phenomenon influencing consumption.

On the same day the New York soda supersizing was upheld, the UK's Scientific Advisory Committee on Nutrition released a consultation document and scientific literature review which proposes renaming added sugars (or non-milk extrinsic sugars) 'free sugars' (SACN 2014). This would include sugars added during food processing. The committee also recommends lowering daily intakes of such sugars and raising intakes of dietary fibre, citing evidence that this would lower rates of 'cardiovascular disease, type II diabetes and bowel cancer' (ibid). This dimension of nutrition policy had not been considered since the early 1990s.

Another report the same day, by Public Health England, also considered sugar consumption. While set to issue formal recommendations to the Department of Health in 2015, which will also build on the SACN research and recommendations, PHE is taking immediate health promotion measures and will be reviewing research on a range of topics including the role of the food industry in sugar consumption (PHE 2014b).

Industry activities will need to be closely monitored. In the UK, minimum alcohol pricing had been mooted by the Coalition government, for which it was criticised by one marketer who observed, 'Cameron has become the teacher who makes the entire class stay behind after school, in the hope that the perpetrator of some misdemeanour will confess'; the government is risking 'a confrontation with the drinks industry' (*Marketing Magazine* 04/04/11). Plans to introduce such pricing were announced in March 2012. But a few months later, the government dropped these plans, instead introducing in May 1914 a ban on 'deep discounting' of alcoholic drinks (in which beverages are sold at below cost price) (*Guardian* 10/02/14; Parliamentary Business 2014). Campaigns and research in support of minimum pricing continue. Resistance to regulation from industry will not disappear, as it adapts to new challenges regarding health, ethics and sustainability, and develops new tactics to influence policy, not all of them overt (Miller and Harkins 2010; Miller and Mooney 2010).

An emerging standard for a healthy diet is the Alternative Healthy Eating Index (AHEI), developed and studied by Akbaraly *et al.* (2011). It shows the importance of fruit, vegetables, fish, nuts and soy foods for avoiding cardiovascular disease. Few of these foods require much value added by the industry. Some social groups have the information, social and economic resources to locate, purchase, prepare and absorb these foods into their diets. The question for social, nutritional and health scientists, for political leaders, policymakers and food providers alike is this: in a foodscape much more likely to feature crisps and soft drinks than raw nuts and fresh fruit, how do we set about restructuring the supply and retailing of food to provide healthy options accessible to all to purchase, prepare and consume? A healthy diet makes a strong contribution to better lifelong health and longer lives; the AHEI study provides strong evidence for this. Can the food industry carry on blanketing public space with a preponderance of unhealthy foods in the face of evidence such as this? Can government maintain its resistance to implementing higher standards for the food supply, and continue its voluntary reductions policy, given its expressed concern about obesity and its health effects? The answer to both questions, at least for the foreseeable future, seems to be: yes.

As long as the discourse surrounding diet-related health remains powerfully centred on a reflexive, choosing, conscious individual, decisive change in food–health policy or industry practice is unlikely. This discourse is rooted in neoliberal ideas that have become so pervasive that they are seen as a matter of common sense; as Harvey stated, 'We're all neoliberals now, without altogether knowing it' (Harvey 2010). In tracing the role of social class and habituation of food consumption from the overlapping perspectives of sociology, history, epidemiology, nutrition, food systems, psychology, economics, geodemographics, food science, product development and marketing, it becomes clear that these fundamental industry influences on diets need to be taken into account as a matter of course, challenging accounts of irresponsible food 'choice'. The similarity of findings in this range of disciplines makes a cumulatively strong case for the limits of the individual choice model, and the need to understand the nature of consumption and the food supply itself, while monitoring the activities of industry more closely.

By setting the structuring influences driving food consumption in the context of global neoliberal industrial and economic forces, a deep, interlocking context for understanding unbalanced food consumption, large bodyweights and high rates of metabolic and other diet-related illness has been revealed. There is a strong case to be made for investigating the commercial forces which are inscribed onto the social landscape in which we live, and which shape our diets and our bodies, via our social status, throughout our lives. From agriculture to arteries, the strategic production, processing, retailing, marketing and consumption of food is indissolubly linked to questions of industry strategies, technologies and goals, but also – as the food is designed, packaged and delivered to where consumers purchase it – social status and class. Health outcomes are also connected to these processes going back to agriculture, and to neoliberal influences on agriculture and on industry activity throughout the food chain.

Paradoxically, inadequate nutrition is often experienced, even in an omnipresent foodscape. Even healthy eaters encounter environments in which it is not easy to locate healthy food. But those who are routinely targeted with unhealthy foods are often multiply disadvantaged, and more likely to face the long-term health consequences of poor diet than if they were more prosperous, higher status people. Indeed, the King's Fund study showed that multiple disadvantage and multiple unhealthy behaviours including poor diet are linked – and increasing in prevalence among the lowest status groups (Buck and Frosini 2012). The present analysis of the complex role of the food industry in structuring consumption aimed to help shift the focus away from the individual's assumed capacity to make good choices, and towards the realm of production and governance, where decisive power to improve population dietary health in a class-structured society rightfully rests.

References

Abraham, J. (1997) 'The science and politics of medicines regulation', in M. A. Elston (ed.) *The Sociology of Medical Science & Technology*, Oxford: Blackwell, pp. 153–83.

Abraham, J. and Davis, C. (2005) 'A comparative analysis of drug safety withdrawals in the UK and the US (1971–1992)', *Social Science & Medicine*, 61(5) pp. 881–92.

Abraham, J. and Davis, C. (2006) 'Testing times: the emergence of the Practolol disaster and its challenge to Britain drug regulation in the modern period', *Social History of Medicine*, 19(1) pp. 127–47.

Abraham, J. and Lewis, G. (1999) 'Harmonising and competing for medicines regulation: how healthy are the European Union's systems of drug approval?', *Social Science & Medicine*, 48(11) pp. 1655–67.

Academy of Medical Royal Colleges (2013) *Measuring Up: The Medical Profession's Prescription for the Nation's Obesity Crisis*, London: Academy of Medical Royal Colleges.

Adams, J. and White, M. (2009) 'Socio-economic and gender differences in nutritional content of foods advertised in popular UK weekly magazines', *European Journal of Public Health*, 19(2) pp. 144–9.

Aggarwal, A., Monsivais, P. and Drewnowski, A. (2012) 'Nutrient intakes linked to better health outcomes are associated with higher diet costs in the US', *Plos One* (Public Library of Science) 7(5), e37533.

Akbaraly, T. N., Ferrie, J. E., Berr, C., Brunner, E. J., Head, J., Marmot, M. G., Singh-Manoux, A., Ritchie, Shipley, M. J. and Kivimaki, M. (2011) 'Alternative healthy eating index and mortality over 18 years of follow-up: results from the Whitehall II cohort', *American Journal of Clinical Nutrition*, 94(i) pp. 247–53.

Ames, B. (2006) 'Low micronutrient intake may accelerate the degenerative diseases of aging through allocation of scarce micronutrients by triage', *PNAS* (*Proceedings of the National Academy of Science of the United States of America*), 103(47) pp. 17589–94.

AMRC: see Academy of Medical Royal Colleges.

Annandale, E. (1998) *The Sociology of Health & Medicine: A Critical Introduction*, Cambridge: Polity Press.

Aphramor, L. (2005) 'Is a weight-centred health framework salutogenic? Some thoughts on unhinging certain dietary ideologies', *Social Theory and Health*, 3(4) pp. 302–14.

Archer, M. (1998) 'Introduction: realism in the social sciences', in M. Archer, R. Bhaskar, A. Collier, T. Lawson and A. Norrie (eds) *Critical Realism: Essential Readings*, London: Routledge, pp. 189–206.

Armand, M., Pasquier, B., André, M., Borel, P., Senft, M., Peyrot, J., Salducci, J., Portugal, H., Jaussan, V. and Lairon, D. (1999) 'Digestion and absorption of 2 fat emulsions with different droplet sizes in the human digestive tract', *American Journal of Clinical Nutrition*, 70(6) pp. 1096–106.

Arthritis Care (2010) 'Living with Arthritis', www.arthritiscare.org.uk/ LivingwithArthritis/Self-management/Eatingwell/ (accessed 19/02/10).

Ashton, J. R., Middleton, J. and Lang, T. (on behalf of 170 signatories) (2014) 'Open letter to Prime Minister David Cameron on food poverty in the UK', *The Lancet*, 383, 10 May.

Atkinson, W. (2007) 'Anthony Giddens as adversary of class analysis', *Sociology*, 41(3).

Backett-Milburn, K. C., Wills, W. J., Roberts, M., and Lawton, J. (2010) 'Food, eating and taste: parents' perspectives on the making of the middle class teenager', *Social Science and Medicine*, 71(7) pp. 1316–23.

Bacon, L. (2008) *Health at Every Size: The Surprising Truth About Your Weight*, Dallas: Benbella Books.

Bacon, L. and Aphramor, L. (2011) 'Weight science: evaluating the evidence for a paradigm shift', *Nutrition Journal*, 10(9) pp. 1–13.

Bagwell, S. (2011) 'The role of independent fast-food outlets in obesogenic environments: a case study of East London in the UK', *Environment and Planning*, 43(9) pp. 2217–36.

Bambra, C. L., Hillier, F. C., Moore, H. J. and Summerbell, C. D. (2012) 'Tackling inequalities in obesity: a protocol for a systematic review of the effectiveness of public health interventions at reducing socioeconomic inequalities in obesity amongst children', *Systematic Reviews*, 1(16) pp. 1–7.

BBC: see British Broadcasting Corporation.

BBSRC (Biotechnology and Biological Sciences Research Council), Swindon, www.bbsrc.ac.uk/business/collaborative-research/industry-clubs/drinc/drinc-background.aspx Swindon (accessed 19/05/12).

Beckley, J. H. and Ramsey, C. A. (2009) 'Observing the consumer in context', in H. R. Moskowitz, I. S. Saguy and T. Straus (eds) *An Integrated Approach to New Food Product Development*, Boca Raton: CRC Press, pp. 233–46.

Bennett, T. (2010) 'Introduction to the Routledge Classics Edition', in P. Bourdieu, *Distinction*, Abingdon: Routledge Classics.

Bennett, T., Savage, M., Silva, E. B., Warde, A., Gayo-Cal, M. and Wright, D. (2009) *Culture, Class, Distinction: Culture, Economy and the Social*, Abingdon: Routledge.

Bentham, J. (1789) *Introduction to the Principles of Morals and Legislation* (www. utilitarianism.com/hedcalc.htm, citing *Penguin Dictionary of Philosophy*, quoting Bentham).

Bhaskar, R. (1979) 'Transcendental realism and the problem of naturalism', in G. Delanty and P. Strydom (eds) (2003) *Philosophies of Social Sciences: The Classic and Contemporary Readings*, Maidenhead: Open University Press, pp. 442–7.

Bhaskar, R. (1989) 'Societies', in M. Archer, R. Bhaskar, A. Collier, T. Lawson and A. Norrie (eds) (1998) *Critical Realism: Essential Readings*, London: Routledge, pp. 206–58.

Bhaskar, R. (1997) 'Philosophy and scientific realism', M. Archer, R. Bhaskar, A. Collier, T. Lawson and A. Norrie (eds) (1998) *Critical Realism: Essential Readings*, London: Routledge, pp. 16–48.

Bhaskar, R. (1998) 'General introduction', in M. Archer, R. Bhaskar, A. Collier, T. Lawson and A. Norrie (eds) *Critical Realism: Essential Readings*, London: Routledge, p. ix.

Bhaskar, R. and Collier, A. (1998) 'Introduction: explanatory critiques', in M. Archer, R. Bhaskar, A. Collier, T. Lawson and A. Norrie (eds) *Critical Realism: Essential Readings*, London: Routledge, pp. 385–95.

Bhaskar, R. and Lawson, T. (1998) 'Introduction: basic texts and development', in M. Archer, R. Bhaskar, A. Collier, T. Lawson and A. Norrie (eds) *Critical Realism: Essential Readings*, London: Routledge, pp. 3–16.

BHF: see British Heart Foundation.

Bhopal, R. (1997) 'Is research into ethnicity and health racist, unsound, or important science?', in T. Heller, R. Muston, M. Sidell and C. Lloyd (eds) (2001) *Working for Health*, London: Sage, pp. 168–80.

Blaxter, M. (2003) 'Biology, social class and inequalities in health', in J. Williams, L. Birke and G. Bendelow (eds) *Debating Biology: Sociological Reflections on Health, Medicine and Society*, London: Routledge, pp. 69–83.

Blythe, J. (2006) *A Very Short, Fairly Interesting and Reasonably Cheap Book About Studying Marketing*, London: Sage.

Bohman, J. (2003) 'Critical theory as practical knowledge: participants, observers and critics', in S. Turner and P. Roth (eds) *The Blackwell Guide to the Philosophy of the Social Sciences*, Oxford: Blackwell, pp. 89–109.

Bourdieu, P. (1990) *The Logic of Practice*, Stanford: Stanford University Press.

Bourdieu, P. (2003) *Firing Back: Against the Tyranny of the Market 2*, London: New Press.

Bourdieu, P. ([1984]2010) *Distinction*, Abingdon: Routledge Classics (first published in English in 1984 by Routledge, Kegan & Paul).

Bovey, S. (ed.) (2008) *Sizable Reflections: Big Women Living Full Lives*, London: Women's Press.

Boyce, T., Robertson, R. and Dixon, A. (2008) *Commissioning and Behaviour Change: Kicking Bad Habits Final Report*, London: King's Fund.

Branagan, B. and Holt, G. (2009) Artists of image appearing in *RANK: Picturing the Social Order 1516–2009*, ed. A. Robinson, Northern Gallery for Contemporary Art, Sunderland, p. 101.

Braziel, J. E. and LeBesco, K. (2001) *Bodies out of Bounds: Fatness and Transgression*, Berkeley: University of California Press.

BritainThinks (2011) 'Speaking Middle English: A study on the middle classes by BritainThinks', London (report not dated – this was the year *Marketing Magazine* reported on it, though it is based on 2003 data), http://britainthinks.com/sites/default/files/reports/SpeakingMiddleEngish_Report.pdf; 'What about the workers?: A new study on the working class by BritainThinks', London, http://britainthinks.com/sites/default/files/reports/WorkingClassReport.pdf (accessed 20/07/11).

British Broadcasting Corporation (2003) 'The rise and fall of Sunny Delight' (03/12), by J. Clayton, http://news.bbc.co.uk/1/hi/business/3257820.stm (accessed 19/08/10).

British Broadcasting Corporation (2005) TV programme, *Honey, We're Killing the Kids*, www.bbc.co.uk/programmes/b006mvr0.

British Broadcasting Corporation (2010) 'Nick Clegg proposes to overhaul social mobility', www.bbc.co.uk/news/uk-politics-11013291 (accessed 18/08/10).

British Broadcasting Corporation (2011a) TV programme, *Business Nightmares with Evan Davis: Marketing Mess-ups.*

British Broadcasting Corporation (2011b) Radio 4, *PM*, 'Behind closed doors in the Downing Street nudge unit' (18/10), by B. Milligan.

British Broadcasting Corporation (2011c) Radio 4, *Nudge Psychology v Nanny State: An All in the Mind Special* (01/11), presenter C. Hammond.

British Broadcasting Corporation (2012) *The Food Programme*, February.

British Broadcasting Corporation (2014) 'US Court rejects New York supersize soda ban' (26/06), www.bbc.com/news/world-us-canada-28049973.

British Heart Foundation (2011) 'The real 5-a-day' (23/11), www.bhf.org.uk/media/news-from-the-bhf/the-real-five-a-day.aspx (accessed 10/04/14).

British Heart Foundation (2014) 'Report shows how junk food makers target children online', www.bhf.org.uk/get-involved/campaigning/food4thought/lardbar/index.aspx (accessed 09/06/14).

British Soft Drinks Association (2013) 'Refreshing the nation: the 2013 UK soft drinks report', www.britishsoftdrinks.com/PDF/2013UKsoftdrinksreport.pdf.

British Soft Drinks Association (2014) 'Creating new choices: the 2014 UK soft drinks report', www.britishsoftdrinks.com/PDF/BSDA%20annual%20report%202014.pdf.

Brooks, D. (2011) *The Social Animal: A Story of How Success Happens*, New York: Random House.

Brown, M., Byatt, T., Marsh, T. and McPherson, K. (2010) *A Prediction of Obesity Trends for Adults and their Associated Diseases: Analysis from the Health Survey for England 1993–2007*, London: National Heart Forum.

Brownell, K. D. and Horgen, K. B. (2004) *Food Fight: The Inside Story of the Food Industry, America's Obesity Crisis & What We Can Do About It*, New York: McGraw Hill.

BSDA: see British Soft Drinks Association.

Buck, D. and Frosini, F. (2012) *Clustering of Unhealthy Behaviours Over Time: Implications for Policy and Practice*, London: King's Fund.

Bunton, R. and Burrows, R. (1995) 'Consumption and health in the "epidemiological" clinic of late modern medicine', in R. Bunton, S. Nettleton and R. Burrows (eds) *The Sociology of Health Promotion*, London: Routledge, pp. 203–18.

Burch, D. and Lawrence, G. (2005) 'Supermarket own brands, supply chains and the transformation of the agri-food system', *International Journal of Sociology of Agriculture and Food*, 13(1) pp. 1–8.

Burnett, J. (1989) *Plenty and Want: A Social History of Food in England from 1815 to the Present Day*, London: Routledge.

Burrows, R. and Gane, N. (2006) 'Geodemographics, software and class', *Sociology*, 40(5) pp. 793–812.

Bury, M. (1997) *Health and Illness in a Changing Society*, London: Routledge.

Buse, K. (2005) 'The commercial sector and global health governance', in K. Lee and J. Collin (eds) *Global Change and Health*, Maidenhead: Open University Press, pp. 178–94.

Business Insights (2011) brief description of report in *Frozen, Chilled & Ready Made Foods Industry Guide*, compiled by British Library Business and IP Centre (updated 05/01).

Cabinet Office (2008) *Food Matters: Towards a Strategy for the 21st Century* (Executive Summary), London: Cabinet Office Strategy Unit.

Cabinet Office (2009) *Report by the Panel on Fair Access to the Professions*, London: Cabinet Office, www.cabinetoffice.gov.uk/strategy/work_areas/access-professions.aspx (accessed 24/07/09).

Cabinet Office (2010) *Applying Behavioural Insight to Health*, London: Cabinet Office Behavioural Insights Team.

CACI (2009) ACORN user guide, www.caci.co.uk/acorn2009/CACI.htm.

CACI (2011) www.caci.co.uk/HealthACORN.aspx (accessed 20/07/11).

CACI (2012) HealthACORN user guide, www.caci.co.uk/HealthACORN.aspx p. 11 (accessed 16/08/12).

CACI (2014) HealthACORN user guide, www.yhpho.org.uk/resource/item.aspx?RID=10140 (accessed 19/06/14).

Campos, P. (2004) *The Obesity Myth: Why America's Obsession with Weight is Hazardous to your Health*, New York: Gotham Books.

Canoy, D. and Buchan, I. (2007) 'Challenges in obesity epidemiology', *Obesity Reviews*, 8(Suppl.1) pp. 1–11.

Carolan, M. (2012) *The Sociology of Food and Agriculture*, Abingdon: Routledge.

CASH: see Consensus Action on Salt and Health.

Change4Life, www.nhs.uk/Change4Life/Pages/change-for-life.aspx (accessed 02/06/12).

Charles, N. and Kerr, M. (1986) 'Eating properly, the family and state benefit', *Sociology*, 20(3) pp. 412–29.

Cherrier, H. and Murray, J. (2004) 'The sociology of consumption: the hidden facet of marketing', *Journal of Marketing Management*, 20(5–6) pp. 509–25.

Christakis, N. and Fowler, J. (2007) 'The spread of obesity in a large social network over 32 years', *New England Journal of Medicine*, 357(4) pp. 370–9.

Christakis, N. and Fowler, J. (2010) *Connected: The Amazing Power of Social Networks and How They Shape Our Lives*, London: Harper Press.

CI: see Consumers International.

Cohen-Cole, E. and Fletcher, J. (2008a) 'Is obesity contagious? Social networks vs. environmental factors in the obesity epidemic', *Journal of Health Economics*, 27(5) pp. 1382–7.

Cohen-Cole, E. and Fletcher, J. (2008b) 'Detecting implausible social network effects in acne, height, and headaches: longitudinal analysis', *British Medical Journal*, 337, a2533, pp. 1–5.

Collier, A. (1998) 'Stratified explanation and Marx's conception of history', in M. Archer, R. Bhaskar, A. Collier, T. Lawson and A. Norrie (eds) *Critical Realism: Essential Readings*, London: Routledge, pp. 258–81.

Consensus Action on Salt and Health (2010) 'Survey reveals shocking levels of salt in your curry night', www.actiononsalt.org.uk/news/surveys/2010/curries/index.html.

Consensus Action on Salt and Health (2010 and 2012) 'Salt and your health factsheets', www.actiononsalt.org.uk/salthealth/factsheets/index.html (accessed 25/05/12).

Consensus Action on Salt and Health (2011a) 'Salt Awareness Week research finds high salt levels in pies', www.actiononsalt.org.uk/less/surveys/2011/Pies/46041.html (accessed 20/03/11).

Consensus Action on Salt and Health (2011b) 'Dangerous levels of salt found in Great British Bangers', www.actiononsalt.org.uk/news/surveys/2011/Sausages/index.html.

Consensus Action on Salt and Health (2012) 'Salt recommendations in the UK', www.actiononsalt.org.uk/salthealth/Recommendations%20on%20salt/index. html (accessed 13/05/12).

Consumer Futures (2014) www.consumerfutures.org.uk/feature/this-website-is-now-closed (accessed 28/04/14).

Consumers International (2011) 'Manual for monitoring food marketing to children', http://issuu.com/consumersinternational/docs/manual_for_monitoring_food_marketing_to_children?e=0/2252232#search (accessed 09/06/14).

Consumers International and World Obesity Federation (2014) 'Recommendations toward a Global Convention to protect and promote healthy diets', http://issuu.com/consint/docs/global_obesity_report.

Cooper, C. (1998) *Fat and Proud: Politics of Size*, London: Women's Press.

Cooper, C. (2011) 'Chubsters and fat studies: developing new models for understanding "the obese"', BSA Conference (07/04).

Coveney, J. and Bunton, R. (2003) 'In pursuit of the study of pleasure: implications for health research and practice', *Health: An Interdisciplinary Journal for the Social Study of Health, Illness and Medicine*, 7(2) pp. 161–79.

Cox, S. A. and Delaney, R. (2009) 'Evolution of sensory evaluation: how product research is being integrated into the product design process', in H. R. Moskowitz, I. S. Saguy and T. Straus (eds) *An Integrated Approach to New Food Product Development*, Boca Raton: CRC Press, pp. 277–90.

Crompton, R. (2008a) 'Forty years of sociology', *Sociology*, 42(6) pp. 1218–27.

Crompton, R. (2008b) *Class and Stratification*, 3rd edn, Cambridge: Polity Press.

Crossley, N. (2004) 'Fat is a sociological issue: obesity rates in late modern "body-conscious" societies', *Social Theory and Health*, 2(3) pp. 222–53.

Crossley, N. (2005) *Key Concepts in Critical Social Theory*, London: Sage.

Crossley, N. (2008) 'Small-world networks, complex systems and sociology', *Sociology*, 42(2) pp. 261–77.

Cunningham, S. A., Kramer, M. R. and Narayan, K. V. (2014) 'Incidence of childhood obesity in the United States', *New England Journal of Medicine*, 370(5), pp. 403–11.

Cutler, D. M., Glaeser, E. L. and Shapiro, J. M. (2003) 'Why have Americans become more obese?', *Journal of Economic Perspectives*, 17(3) pp. 93–118.

Darmon, N. and Drewnowski, A. (2008) 'Does social class predict diet quality?', *American Journal of Clinical Nutrition*, 87(5) pp. 1107–17.

Davis, A., Hirsch, D. and Padley, M. (2014) *A Minimum Income Standard for the UK in 2014*, York: Joseph Rowntree Foundation, www.jrf.org.uk/sites/files/jrf/Minimum-income-standards-2014-FULL.pdf.

Defra: see Department for Environment, Food and Rural Affairs.

Delanty, G. and Strydom, P. (2003) 'The critical tradition', in G. Delanty and P. Strydom (eds) *Philosophies of Social Sciences: The Classic and Contemporary Readings*, Maidenhead: Open University Press, pp. 207–17.

Department for Environment, Food and Rural Affairs (2011) 'Food and drink purchases by UK households in 2010 with derived energy and nutrient intakes', www.defra.gov.uk/statistics/files/defra-stats-foodfarm-food-familyfood-purchases-1112131.pdf.

Department for Environment, Food and Rural Affairs (2012) *Family Food 2011*, London: Defra, www.gov.uk/government/uploads/system/uploads/attachment_data/file/193804/familyfood-2011report.pdf.

Department for Environment, Food and Rural Affairs (2013) *Family Food 2012*, London: Defra, www.gov.uk/government/uploads/system/uploads/attachment_ data/file/265243/familyfood-2012report-12dec13.pdf.

Department of Health (2004) *Choosing Health: Making Healthy Choices Easier*, London: DoH.

Department of Health (2007) *Choosing a Better Diet: A Food and Health Action Plan*, London: DoH, www.dh.gov.uk/prod_consum_dh/groups/dh_digitalas-sets/@dh/@en/documents/digitalasset/dh_4105709.pdf.

Department of Health (2010a) *Healthy Lives, Healthy People: Our Strategy for Public Health in England*, London: DoH, www.dh.gov.uk/prod_consum_dh/ groups/dh_digitalassets/documents/digitalasset/dh_127424.pdf.

Department of Health (2010b) *National Child Measurement Programme: England 2009/10 School Year*, London: Health and Social Care Information Centre, www. ic.nhs.uk/webfiles/publications/003_Health_Lifestyles/ncmp/NCMP_2009-10_ report.pdf.

Department of Health (2011a) *Public Health Responsibility Deal*, London: COI for DoH, www.dh.gov.uk/prod_consum_dh/groups/dh_digitalassets/documents/ digitalasset/dh_125237.pdf; www.dh.gov.uk/prod_consum_dh/groups/ dh_digitalassets/documents/digitalasset/dh_130511.pdf (p. 14); press release: http://mediacentre.dh.gov.uk/2011/10/13/government-calls-time-on-obesity/ (accessed 13/10/11).

Department of Health (2011b) *Healthy Lives, Healthy People: A Call to Action on Obesity in England*, London: DoH, www.dh.gov.uk/prod_consum_dh/groups/ dh_digitalassets/documents/digitalasset/dh_130487.pdf.

Diamond, J. (1999) *Guns, Germs, and Steel: The Fates of Human Societies*, New York: Norton.

Diabetes UK (2004) *Diabetes in the UK 2004*, London: Diabetes UK.

Diabetes UK (2006) *Diabetes and the Disadvantaged*, London: All Parliamentary Group for Diabetes and Diabetes UK, www.diabetes.org.uk/Professionals/ Publications-reports-and-resources/Reports-statistics-and-case-studies/Reports/ Diabetes_and_the_disadvantaged/.

Diabetes UK (2012) *Diabetes in the UK 2012*, London: Diabetes UK, www.diabetes. org.uk/Documents/Reports/Diabetes-in-the-UK-2012.pdf.

Diabetes UK (2013) 'Number of people diagnosed with diabetes reaches three million' (04/03), www.diabetes.org.uk/About_us/News_Landing_Page/Number-of-people-diagnosed-with-diabetes-reaches-three-million/.

Dibb, S. and Simkin, L. (2009) *Marketing Essentials*, London: South-Western Cengage Learning.

Donini, L. M., Savina, C., Gennaro, E., De Felice, M. R., Rosano, A., Pandolfo, M. M., Del Balzo, V., Cannella, C., Ritz, P. and Chumlea, W. C. (2012) 'A systematic review of the literature concerning the relationship between obesity and mortality in the elderly', *Journal of Nutrition, Health & Aging*, 16(1) pp. 89–98.

DoH: see Department of Health.

Dowler, E. (2003) 'Food and poverty: insights from the "north"', *Development Policy Review*, 21(5–6) pp. 569–80.

Dowler, E. (2008a) 'Food and health inequalities: the challenge of sustaining just consumption', *Local Environment*, 13(8) pp. 759–72.

Dowler, E. (2008b) 'Policy initiatives to address low-income households' nutritional needs in the UK', *Proceedings of the Nutrition Society*, 67(3) pp. 289–300.

Dowler, E. and O'Connor, D. (2012) 'Rights-based approaches to addressing food poverty and food insecurity in Ireland and UK', *Social Science and Medicine*, 74(1) pp. 44–51.

Dowler, E., Turner, S. and Dobson, B. (2001) *Poverty Bites: Food, Health and Poor Families*, London: Child Poverty Action Group.

Dowler, E., Kneafsey, M., Cox, R. and Holloway, L. (2009) 'Doing food differently: reconnecting biological and social relationships through care for food', *Sociological Review*, 57(Suppl.2) pp. 200–21.

Downward, P. and Mearman, A. (2007) 'Retroduction as mixed-methods triangulation in economic research', *Cambridge Journal of Economics*, 31(1) pp. 77–99.

Drewnowski, A., Hanks, A. S. and Smith, T. G. (2010) 'International trade, food and diet costs, and the global obesity epidemic', in C. Hawkes, C. Blouin, S. Henson and N. Drager (eds) *Trade, Food, Diet and Health: Perspectives and Policy Options*, Oxford: Blackwell, pp. 77–90.

Earls, M. (2009) *Herd: How to Change Mass Behaviour by Harnessing our True Nature*, Chichester: John Wiley.

Economist (2011) 'Retail therapy: how Ernest Dichter, an acolyte of Sigmund Freud, revolutionised marketing' (17/12), 401(8764) pp. 119–23.

Edwards, T. (2000) *Contradictions of Consumption: Concepts, Practices and Politics in Consumer Society*, Maidenhead: Open University Press.

Egan, J. (2008) 'A century of marketing', *Marketing Review*, 8(1) pp. 3–23.

El-Sayed, A. M., Scarborough, P. and Galea, S. (2012) 'Unevenly distributed: a systematic review of the health literature about socioeconomic inequalities in adult obesity in the United Kingdom', *BMC Public Health*, 12(18) pp. 1–12.

Elliott, J. and Vaitilingam, R. (2008) 'Now we are 50: key findings from the 1958 National Child Development Study', London: Centre for Longitudinal Studies, ESRC.

Experian (2011) www.experian.co.uk/business-strategies/mosaic-grocery.html; http://publicsector.experian.co.uk/Products/Mosaic%20Public%20Sector.aspx (accessed 20/07/11).

Exworthy, M., Stuart, M., Blane, D. and Marmot, M. (2003) *Tackling Health Inequalities Since the Acheson Inquiry*, London: Joseph Rowntree Foundation/ Policy Press, www.jrf.org.uk/sites/files/jrf/jr140-health-inequalities-acheson.pdf.

Fairclough, N. (1993) 'Critical discourse analysis and the marketization of public discourse: the universities', *Discourse & Society*, 4(2) pp. 133–68.

Fairclough, N. (2010) *Critical Discourse Analysis: The Critical Study of Language*, 2nd edn, Harlow: Longman.

Farr, M., Wardlaw, J. and Jones, C. (2008) 'Tackling health inequalities using geodemographics: a social marketing approach', *International Journal of Market Research*, 50(4) pp. 449–67.

Ferguson, N. (2002) *Empire: The Rise and Demise of the British World Order and the Lessons for Global Power*, New York: Basic Books.

Fine, B. (2006) 'Addressing the consumer', in F. Trentmann (ed.) *The Making of the Consumer: Knowledge, Power and Identity in the Modern World*, Oxford: Berg, pp. 291–311.

Fine, B., Heasman, M. and Wright, J. (1996) *Consumption in the Age of Affluence*, London: Routledge.

Fine, B., Heasman, M. and Wright, J. (1998) 'What we eat and why: social norms and systems of provision', in A. Murcott (ed.) *The Nation's Diet: The Social Science of Food Choice*, Harlow: Addison Wesley Longman, pp. 95–111.

Flicker, L., McCaul, K. A., Hankey, G. J., Jamrozik, K., Brown, W. J., Byles, J. E. and Almeida, O. P. (2010) 'Body mass index and survival in men and women aged 70 to 75', *Journal of the American Geriatrics Society*, 58(2) pp. 234–41.

Fogelholm, M. (2010) 'Physical activity, fitness and fatness: relations to mortality, morbidity and disease risk factors. A systematic review', *Obesity Reviews*, 11(3) pp. 202–21.

Food Standards Agency (2007a) *Low Income Diet and Nutrition Survey (LIDNS)*, Summary of Key Findings, London: FSA.

Food Standards Agency (2007b) *Low Income Diet and Nutrition Survey (LIDNS)*, Vol. 2, Food Consumption and Nutrient Intake, London: FSA.

Food Standards Agency and Department of Health (2008/09) *National Diet and Nutrition Survey: Headline Results from Year 1 of the Rolling Programme*, London: FSA/DoH.

Foresight (2007) *Tackling Obesities: Future Choices – Summary of Key Messages*, London: Government Office for Science. For other Foresight reports on obesity cited in this book see Maio et al. (2007) and Paterson (2007).

Foucault, M. (1972–77) 'Truth and Power', in *Power/Knowledge: Selected Interviews and Other Writings 1972–1977*, ed. C. Gordon, Harvester Press, reprinted in P. Rabinow (1984) *The Foucault Reader: An Introduction to Foucault's Thought*, London: Penguin, pp. 51–75.

Foucault, M. (1975) 'Docile Bodies', in *Discipline and Punish*, reprinted in P. Rabinow (1984) *The Foucault Reader: An Introduction to Foucault's Thought*, London: Penguin, pp. 179–87.

Fowler, J. and Christakis, N. (2008) 'Estimating peer effects on health in social networks: a response to Cohen-Cole and Fletcher; and Trogdon, Nonnemaker, and Pais', *Journal of Health Economics*, 27, pp. 1400–5.

Foxall, G. (2010) *Interpreting Consumer Choice: The Behavioural Perspective Model*, Abingdon: Routledge.

Frederick, C. B., Snellman, K. and Putnam, R. D. (2014) 'Increasing socioeconomic disparities in adolescent obesity', *Proceedings of the National Academy of Sciences of the United States of America*, 111(4) pp. 1338–42.

French, J., Blair-Stevens, C., McVey, D. and Merritt, R. (2010) *Social Marketing and Public Health: Theory and Practice*, Oxford: Oxford University Press.

Friedmann, H. (2009) 'Discussion: moving food regimes forward: reflections on symposium essays', *Agriculture and Human Values*, 26, pp. 335–44.

FSA: see Food Standards Agency.

Fuller, G. W. (2001) *Food, Consumers and the Food Industry: Catastrophe or Opportunity?* Boca Raton: CRC Press.

Fuller, G. W. (2005) *New Food Product Development: From Concept to Marketplace*, 2nd edn, Boca Raton: CRC Press.

Gaesser, G. (2002) *Big Fat Lies: The Truth about Your Weight and Your Health*, Carlsbad: Gurze Books.

Gard, M. (2009) 'Friends, enemies and the cultural politics of critical obesity research', in J. Wright and V. Harwood (eds) *Biopolitics and the Obesity Epidemic: Governing Bodies*, Abingdon: Routledge, pp. 31–44.

Gaskell, E. ([1848]1970) *Mary Barton*, London: Penguin.

Gaskell, E. ([1854]1994) *North and South*, London: Penguin.

Gatfield, T. (2006) 'Australia's gone chicken! An examination of consumer behaviour and trends related to chicken and beef meats in Australia', *Journal of Food Products Marketing*, 12(3) pp. 29–43.

Geyskens, K., Pandelaere, M., Dewitte, S. and Warlop, L. (2007) 'The backdoor to overconsumption: the effect of associating "low-fat" food with health references', *Journal of Public Policy & Marketing*, 26(1) pp. 118–25.

Giddens, A. (1982) 'Class structuration and class consciousness', in A. Giddens and D. Held (eds) *Classes, Power and Conflict: Classical and Contemporary Debates*, Basingstoke: Macmillan.

Giddens, A. (1991) *Modernity and Self Identity: Self and Society in the Late Modern Age*, Cambridge: Polity Press.

Giddens, A. (1994) *Beyond Right and Left*, Cambridge: Polity Press.

Giddens, A. (1995) *Politics, Sociology and Social Theory: Encounters in Classical and Contemporary Social Thought*, Cambridge: Polity Press.

Giddens, A. (2007) *Over to You, Mr Brown*, Cambridge: Polity Press.

Golding, M. and Wooster, T. J. (2010) 'The influence of emulsion structure and stability on lipid digestion', *Current Opinion in Colloid & Interface Science*, 15(1–2) pp. 90–101.

Gonzalez-Benito, O. and Gonzalez-Benito, J. (2005) 'The role of geodemographic segmentation in retail location strategy', *International Journal of Market Research*, 47(3) pp. 295–316.

Goss, J. (1995) 'Marketing the new marketing: the strategic discourse of geographic information systems', in J. Pickles (ed.) *Ground Truth: The Social Implications of Geographic Information Systems*, New York: Guilford Press, pp. 130–70.

Graham, H. (2007) *Unequal Lives: Health and Socioeconomic Inequalities*, Maidenhead: Open University Press.

Graves, P. (2010) *Consumerology: The Market Research Myth, the Truth about Consumer Behaviour and the Psychology of Shopping*, London: Nicholas Brealey.

Grier, S. A., Mensinger, J., Huang, S. H., Kumanyika, S. K. and Stettler, N. (2007) 'Fast-food marketing and children's fast-food consumption: exploring parents' influences in an ethnically diverse sample', *Journal of Public Policy and Marketing*, 26(2) pp. 221–35.

The Guardian newspaper (London): see news reports listed by date at the end of the References; investigative and commentary articles are listed by author in this section.

Guthman, J. (2008) 'Neoliberalism and the making of food politics in California', *Geoforum*, 39, pp. 1171–83.

Guthman, J. (2009) 'Teaching the politics of obesity: insights into neoliberal embodiment and contemporary biopolitics', *Antipode*, 41(5) pp. 1110–33.

Guthman, J. (2011) *Weighing In: Obesity, Food Justice and the Limits of Capitalism*, Berkeley: University of California Press.

Guthman, J. and Dupuis, M. (2006) 'Embodying neoliberalism: economy, culture, and the politics of fat', *Environment and Planning D: Society and Space*, 24, pp. 427–48.

Habermas, J. (1987) *Toward a Rational Society*, English translation (originally published 1969 in German), Cambridge: Polity Press.

Habermas, J., various excerpts in W. Outhwaite (ed.) (1996) *The Habermas Reader*, Cambridge: Polity Press:

- (1962) 'The transformation of the public sphere's political function', from *The Structural Transformation of the Public Sphere* (English translation 1989), pp. 28–31.
- (1968) 'Knowledge and human interests: a general perspective', from *Knowledge and Human Interests* (English translation 1971), pp. 96–104.
- (1973) 'Social principles of organization', from *Legitimation Crisis* (English translation 1976), pp. 240–5.
- (1976) 'Legitimation problems in the modern state', from *Communication and the Evolution of Society* (English translation 1979), pp. 248–65.
- (1981) 'Relations to the world and aspects of rationality in four sociological concepts of action', from *Theory of Communicative Action*, Vol. 1 (English translation 1984), pp. 132–50; 'The uncoupling of system and lifeworld', 'Marx and the thesis of internal colonization' and 'The tasks of a critical theory of society', from *Theory of Communicative Action*, Vol. 2 (English translation 1987), pp. 278–282, 283–303 and 309–36.
- (1983) 'Discourse ethics', from *Moral Consciousness and Communicative Action* (English translation 1989), pp. 180–92.
- (1985) 'The normative content of modernity', from *The Philosophical Discourse of Modernity* (English translation 1987), pp. 341–65.

Habermas, J. ([1965]2003) 'Knowledge and human interests', in G. Delanty and P. Strydom (eds) *Philosophies of Social Sciences: The Classic and Contemporary Readings*, Maidenhead: Open University Press, pp. 234–9.

Hackley, C. (2001) *Marketing and Social Construction: Exploring the Rhetorics of Managed Consumption*, London: Routledge.

Hackley, C. (2009) *Marketing: A Critical Introduction*, London: Sage.

Hackley, C. (2010) *Advertising and Promotion: An Integrated Marketing Communications Approach*, 2nd edn, London: Sage.

Hammersley, M. (1995) *The Politics of Social Research*, London: Sage.

Harding, K. and Kirby, M. (2009) *Lessons from the Fat-O-Sphere*, New York: Penguin.

Harper, S., Lynch, J. and Davey Smith, G. (2011) 'Social determinants and the decline of cardiovascular diseases', *Annual Review of Public Health*, 32, pp. 39–69.

Harvard School of Public Health (2012) 'Fats and cholesterol: the bottom line', www.hsph.harvard.edu/nutritionsource/what-should-you-eat/fats-and-cholesterol/index.html (accessed 10/04/12).

Harvey, D. (2005) *A Brief History of Neoliberalism*, Oxford: Oxford University Press.

Harvey, D. (2007) 'Neoliberalism as creative destruction', *ANNALS, AAPSS*, 610, March, pp. 22–44.

Harvey, D. (2010) 'The enigma of capital', lecture at the London School of Economics (26/04), www2.lse.ac.uk/newsAndMedia/videoAndAudio/channels/publicLecturesAndEvents/player.aspx?id=629.

Harvey, L. (1990) *Critical Social Research*, London: Unwin Hyman.

Hautvast, J., Elmadva, I. and Rayner, M. (2000) 'Policy, trade, economic, and technological aspects of improving nutrient intake and lifestyles in the European Union', *Public Health Nutrition*, 4(2A) pp. 325–36.

Hawkes, C. (2006) 'Uneven dietary development: linking the policies and processes of globalization with the nutrition transition, obesity and diet-related chronic diseases', *Globalization and Health*, 2(4) pp. 1–18.

Hawkes, C. (2007) 'Regulating food marketing to young people worldwide', *American Journal of Public Health*, 97(11) pp. 1962–73.

Hawkes, C. (2008) 'Dietary implications of supermarket development: a global perspective', *Development Policy Review*, 26(6) pp. 657–92.

Hawkes, C. (2009) 'Identifying innovative interventions to promote healthy eating using consumption-oriented food supply chain analysis', *Journal of Hunger & Environmental Nutrition*, 4(3–4) pp. 336–56.

Hawkes, C. (2010) 'The influence of trade liberalisation and global dietary change', in C. Hawkes, C. Blouin, S. Henson and N. Drager (eds) *Trade, Food, Diet and Health: Perspectives and Policy Options*, Oxford: Blackwell, pp. 35–59.

Hawkes, C. and Murphy, S. (2010) 'An overview of global food trade', in C. Hawkes, C. Blouin, S. Henson and N. Drager (eds) *Trade, Food, Diet and Health: Perspectives and Policy Options*, Oxford: Blackwell, pp. 16–34.

Hawkes, C. and Ruel, M. (2006) 'The links between agriculture and health: an intersectoral opportunity to improve the health and livelihoods of the poor', *Bulletin of the World Health Organization*, 84(12) pp. 984–90.

Hawkes, C., Blouin, C., Henson, S. and Drager, N. (eds) (2010) *Trade, Food, Diet and Health: Perspectives and Policy Options*, Oxford: Blackwell.

Hawkes, C., Friel, S., Lobstein, L. and Lang, T. (2012) 'Linking agricultural policies with obesity and noncommunicable diseases: a new perspective for a globalising world', *Food Policy*, 37, pp. 343–53.

Health Committee (2004) *Obesity: Third Report of Session 2003–04*, Vol. 1, London: House of Commons Health Committee.

Health Committee (2011) *Public Health: Twelfth Report of Session 2010–12*, Vol. 1, London: House of Commons Health Committee, www.publications. parliament.uk/pa/cm201012/cmselect/cmhealth/1048/1048.pdf.

Health Survey for England (2008) Vol. 1, 'Physical activity and fitness', by M. Roth, www.hscic.gov.uk/catalogue/PUB00430/heal-surv-phys-acti-fitn-eng-2008-rep-v2.pdf.

Health Survey for England (2011), Vol. 1, Chapter 4, 'Diabetes and hyperglycemia', by A. Moody, www.hscic.gov.uk/catalogue/PUB09300/HSE2011-Ch4-Diabetes. pdf (accessed 14 May 2014).

Health Survey for England (2012a), Vol. 1, Chapter 2, 'Physical activity in adults', by S. Scholes and J. Mindell, http://healthsurvey.hscic.gov.uk/media/1022/chpt-2_physical-activity-in-adults.pdf (accessed 09/06/14).

Health Survey for England (2012b), Vol. 1, Chapter 10, 'Adult anthropometric measures, overweight and obesity', by A. Moody, http://healthsurvey.hscic.gov. uk/media/1021/chpt-10_adult-measures.pdf (accessed 09/06/14).

HealthACORN: see CACI.

Henley, J. (2010) 'Crunch time: they're fried in fat and smothered in salt, but still we eat a heart-stopping 6bn packets of them a year', *Guardian* (01/09), pp. 4–7.

Henry, P. C. (2005) 'Social class, market situation and consumers' metaphors of (dis)empowerment', *Journal of Consumer Research*, 31(4) pp. 766–78.

Henry, P. C. and Caldwell, M. (2008) 'Spinning the proverbial wheel? Social class and marketing', *Marketing Theory*, 8(4) pp. 387–405.

Herrick, C. (2009) 'Shifting blame/selling health: corporate social responsibility in the age of obesity', *Sociology of Health and Illness*, 31(1) pp. 51–65.

Hex, N., Bartlett, C., Wright, D., Taylor, M. and Varley, D. (2012) 'Estimating the current and future costs of Type 1 and Type 2 diabetes in the UK', *Diabetic Medicine*, 29(7) pp. 855–62.

Hitchman, C., Christie, I., Harrison, M. and Lang, T. (2002) *Inconvenience Food: The Struggle to Eat Well on a Low Income*, London: Demos.

Hobsbawm, E. (1979) 'The influence of Marxism 1945–83', in E. Hobsbawm (2011) *How to Change the World: Tales of Marx and Marxism*, London: Little, Brown, pp. 344–84.

Hoek, J. and Gendall, P. (2006) 'Advertising and obesity: a behavioural perspective', *Journal of Health Communication*, 11(4) pp. 409–23.

Holloway, L., Kneafsey, M., Venn, L., Cox, R., Dowler, E. and Tuomainen, H. (2007) 'Possible food economies: a methodological framework for exploring food production–consumption relationships', *Sociologia Ruralis*, 47(1) pp. 1–19.

Holt, D. B. (1998) 'Does cultural capital structure American consumption?', *Journal of Consumer Research*, 25(1) pp. 1–25.

Houpt, S. (2011) 'A repentant marketer confesses his sins: branding expert Martin Lindstrom dishes the dirt on an industry that's kept him fed for more than two decades', *The Globe and Mail* (23/09), Toronto.

House of Lords (2011) *Behaviour Change: Report*, London: House of Lords Science and Technology Committee, www.publications.parliament.uk/pa/ld201012/ldselect/ldsctech/179/179.pdf.

HSE: see Health Survey for England.

Hu, F. B., Willett, W. C., Li, T., Stampfer, M. J., Colditz, G. A. and Manson, J. E. (2004) 'Adiposity as compared with physical activity in predicting mortality among women', *New England Journal of Medicine*, 351(26) pp. 2694–703.

Huda, M. S. B., Wilding, J. P. H. and Pinkney, J. H. (2006) 'Gut peptides and the regulation of appetite', *Obesity Reviews*, 7(2) pp. 163–82.

Hughes, K. (2014) 'Don't look down on those who eat fast food', *Guardian* (08/06), www.theguardian.com/commentisfree/2014/jun/08/fast-food-mcdonalds-kfc-jamie-oliver.

Huizinga, M. M., Cooper, L. A., Bleich, S. N., Clark, J. M. and Beach, M. C. (2009) 'Physician respect for patients with obesity', *Journal of General Internal Medicine*, 24(11) pp. 1236–9.

IAB: see Internet Advertising Bureau.

Iacobellis, G. and Sharma, A. M. (2007) 'Obesity and the heart: redefinition of the relationship', *Obesity Reviews*, 8(1) pp. 35–9.

Internet Advertising Bureau (2013) 'UK digital adspend hits record 6 month high of £3bn', www.iabuk.net/about/press/archive/uk-digital-adspend-hits-record-6-month-high-of-3bn.

Joffe, M. (1993) 'Future of European Community (EC) activities in the area of public health', *Health Promotion International*, 8(1) pp. 53–61.

Johnson, S. (2010) *Where Good Ideas Come From: The Natural History of Innovation*, London: Allen Lane.

Jutel, A. (2006) 'The emergence of overweight as a disease entity: measuring up normality', *Social Science and Medicine*, 63(9) pp. 2268–79.

Kahnemann, D. (2010) 'Daniel Kahnemann – autobiography', www.nobelprize.org/nobel_prizes/economics/laureates/2002/kahneman-autobio.html (accessed 10/06/12).

Kant, A. K. and Graubard, B. I. (2013) 'Family income and education were related with 30-year time trends in dietary and meal behaviors of American children and adolescents', *Journal of Nutrition*, 143(5) pp. 690–700.

Kantar (2011) 'Nutritional purchasing: spotlight on saturates', London: Kantar Worldpanel, PowerPoint presentation supplied to author May 2012.

Kaufmann, D., Kraay, A. and Mastruzzi, M. (2009) *Governance Matters 2009: Learning from over a decade of the Worldwide Governance Indicators*, Washington: Brookings Institution, www.brookings.edu/opinions/2009/0629_governance_indicators_kaufmann.aspx (accessed 30/03/13).

Kelly, M. P. and Charlton, B. (1995) 'The modern and the postmodern in health promotion', in R. Bunton, S. Nettleton and R. Burrows (eds) *The Sociology of Health Promotion*, London: Routledge, pp. 77–90.

Kessler, D. (2009) *The End of Overeating: Taking Control of the Insatiable North American Appetite*, Toronto: McLelland & Stewart.

Key, T. (2011) 'Fruit and vegetables and cancer risk', *British Journal of Cancer*, 104(1) pp. 6–11.

Key, T. J., Appleby, P. N., Reeves, G. K., and Roddam, A. W. (2011) (Endogenous Hormones and Breast Cancer Collaborative Group; authors cited are UK representatives of this group, which has dozens of participants worldwide) 'Circulating sex hormones and breast cancer risk factors in postmenopausal women: reanalysis of 13 studies', *British Journal of Cancer*, 105(5) pp. 709–22.

Knauper, B., McCollam, A., Rosen-Brown, A., Lacaille, J., Kelso, E. and Roseman, M. (2011) 'Fruitful plans: adding targeted mental imagery to implementation intentions increases fruit consumption', *Psychology and Health*, 26(5) pp. 601–17.

Koster, E. P. (2009) 'Diversity in the determinants of food choice: a psychological perspective', *Food Quality and Preference*, 20(2) pp. 70–82.

Laberge, Y. (2010) 'Habitus and social capital: from Pierre Bourdieu and beyond', *Sociology*, 44(4) pp. 770–77.

Lang, T. (2009) 'Reshaping the food system for ecological public health', *Journal of Hunger and Environmental Nutrition*, 4(3–4) pp. 315–35.

Lang, T. and Rayner, G. (2005) 'Obesity: a growing issue for European policy?', *Journal of European Social Policy*, 15(4) pp. 301–27.

Lang, T., Barling, D. and Caraher, M. (2009) *Food Policy: Integrating Health, Environment and Society*, Oxford: Oxford University Press.

Laurence, A. (2002) *Women in England 1500–1960: A Social History*, London: Phoenix Press.

Lawrence, F. (2008a) *Eat Your Heart Out: Why the Food Business is Bad for the Planet and Your Health*, London: Penguin.

Lawrence, F. (2008b) 'Our diet of destruction', *Guardian* (16/06).

Lawrence, F. (2008c) 'Britain on a plate', *Guardian* (01/10), www.theguardian.com/lifeandstyle/2008/oct/01/foodanddrink.oliver.

Lawson, N. (2009) *All Consuming: How Shopping Got Us into this Mess and How We Can Find Our Way Out*, London: Penguin.

Lawson, T. (1997) 'Economic science without experimentation', in *Economics and Reality*, London: Routledge; reprinted in M. Archer, R. Bhaskar, A. Collier, T. Lawson and A. Norrie (eds) (1998) *Critical Realism: Essential Readings*, London: Routledge, pp. 144–87.

Lea, S. E. G. (1978) 'The psychology and economics of demand', *Psychological Bulletin*, 85(3) pp. 441–66.

Leblanc, A. G. W. and Janssen, I. (2010) 'Difference between self-reported and accelerometer measured moderate-to-vigorous physical activity in youth', *Pediatric Exercise Science*, 2(4) pp. 523–34.

Lee, H. (2011) 'Inequality and obesity in the United States', *Sociology Compass*, 5(3) pp. 215–32.

Lee, K. and Goodman, H. (2002) 'Global policy networks: the propagation of health care financing reform since the 1980s', in K. Lee, K. Buse and S. Fustukian (eds) *Health Policy in a Globalising World*, Cambridge: Cambridge University Press, pp. 97–119.

Leisure Database Company (2013) www.theleisuredatabase.com/news/news-archive/fitness-industry-improves-growth-at-a-price.

Lloyd-Williams, F., O'Flaherty, M., Mwatsama, M., Birt, C., Ireland, R. and Capewell, S. (2008) 'Estimating the cardiovascular mortality burden attributable to the European Common Agricultural Policy on dietary saturated fats', *Bulletin of the World Health Organisation*, 86(7) pp. 535–42.

Lobstein, T., Baur, L. and Uauy, R. (2004) 'Obesity in children and young people: a crisis in public health', *Obesity Reviews*, 5(Suppl. S1) pp. 4–85.

Lobstein, T., Millstone, E., Jacobs, M., Stirling, A. and Mohebati, L. (2006) *Policy Options for Responding to Obesity: UK National Report of the PorGrow Project*, Brighton: SPRU (Science and Technology Policy Research), University of Sussex.

Lock, K., Smith, R. D., Dangour, A. D., Keogh-Brown, M., Pigatto, G., Hawkes, C., Fisberg, R. M. and Chalabi, Z. (2010) 'Health, agricultural, and economic effects of adoption of healthy diet recommendations', *The Lancet*, 376(9753) pp. 1699–709.

Longley, P. A. and Goodchild, M. F. (2008) 'The use of geodemographics to improve public service delivery', in J. Hartley, C. Donaldson, C. Skelcher and M. Wallace (eds) *Managing to Improve Public Services*, Cambridge: Cambridge University Press, pp. 176–94.

Low Income Diet and Nutrition Survey (2007): see Food Standards Agency.

Lupton, D. (2003) *Medicine as Culture: Illness, Disease and the Body in Western Societies*, 2nd edn, London: Sage.

Lustig, R. (2009) 'Sugar: the bitter truth', television lecture, University of California, www.youtube.com/watch?v=dBnniua6-oM (accessed 15/06/14).

Lustig, R. (2014) *Fat Chance: The Hidden Truth about Sugar, Obesity and Disease*, London: Fourth Estate.

Lyon, D. (2003) 'Surveillance as social sorting: computer codes and mobile bodies', in D. Lyon (ed.) *Surveillance as Social Sorting: Privacy, Risk and Digital Discrimination*, London: Routledge, pp. 13–30.

Malik, V. S., Popkin, B. M., Bray, G. A., Despres, J. P., Willett, W. C. and Hu, F. B. (2010) 'Sugar-sweetened beverages and risk of metabolic syndrome and Type 2 diabetes', *Diabetes Care*, 33(11) pp. 2477–83.

Mail Media Centre (2009) www.mmc.co.uk/Knowledge-centre/Research/How-brands-can-engage-consumers-neuroscience/?campaignid=TMW_LCH_MMCHP-OMD-Google-neuromarketing (accessed 16/03/11).

Maio, G. R., Manstead, A. S. R., Verplanken, B., Stroebe, W., Abraham, C., Sheeran, P. and Conner, M. (2007) *Foresight: Tackling Obesities: Future Choices – Lifestyle Change – Evidence Review*, London: Government Office for Science.

Mann, T., Tomiyama, A. J., Westling, E., Lew, A. M., Samuels, B. and Chatman, J. (2007) 'Medicare's search for effective obesity treatments: diets are not the answer', *American Psychologist*, 62(3) pp. 220–33.

Marketing Magazine (London: Haymarket): see articles listed by date at the end of the References.

Marmot, M. (2004) 'Social causes of social inequalities in health', in S. Anand, F. Peter and A. Sen (eds) *Public Health, Ethics and Equity*, Oxford: Oxford University Press, pp. 37–62.

Marmot, M. and Mustard, J. F. (1994) 'Coronary heart disease from a population perspective', in R. G. Evans, M. L. Barer and T. R. Marmor (eds) *Why are Some People Healthy and Others Not? The Determinants of Health of Populations*, New York: Aldine de Gruyter, pp. 189–216.

Marmot, M., Allen, J., Goldblatt, P., Boyce, T., McNeish, D., Grady, M. and Geddes, I. (2010) *Fair Society, Healthy Lives: Strategy Review of Health Inequalities in England Post-2010*, London: Marmot Review (executive summary and full report).

Marx, K., various excerpts in C. Pierson (ed.) (1997) *The Marx Reader*, London: Polity Press:

- (1845) *The German Ideology* (unpublished until the 1930s), pp. 94–118.
- (1846) *Letter to Annenkov*, pp. 121–7.
- (1852) *The Eighteenth Brumaire of Louis Bonaparte*, pp. 156–76.
- (1857) *Grundrisse*, pp. 182–202.
- (1859) *Preface to a Contribution to the Critique of Political Economy*, pp. 119–20.
- (1867) *Capital*, pp. 203–48.

Mayhew, H. ([1851]2008), *London Labour and the London Poor*, Ware: Wordsworth Editions.

McCullough, M. L. and Willett, W. C. (2006) 'Evaluating adherence to recommended diets in adults: the Alternate Healthy Eating Index', *Public Health Nutrition*, 9(1A) pp. 152–7.

McDonald, S. D., Han, Z., Mulla, S. and Beyene, J. (2010) 'Overweight and obesity in mothers and risk of preterm birth and low birth weight infants', *BMJ Online*, 341(7765) c3428 (pp. 1–20 in pdf).

McMichael, P. (2000) 'The power of food', *Agriculture and Human Values*, 17, pp. 21–33.

McMichael, P. (2005) 'Global development and the corporate food regime', *Research in Rural Sociology and Development*, 11, pp. 265–99.

McMichael, P. (2009) 'A food regime analysis of the "world food crisis"', *Agriculture and Human Values*, 26, pp. 281–95.

McNaughton, S. A., Mishra, G. D. and Brunner, E. J. (2008) 'Dietary patterns, iInsulin resistance, and incidence of Type 2 diabetes in the Whitehall II study', *Diabetes Care*, 31(7) pp. 1343–8.

Meiselman, H. L. (2009) 'Recent developments in consumer research of food', in H. R. Moskowitz, I. S. Saguy and T. Straus (eds) *An Integrated Approach to New Food Product Development*, Boca Raton: CRC Press, pp. 345–69.

Metcalf, B. S., Voss, L. D., Hosking, J., Jeffery, A. N. and Wilkin, T. J. (2008) 'Physical activity at the government-recommended level and obesity-related health outcomes: a longitudinal study (Early Bird 37)', *Archives of Disease in Childhood*, 93(9) pp. 772–7.

Metcalf, B. S., Hosking, J., Jeffery, A. N., Voss, L. D., Henley, W. and Wilkin, T. J. (2011) 'Fatness leads to inactivity, but inactivity does not lead to fatness: a longitudinal study in children; Early Bird 45', *Archives of Disease in Childhood*, 96(10) pp. 942–7.

Michman, R. D. and Mazze, E. M. (1998) *The Food Industry Wars: Marketing Triumphs and Blunders*, Westport, Quorum Books.

Mick, D. G. (2007) 'The ends of marketing and the neglect of moral responsibility by the American Marketing Association', *Journal of Public Policy and Marketing*, 26(2) pp. 289–92.

Mikkelson, B. E. (2011) 'Foodscape studies: a powerful tool to improve our understanding of the impact of food environments on our behaviour', *Perspectives in Public Health*, 131(5) p. 206.

Milburn, A. (2012) *Fair Access to the Professions: A Progress Report by the Independent Reviewer on Social Mobility and Child Poverty*, London: Cabinet Office.

Miller, D. and Harkins, C. (2010) 'Corporate strategy, corporate capture: food and alcohol industry lobbying and public health', *Critical Social Policy*, 30(4) pp. 564–89.

Miller, D. and Mooney, G. (2010) 'Introduction to the themed issue. Corporate power: agency, communication, influence and social policy', *Critical Social Policy*, 30(4) pp. 459–571.

Millstone, E. (2009) 'Science, risk and governance: radical rhetorics and the realities of reform in food safety governance', *Research Policy*, 38(4) pp. 624–36.

Millstone, E. (2010) 'Can science and politics keep each other honest?', professorial lecture (11/05), University of Sussex, Brighton, www.sussex.ac.uk/newsandevents/sussexlectures/2010?lecture=50&fmt=qt (accessed January 2012).

Millstone, E. and Lang, T. (2008) 'Risking regulatory capture at the UK's Food Standards Agency?', *The Lancet*, 372(9633).

Milton, A. (2010) Speech to the World Health Organisation Forum on Salt by the Parliamentary Under Secretary of State for Public Health, www.dh.gov.uk/en/MediaCentre/Speeches/DH_117312.

Monaghan, L. (2005) 'Discussion piece: a critical take on the obesity debate', *Social Theory and Health*, 3(4) pp. 302–14.

Moore, E. A. (2007) 'Perspectives on food marketing and childhood obesity', *Journal of Public Policy and Marketing*, 26(2) pp. 157–61.

Moore, E. A. and Rideout, V. (2007) 'The online marketing of food to children: is it just fun and games?', *Journal of Public Policy and Marketing*, 26(2) pp. 202–20.

Moore, K. and Sheron, N. (2009) 'Why we need a national strategy for liver disease', *British Journal for Hospital Medicine*, 70(12) pp. 674–5.

Moore, L. V., Diez Roux, A. V., Nettleton, J. A., Jacobs, D. R. and Franco, M. (2009) 'Fast-food consumption, diet quality, and neighborhood exposure to fast food: the multi-ethnic study of atherosclerosis', *American Journal of Epidemiology*, 170(1) pp. 29–36.

Moran, J. (2007) *Queuing for Beginners: The Story of Daily Life from Breakfast to Bedtime*, London: Profile Books.

Munro-Wild, H. and Fellows, C. (2009) 'The London findings of the National Child Measurement Programme 2006 to 2008', London: London Health Observatory.

Murcott, A. (ed.) (1998) *The Nation's Diet: The Social Science of Food Choice*, London: Addison Wesley Longman.

Murcott, A. (2000) 'Understanding life-style and food use: contributions from the social sciences', *British Medical Bulletin*, 56(1) pp. 121–32, London: Routledge.

Murcott, A. (2011) 'The BSA and the emergence of a "sociology of food": a personal view', *Sociological Research Online*, 16(3) 14, www.socresonline.org.uk/16/3/14.html.

Murray, C. J. L., Richards, M. A. and Newton, J. N. (and 39 others) (2013) 'UK health performance: findings of the Global Burden of Disease Study 2010', *The Lancet*, http://download.thelancet.com/pdfs/journals/lancet/PIIS0140673613603554.pdf?id=5bbe37e152166496:4555a725:13d3abc88a2:1d401362493966118.

Naaz, A., Holsberger, D. R., Iwamoto, G. A., Nelson, A., Kiyokawa, H. and Cooke, P. S. (2004) 'Loss of cyclin-dependent kinase inhibitors produces adipocyte hyperplasia and obesity', *Journal of Federation of American Societies for Experimental Biology*, 18(15) pp. 1925–7.

Narkiewicz, K. (2006) 'Diagnosis and management of hypertension in obesity', *Obesity Reviews*, 7(2) pp. 155–62.

National Centre for Social Research/Medical Research Council (2008) 'An assessment of dietary sodium levels among adults (aged 19–64) in the UK general population in 2008, based on analysis of dietary sodium in 24 hour urine samples', www.food.gov.uk/multimedia/pdfs/08sodiumreport.pdf.

National Centre for Social Research (2011) British Social Attitudes 28 http://ir2.flife.de/data/natcen-social-research/igb_html/index.php?bericht_id=1000001&index=&lang=ENG (accessed 7/12/11).

National Child Measurement Programme England (2013) London, Health and Social Care Information Centre, Public Health England, www.hscic.gov.uk/catalogue/PUB13115/nati-chil-meas-prog-eng-2012-2013-rep.pdf.

National Confidential Enquiry into Patient Outcome and Death (2012) 'Bariatric surgery: too lean a service?', www.ncepod.org.uk/2012report2/downloads/BS_report_summary.pdf (accessed 19/06/14).

National Consumer Council (2006) *Short-changed on Health? How Supermarkets Can Affect Your Chances of a Healthy Diet*, by J. Pitt, London: NCC.

National Consumer Council (2008) *Cut Price, What Cost? How Supermarkets Can Affect Your Chances of a Healthy Diet*, by L. Yates, London: NCC.

National Diet and Nutrition Survey: see Food Standards Agency 2010.

National Heart Forum: see Brown *et al.* (2010).

National Obesity Observatory (2010) 'Adult obesity and socioeconomic status', www.noo.org.uk/uploads/doc/vid_7929_Adult%20Socioeco%20Data%20Briefing%20October%202010.pdf (accessed January 2011, rechecked 25/05/12).

National Obesity Observatory (2012a) 'Adult obesity and socioeconomic status', www.noo.org.uk/uploads/doc/vid_16966_AdultSocioeconSep2012.pdf.

National Obesity Observatory (2012b) 'Slide sets for adult and child obesity', www.noo.org.uk/slide_sets (accessed 10/03/13).

NCC: see National Consumer Council.

NCEPOD: see National Confidential Enquiry into Patient Outcomes and Death.

NCMP: see National Child Measurement Programme.

Nelson, M., Erens, E., Bates, B., Church, S. and Boshier, T. (2007) *Low Income Diet and Nutrition Survey*, London: FSA (also see Food Standards Agency above).

Nestle, M. (2002) *Food Politics*, Berkeley: University of California Press.

Ng, M. *et al.* (collaborators number approximately 170) (2014) 'Global, regional, and national prevalence of overweight and obesity in children and adults during 1980–2013: a systematic analysis for the Global Burden of Disease Study 2013', *The Lancet*, early online publication (29/05).

NHS (2008) *Statistics on Physical Activity, Obesity and Diet: England 2008*, The Information Centre, Lifestyles Statistics, www.ic.nhs.uk/webfiles/publications/opan08/OPAD%20Jan%202008%20final%20v7%20with%20links%20and%20buttons%20-%20NS%20logo%20removed%2020112008.pdf (accessed 22/10/10).

NHS (2010) *Statistics on Physical Activity, Obesity and Diet: England 2010*, Health and Social Care Information Centre, www.ic.nhs.uk/webfiles/publications/opad10/Statistics_on_Obesity_Physical_Activity_and_Diet_England_2010.pdf (accessed 23/05/12).

NHS (2012) *Future Forum Summary Report – Second Phase*, London: Department of Health, www.dh.gov.uk/prod_consum_dh/groups/dh_digitalassets/documents/digitalasset/dh_132085.pdf (accessed 23/03/12).

NHS NDA (2011) National Diabetes Audit 2003-04 to 2009-10 (2011) London: NHS Information Centre, www.ic.nhs.uk/news-and-events/news/up-to-24000-people-with-diabetes-suffer-an-avoidable-death-in-england-each-year.

Ni Mhurchu, C. N., Capelin, C., Dunford, E. K., Webster, J., Neal, B. C. and Jebb, S. A. (2011) 'Sodium content of processed foods in the United Kingdom: analysis of 44,000 foods purchased by 21,000 households', *American Journal of Clinical Nutrition*, 93(3) pp. 594–600.

NICE (National Institute for Health and Clinical Excellence) (2006, modified 2010) 'Obesity: guidance on the prevention, identification, assessment and management of overweight and obesity in adults and children', http://publications.nice.org.uk/obesity-cg43/guidance#clinical-recommendations (accessed 2010 and 2012).

NICE (2010) 'Cut salt and saturated fat levels in processed food to save thousands of lives, says NICE', www.nice.org.uk/newsroom/pressreleases/PressRelease CVDPrevention.jsp (accessed 23/05/12).

NICE (2011) 'Behind the headlines: is salt good for you?', www.nice.org.uk/newsroom/features/BehindTheHeadlineIsSaltGoodForYou.jsp (accessed 18/08/12).

NICE (2014a) 'Obesity: guidance on the prevention, identification, assessment and management of overweight and obesity in adults and children' (CG43), http://publications.nice.org.uk/obesity-cg43/guidance (accessed 09/06/14).

NICE (2014b) 'Overweight and obese adults: lifestyle weight management' (PH53), http://guidance.nice.org.uk/ph53 (accessed 09/06/14).

NICE (2014c) Evidence statements for 'Overweight and obese adults: lifestyle weight management', www.nice.org.uk/nicemedia/live/14530/67799/67799.pdf (accessed 09/06/14).

NICE (2014d) 'Managing overweight and obese adults: update review. The clinical effectiveness of long-term weight management schemes for adults (Review 1a)', by J. Hartmann-Boyce, D. Johns, P. Aveyard, I. Onakpoya, S. Jebb, D. Phillips, J. Ogden and C. Summerbell, www.nice.org.uk/nicemedia/live/14530/67812/67812.pdf.

NICE (2014e) Draft guideline for consultation, www.nice.org.uk/guidance/gid-cgwave0682/resources/obesity-update-draft-guideline-nice2.

Nichols, G. A. (2006) 'Syndrome or no syndrome: clustering of metabolic risk factors predicts diabetes and cardiovascular disease', Medscape Diabetes and Endocrinology (07/25), www.medscape.org/viewarticle/540923 (accessed February 2013).

NOO: see National Obesity Observatory.

Oakley, A. (2000) *Experiments in Knowing: Gender and Method in the Social Sciences*, New York: New Press.

The Observer newspaper (London): see news reports listed by date at the end of the References.

OECD: see Organisation for Economic Co-operation and Development.

Ofcom (Office of Communications) (2007) 'Television advertising of food and drink products to children: final statement', http://stakeholders.ofcom.org.uk/binaries/consultations/foodads_new/statement/statement.pdf (accessed 25/05/12).

Offer, A., Pechey, R. and Ulijaszek, S. (2010) 'Obesity under affluence varies by welfare regimes: the effect of fast food, insecurity and inequality', *Economics and Human Biology*, 8(3) pp. 297–308.

Organisation for Economic Co-operation and Development (2011) 'Divided we stand: why inequality keeps rising', www.oecd.org/dataoecd/40/22/49170234.pdf (accessed 6/12/11).

Osborne, G. (2008) 'Nudge, nudge, win, win: why are Conservatives hooked on these new economic-psychological ideas? Because they work', *Guardian* (14/07).

Osborne, G. and Thaler, R. H. (2010) 'We can make you behave: our plan is to embed the insights gleaned from behavioural economics throughout government', *Guardian* (29/01).

Outhwaite, W. (ed.) (1996) *The Habermas Reader*, Cambridge: Polity Press.

Pariser, E. (2011) *The Filter Bubble: What the Internet is Hiding from You*, London: Penguin, excerpted in *Observer* (12/06, pp. 20–21).

Parker, S., Uprichard, E. and Burrows, R. (2007) 'Class places and place classes: geodemographics and the spatialization of class', *Information, Communication and Society*, 10(6) pp. 902–21.

Parkin, D. M. (2011a) 'The fraction of cancer attributed to lifestyle and environmental factors in the UK in 2010', *British Journal of Cancer*, 105(Suppl.2) pp. S77–S81.

Parkin, D. M. (2011b) 'Cancers attributable to dietary factors in the UK in 2010: meat consumption', *British Journal of Cancer*, 105(Suppl.2) pp. S24–S26.

Parkin, D. M. and Boyd, L. (2011) 'Cancers attributable to dietary factors in the UK in 2010: low consumption of fruit and vegetables', *British Journal of Cancer*, 105(Suppl.2) pp. S19–S23.

Parliamentary Business (2014) 'Alcohol: minimum pricing – Commons Library Standard Note', by P. Ward and J. Woodhouse (19/05), www.parliament.uk/business/publications/research/briefing-papers/SN05021/alcohol-minimum-pricing.

Paterson, M. (2007) *Foresight: Tackling Obesities: Future Choices – Food Chain Industries' Perspectives on the Future*, London: Government Office for Science.

Pember Reeves, M. (1913) *Round About a Pound a Week*, London: G. Bell and Sons, republished London: Persephone Books (2008).

PHE: see Public Health England.

Phillips, D. and Curry, M. (2003) 'Privacy and the phenetic urge: geodemographics and the changing spatiality of local practice', in D. Lyon (ed.) *Surveillance as*

Social Sorting: Privacy, Risk and Digital Discrimination, London: Routledge, pp. 137–52.

Pierson, C. (ed.) (1997) *The Marx Reader*, London: Polity Press.

Pietrykowski, B. (2009) *The Political Economy of Consumer Behaviour*, Abingdon: Routledge.

Pitts, M., Dorling, D. and Pattie, C. (2007) 'Oil for food: the global story of edible lipids', *Journal of World-Systems Research*, XIII(1) pp. 12–32.

Pollock, A. (2005) *NHS plc: The Privatisation of Our Health Care*, London: Verso.

Porter, R. (1999) *The Greatest Benefit to Mankind: A Medical History of Humanity from Antiquity to the Present*, London: Fontana.

Public Health England (2014a) Note accompanying slide portraying 'trend in adult obesity prevalence by social class' (PHE_Obesity_AdultSlideSet), see www.noo.org.uk/slide_sets (accessed 11/06/14).

Public Health England (2014b) 'About obesity: health inequalities', www.noo.org.uk/NOO_about_obesity/inequalities#d6888 (accessed 11/06/14).

Public Health England (June 2014c) 'Sugar reduction: responding to the challenge', www.gov.uk/government/uploads/system/uploads/attachment_data/file/324043/Sugar_Reduction_Responding_to_the_Challenge_26_June.pdf.

Rayner, G. and Lang, T. (2011) 'Is nudge an effective public health strategy to tackle obesity? No', *BMJ*, 342, d2177, pp. 1–2.

Rayner, G., Hawkes, C., Lang, T. and Bello, W. (2007) 'Globalization for health: trade liberalization and the diet transition: a public health response', *Health Promotion International*, 21(S1), pp. 67–74.

Rayner, M., Scarborough, P. and Stockley, L. (2004) *Nutrient Profiles: Options for Definitions for Use in Relation to Food Promotion and Children's Diets: Final Report*, Oxford: British Heart Foundation Health Promotion Research Group, Department of Public Health, University of Oxford.

Real Food, Tesco Magazine (Spring 2011) London: Cedar Communications.

Reuters (2013) 'New York court to hear Bloomberg's appeal to restore soda ban', www.reuters.com/article/2013/10/17/us-nycsodaban-appeal-idUSBRE99G0T620131017 (accessed 28/05/14).

Reyes, O. (2005) 'New Labour's politics of the hard-working family', in D. Howarth and J. Torfing (eds) *Discourse Theory in European Politics*, Basingstoke, Palgrave Macmillan, pp. 231–51.

Rich, E. and Evans, J. (2005) '"Fat ethics": the obesity discourse and body politics', *Social Theory and Health*, 3(4) pp. 341–58.

Rich, E., Monaghan, L. F. and Aphramor, L. (eds) (2011) *Debating Obesity: Critical Perspectives*, Basingstoke: Palgrave Macmillan.

Richards, C., Bjørkhaug, H., Lawrence, G. and Hickman, E. (2013) 'Retailer-driven agricultural restructuring: Australia, the UK and Norway in comparison', *Agriculture and Human Values*, 30(2) pp. 235–45.

Rigby, N. J., Kumanyika, S. and James, W. P. T. (2004) 'Confronting the epidemic: the need for global solutions', *Journal of Public Health Policy*, 25(3/4) pp. 418–34.

Rose, N. and Miller, P. ([1992]2010) 'Political power beyond the state: problematics of government', *British Journal of Sociology*, 61 (60th anniversary issue) pp. 271–303.

Saberi, H. (ed.) (2011) *Cured, Fermented and Smoked Foods: Proceedings of the Oxford Symposium on Food and Cookery 2010*, Totnes: Prospect Books.

SACN: see Scientific Advisory Committee on Nutrition.

Sandwich News website, www.sandwichnews.com/sandwich-facts-and-trivia (accessed 10/04/14).

Savage, M. (2000) *Class Analysis and Social Transformation*, Buckingham: Open University Press.

Savage, M. and Burrows, R. (2007) 'The coming crisis of empirical sociology', *Sociology*, 41(5) pp. 885–99.

Savage, M. and Williams, K. (2008) 'Elites: remembered in capitalism and forgotten by social sciences', in M. Savage and K. Williams (eds) *Remembering Elites*, Oxford: Blackwell, pp. 1–24.

Savage, M., Devine, F., Cunningham, N., Taylor, M., Li, Y., Hjellbrekke, J., Le Roux, B., Friedman, S. and Miles, A. (2013) 'A new model of social class? Findings from the BBC's Great British Class Survey Experiment', *Sociology*, 47(2) pp. 219–50.

Scambler, G. (2001) 'Class, power and the durability of health inequalities', in G. Scambler (ed.) *Habermas, Critical Theory and Health*, London: Routledge.

Scambler, G. and Higgs, P. (2001) '"The dog that didn't bark": taking class seriously in the health inequalities debate', *Social Science & Medicine*, 52(1) pp. 157–9.

Scambler, G. (2002) *Health and Social Change: A Critical Theory*, Buckingham: Open University Press.

Scambler, G. (2007) 'Social structure and the production, reproduction and durability of health inequalities', *Social Theory & Health*, 5(4) pp. 297–315.

Scambler, G. (2012) 'Review article: health inequalities', *Sociology of Health and Illness*, 34(1) pp. 130–46.

Scambler, G. and Scambler, S. (2013) 'Marx, critical realism and health inequalities', in W. Cockerham (ed.), *Medical Sociology on the Move: New Directions in Theory*, New York: Springer.

Scammel-Katz, S. (2012) *The Art of Shopping: How We Shop and Why We Buy*, London: LID Publishing.

Scarborough, P., Bhatnagar, P., Wickramasinghe, K., Smolina, K., Mitchell, C. and Rayner, M. (2010) *Coronary Heart Disease Statistics*, Oxford: British Heart Foundation Health Promotion Research Group.

Scarborough, P., Bhatnagar, P., Wickramasinghe, K., Allender, S., Foster, C. and Rayner, M. (2011) 'The economic burden of ill health due to diet, physical inactivity, smoking, alcohol and obesity in the UK', *Journal of Public Health*, 33(4) pp. 527–35.

Scarborough, P., Nnoaham, K. E., Clarke, D., Capewell, S. and Rayner, M. (2012) 'Modelling the impact of a healthy diet on cardiovascular disease and cancer mortality', *Journal of Epidemiology and Community Health*, 66(5) pp. 420–6.

Schmidt, C. (2009) 'Defining and meeting customer needs: beyond hearing the voice', in H. R. Moskowitz, I. S. Saguy and T. Straus (eds) *An Integrated Approach to New Food Product Development*, Boca Raton: CRC Press, pp. 217–32.

Schmidt, V. A. (2000) 'Democracy and discourse in an integrating Europe and a globalising world', *European Law Journal*, 6(3) pp. 277–300.

Scientific Advisory Committee on Nutrition (2003) *Salt and Health*, London: The Stationery Office for the Food Standards Agency and Department of Health.

Scientific Advisory Committee on Nutrition (2014) 'New draft report from the Scientific Advisory Committee on Nutrition recommends more fibre and less sugar in diet', www.sacn.gov.uk/pdfs/sacn_press_release_carbohydrates_and_health.pdf.

Scully, P., Reid, O., Macken, A., Healy, M., Saunders, J., Leddin, D., Cullen, W., Dunne, C. and O'Gorman, C. S. (2014) 'Food and beverage cues in UK and Irish children: television programming', *Archives of Disease in Childhood* (published online 01/07).

Seifert, S. M., Schaechter, J. L., Hershorin, E. R. and Lipshultz, S. E. (2011) 'Health effects of energy drinks on children, adolescents, and young adults', *Pediatrics*, 127(3) pp. 511–28.

Seldon, A. (2012) 'The big society must be grounded in goodness', *Guardian* (03/01), www.guardian.co.uk/commentisfree/2012/jan/03/big-society-goodness-government-morality?INTCMP=SRCH (accessed 25/01/12).

Sen, A. (2004) 'Why health equity?', in S. Anand, F. Peter and A. Sen (eds) *Public Health, Ethics and Equity*, Oxford: Oxford University Press.

Sesame (Open University alumni magazine) (2010) 'Brand appeal', interview with Fiona Ellis-Chadwick, Senior Lecturer, Retail Management, issue 246 (autumn) pp. 40–2.

Shaheen, S. O., Jameson, K. A., Syddall, H. E., Aihie Sayer, A., Dennison, E. M., Cooper, C., Robinson, S. M. and The Hertfordshire Cohort Study Group (2010) 'The relationship of dietary patterns with adult lung function and COPD', *European Respiratory Journal*, 36(2) pp. 277–84.

Sharpe, K. M., Staelin, R. and Huber, J. (2008) 'Using extremeness aversion to right obesity: policy implications of context-dependent demand', *Journal of Consumer Research*, 35(3) pp. 406–22.

Shilling, C. (2003) *The Body and Social Theory*, 2nd edn, London: Sage.

Singh, G. K., Siahpush, M., Hiatt, R. A. and Timsina, L. R. (2011) 'Dramatic increases in obesity and overweight prevalence and body mass index among ethnic-immigrant and social class groups in the United States, 1976–2008', *Journal of Community Health*, 36, pp. 94–110.

Skalen, P., Fougere, M. and Felleson, M. (2008) *Marketing Discourse: A Critical Perspective*, Abingdon: Routledge.

Skeggs, B. (2004) *Class, Self, Culture*, London: Routledge.

Skidmore, P. M. L., Hardy, R. J., Kuh, D. J., Langenberg, C. and Wadsworth, M. E. J. (2007) 'Life course body size and lipid levels at 53 years in a British birth cohort', *Journal of Epidemiology and Community Health*, 61(3) pp. 215–20.

Sklair, L. and Miller, D. (2010) 'Capitalist globalization, corporate social responsibility and social policy', *Critical Social Policy*, 30(4) pp. 472–95.

Soil Association (2012) 'Organic market report 2012' (summary), www.soilassociation.org/marketreport (accessed 26/05/12).

Soil Association (2014) 'Organic market report 2014', www.soilassociation.org/marketreport (accessed 14/04/14).

Steel, C. (2009) *Hungry City: How Food Shapes Our Lives*, London: Vintage.

Steinbach, S. (2004) *Women in England 1760–1914: A Social History*, London: Phoenix.

Stern, B. (2004) 'The importance of being Ernest: commemorating Dichter's contribution to advertising research', *Journal of Advertising Research*, 44(2) pp. 165–69.

Su, D., Esqueda, O. A., Li, L. and Pagan, J. A. (2012) 'Income inequality and obesity prevalence among OECD countries', *Journal of Biosocial Science*, 44, pp. 417–32.

Sui, X., LaMonte, M. J., Laditka, J. N., Hardin, J. W., Chase, N., Hooker, S. P., Blair, S. N. (2007) 'Cardiorespiratory fitness and adiposity as mortality predictors in older adults', *Journal of the American Medical Association*, 298(21) pp. 2507–16.

Sustain (2012) 'Asda, Morrisons and Iceland named as "worst offenders for undermining children's healthy eating"', www.sustainweb.org/news/apr12_checkouts_checked_out_survey_report/ (accessed 26/04/12).

Thaler, R. H. and Sunstein, C. R. (2009) *Nudge: Improving Decisions about Health, Wealth and Happiness*, London: Penguin.

Thankamony, G. N. A., Williams, R. and Dunger, D. B. (2011) 'Metabolic syndrome in children unravelled', *Pediatrics and Child Health*, 21(7) pp. 301–5.

Thompson, C. (2011) 'Investigating food shopping and food consumption using the "go-along" interview', BSA Conference presentation, London (07/04), transcript provided by C. Thompson.

Tomlinson, M. (2003) 'Lifestyle and social class', *European Sociological Review*, 19(1) pp. 97–111.

Tonkiss, F. (1998) 'Analysing discourse', in C. Seale (ed.) *Researching Society and Culture*, London: Sage, pp. 245–60.

UCL Institute of Health Equity (2012) *The Role of the Health Workforce in Tackling Health Inequalities: Action on the Social Determinants of Health*, London: UCL.

UCL Institute of Health Equity (2013) *Working for Health Equity: The Role of Health Professionals*, by M. Allen, J. Allen, S. Hogarth with M. Marmot, London: UCL.

Urbick, B. (2009) 'Getting the food right for children: how to win with kids', in H. R. Moskowitz, I. S. Saguy and T. Straus (eds) *An Integrated Approach to New Food Product Development*, Boca Raton: CRC Press, pp. 247–62.

Van Aken, G. A. (2010) 'Relating food emulsion structure and composition to the way it is processed in the gastrointestinal tract and physiological responses', *Food Biophysics*, 5(4) pp. 258–83.

Van Boekel, M. A. J. S. (2009) 'Innovation as science' in H. R. Moskowitz, I. S. Saguy and T. Straus (eds) *An Integrated Approach to New Food Product Development*, Boca Raton: CRC Press, pp. 37–52.

Veenstra, G. (2006) 'Neo-Marxist class position and socio-economic status: distinct or complementary determinants of health?', *Critical Public Health*, 16(2) pp. 111–29.

Wang, Y., Beydoun, M. A., Liang, L., Caballero, B. and Kumanyika, S. K. (2008) 'Will all Americans become overweight or obese? Estimating the progression and cost of the US obesity epidemic', *Obesity*, 16(10), pp. 2323–30.

Wann, M. (1998) *Fat! So? Because You Don't Have to Apologise for Your Size*, Berkeley: Ten Speed Press.

Wansink, B. and Chandon, P. (2006) 'Can "low-fat" nutrition labels lead to obesity?', *Journal of Marketing Research*, 43(4) pp. 605–17.

Warde, A. (1997) *Consumption, Food and Taste: Culinary Antinomies and Commodity Culture*, London: Sage.

Watzke, H. J. and German, B. (2009) 'Personalizing foods' in H. R. Moskowitz, I. S. Saguy and T. Straus (eds) *An Integrated Approach to New Food Product Development*, Boca Raton: CRC Press, pp. 133–74.

WCRF: see World Cancer Research Fund.

Wearing, S. C., Hennig, E. M., Byrne, N. M., Steele, J. R. and Hills, A. P. (2006) 'The impact of childhood obesity on musculoskeletal form', *Obesity Reviews*, 7(2) pp. 209–18.

Weaver, D. and Finke, M. (2003) 'The relationship between the use of sugar content information on nutrition labels and the consumption of added sugars', *Food Policy*, 28(3) pp. 213–19.

Webber, R. (2007) 'The metropolitan habitus: its manifestations, locations and consumption profiles', *Environment and Planning*, 39(1) pp. 182–207.

Webster, A. (2007) *Health, Technology and Society*, Basingstoke: Palgrave Macmillan.

Weinstein, A. R., Sesso, H. D., Lee, I. M., Rexrode, K. M., Cook, N. R., Manson, J. E., Buring, J. E., Gaziano, J. M. (2008) 'The joint effects of physical activity and body mass index on coronary heart disease risk in women', *Archives of Internal Medicine*, 168(8) pp. 884–90.

Weissberg, P. (2011) 'Foreword', in *Trends in Coronary Heart Disease, 1961–2011*, London: British Heart Foundation.

Wennstrom, P. and Mellentin, J. (2002) *The Food and Health Marketing Handbook: Five Strategies to Enter the Market and the Four Success Factors to Position your Brand*, Brentford: New Nutrition Business.

Whimster, S. (2011) 'Desert island discourse', *Network: the magazine of the British Sociological Association*, 108, pp. 38–9.

White, R. (2011) 'No fat future? Anti-social queer theory and fat activism', BSA conference presentation, London (07/04).

WHO: see World Health Organisation.

Wilkinson, R. and Pickett, K. (2009) *The Spirit Level: Why More Equal Societies Almost Always Do Better*, London: Allen Lane.

Williams, J. D., Crockett, D., Harrison, R. L. and Thomas, K. D. (2012) 'Commentary: the role of food culture and marketing activity in health disparities', *Preventive Medicine*, 55(5) pp. 382–6.

Williams, S. J. (1995) 'Theorising class, health and lifestyles: can Bourdieu help us?', *Sociology of Health and Illness*, 17(5) pp. 577–604.

Williams, S. J. (2003) 'Beyond meaning, discourse and the empirical world: critical realist reflections on health', *Social Theory & Health*, 1(1) pp. 42–71.

Wills, W., Backett-Milburn, K., Roberts, M. and Lawton, J. (2011) 'The framing of social class distinctions through family food and eating practices', *Sociological Review*, 59(4) pp. 725–40.

Wilson, B. (2009) *Swindled: From Poison Sweets to Counterfeit Coffee – the Dark History of the Food Cheats*, London: John Murray.

Winson, A. (2004) 'Bringing political economy into the debate on the obesity epidemic', *Agriculture and Human Values*, 21(4) pp. 299–312.

Wodak, R. (2007) 'Pragmatics and critical discourse analysis', *Pragmatics & Cognition*, 15(1) pp. 203–25.

World Action on Salt and Health (2009) 'New research reveals huge differences in salt contents in global brands', www.worldactiononsalt.com/less/surveys/2009/international/index.html (accessed 26/07/09).

World Bank (2010) Worldwide governance indicators, http://info.worldbank.org/governance/wgi/mc_chart.asp (accessed 2010 and 14/08/12).

World Cancer Research Fund (2010) 'Cancer charity warns that women more likely to have large waists', www.wcrf-uk.org/audience/media/press_release.php?recid=136 (accessed January 2011).

World Cancer Research Fund/American Institute for Cancer Research (2007) *Food, Nutrition, Physical Activity and the Prevention of Cancer: A Global Perspective*, Washington: AICR, www.dietandcancerreport.org/cancer_resource_center/downloads/Second_Expert_Report_full.pdf (accessed 2010 and May and August 2012).

World Health Organisation (2014) 'Draft guideline: sugars intake for adults and children', www.who.int/nutrition/sugars_public_consultation/en/; www.who.int/mediacentre/news/notes/2014/consultation-sugar-guideline/en/ (accessed 30/06/14).

Xtreme Impact (2011) Marketing, promotions, strategies, www.xtremeimpakt.com/index/Capabilities/Strategic-Services/Consumer-Segmentation (accessed 16/03/11).

Interviews

Interviewee A: consultant, market research firm, June 2011.
Interviewee B: consultant, market research firm, May 2012.

Magazine and newspaper articles

Business Week

- 01/02/13 'Did Pizza Hut really invent the stuffed crust pizza?', by V. Wong, www.businessweek.com/articles/2013-02-01/did-pizza-hut-really-invent-the-stuffed-crust-pizza.

Marketing Magazine

- 02/10/07 (online) www.marketingmagazine.co.uk/news/742967/Quotes/?DCMP=ILC-SEARCH (accessed 09/09/10).
- 18/02/09(a) 'Brand termination: knowing when to swing the axe', by N. Clark, pp. 30–1.
- 18/02/09(b) 'Bringing brands to life', by B. Wilkerson, pp. 35–8.
- 04/03/09 'It's the same difference', by A. Walmsley, p. 12.
- 03/03/10 'Walkers Sensations', by J. Lee, p. 17.
- 'Revolution' supplement 09/10a, 'Facing up to facebook', by T. Clawson, pp. 40–1.
- 'Revolution' supplement 09/10b, 'Smarter digital marketing: case studies – Kellogg's Krave'.
- 22/09/10 'Out of home, top of mind', by S. Bashford, p. 28.
- 27/10/10 'A new consumer champion', by H. Edwards, p. 19.
- 10/11/10 'Sector Insight. Nuts, seeds and dried fruit', by J. Bainbridge, pp. 32–3.
- 17/11/10 'Not only but also: Marks & Spencer's latest strategy has echoes of the brand's past', by R. Barnes and E. Owen, p. 16.
- 11/01/11 'Will sweeteners turn sour? Sprite's roll-out of a drink containing sugar substitutes Truvia is not without its risks', by J. Thomas, p. 16.
- 12/01/11 'Tomorrow's world: cautious and resourceful, tomorrow's consumers will be forced to find ways to live without a floodtide of prosperity', by J. Walker Smith, p. 15.

- 19/01/11 'Brands on location: marketers at three major brands assess the opportunities created by mobile payment', by E. Owen, p. 14.
- 26/01/11 'The perils of virtual stalking', by A. Walmsley, p. 12.
- 02/02/11 'In brief: McCain', p. 4.
- 16/02/11 'A fashionable strategy: Morrisons could add clothing to build on its strength in food', by L. Eleftheriou-Smith, p. 18.
- 23/02/11(a) 'Consumer surveillance: don't let relevance blind you to privacy', by A. Mitchell, p. 26–7.
- 23/02/11(b) 'Thinking inside the box: strict policing of the content of children's food is forcing brands to innovate', by N. Hughes, p. 18.
- 23/02/11(c) 'Kids' health needs NPD agenda', by N. McElhatton, p. 25.
- 23/02/11(d) 'A glass half full kind of guy', by G. Charles, pp. 22–3.
- 02/03/11(a) 'Eyeing up the opposite sex', by J. Reynolds, p. 14.
- 02/03/11(b) 'Lucozade targets social media users via Spotify', by G. Charles, p. 7.
- 09/03/11(a) 'Memo to new CEO: tips from the trade', comment by Tracey Follows, VCCP, p. 14.
- 09/03/11(b) 'Memo to new CEO: tips from the trade', comment by Dave Trott, CST The Gate, p. 15.
- 16/03/11 'Flavour of the month: cash-strapped consumers are skipping healthier options in favour of the affordable indulgence offered by premium crisp brands', by J. Bainbridge, pp. 36–7.
- 23/03/11 'Defining the new middle class', by G. Charles, pp. 14–15.
- 30/03/11 'UK brands splash $4.1bn on online ads', by S. Shearman, p. 1.
- 04/04/11 'David Cameron's plan to curb binge drinking runs contrary to many of the ideas of behavioural "hedonic consumption" theory', by H. Edwards, p. 18.
- 13/04/11 'United we understand: conducting research with, rather than on, people can give incisive glimpses into their behaviour', by H. Edwards, p. 19.
- 04/05/11 'Domino's to integrate behavioural economics', by A. McCormick, p. 5.
- 11/05/11 'Coca-Cola in "meals" push', by L. Eleftheriou-Smith, p. 1.
- 18/05/11(a) 'Analysis – Behavioural Economics: when push comes to nudge', by A. McCormick, pp. 16–17.
- 18/05/11(b) 'Readers say: Coca-Cola encourages mealtime consumption', letter from J. Filmer, p. 27.
- 25/05/11 'Marketing's new mindset: brand marketers can now analyse campaigns in real time, but they need more than logic to succeed', by A. Walmsley, p. 13.
- 08/06/11(a) 'Looking ahead: can your customers become your field-marketing agents?, p. 35.
- 08/06/11(b) 'We know where you live', by B. Bold, p. 17.
- 08/06/11(c) 'Brand revitalisation: Robinsons Fruit Shoot', p. 11.
- 08/06/11(d) 'Ginsters debuts Bara', p. 11.
- 08/06/11(e) 'Winner, Brand: Walkers. Agency: Abbott Mead Vickers BBDO', p. 22.
- 15/06/11(a) 'Sector Insight: biscuits, cookies and crackers', by J. Bainbridge, pp. 38–9.
- 15/06/11(b) 'Consumer behaviour: how to navigate the customer journey', by C. Smith, pp. 28–9.
- 22/06/11 Conference leaflet, 'Appeal to Kids and Sell to Parents', 5th Annual Kids Conference.

- 29/06/11 'Waitrose: the supermarket brand has adopted an "honestly priced" strategy to stand out from the crowd', p. 18.
- July 2011 conference supplement: (a) 'Social media – playtime's over!', letter from Michael Saylor, MicroStrategy Inc.; (b) 'Social CRM – the ultimate customer engagement', by D. Peppers.
- 06/07/11 'Working-class heroes', by G. Charles, pp. 18–19.
- 27/07/11 'Asking the right question', by W. Gordon, p. 9.
- 03/08/11 'Top 10 marketing U-turns', by G. Carson, p. 13.
- 10/08/11 'Changing the recipe at Kraft', by D. Fielding, pp. 22–3.
- 24/08/11(a) 'Greggs: the bakery chain must arrest a drop in profits if it is to realise expansion plans', by R. Barnes, p. 18.
- 24/08/11(b) 'Kids Brand Index 2011', by C. Bussey, p. 26.
- 07/09/11 'Should brands that add to the obesity crisis subsidise healthier food options?', p. 28.
- 14/09/11(a) 'Best behaviour', by K. Benjamin, p. 29.
- 14/09/11(b) 'Going cold turkey on price promotions', by D. Benady, pp. 26–7.
- 14/09/11(c) 'Price gives pizza solid base', by J. Bainbridge, pp. 38–9.
- 19/10/11 'Ticking the healthy box', by J. Bainbridge, pp. 30–1.
- 26/10/11 'Will the plan to cut 5bn calories from the nation's daily diet by 2020 work?', p. 24.
- 07/12/11 'Don't expect a peaceful 2012', by A. Walmsley, p. 12.
- 25/01/12 'Manaaz Akhtar: Subway's UK head of marketing cites health and value as the main selling pts that will broaden the chain's consumer base', by G. Charles, pp. 29–31.
- 15/02/12(a) 'Mars UK to cut calories across chocolate lines', by G. Charles, p. 5.
- 15/02/12(b) 'Twitter's branded adventure', by S. Shearman, pp. 10–11.
- 14/03/12 'Transparently green', by E. Jeffries, pp. 32–3.
- 04/04/12 'Sector insight: crisps and salty snacks', by J. Bainbridge, p. 14.
- 25/04/12 'Red Bull set to roll out Editions offering in UK', by L. Eleftheriou-Smith, p. 4.
- 02/05/12(a) 'Polman: marketers are "losing ground"', by R. Barnes, p. 5.
- 02/05/12(b) 'After years promoting bigger pack sizes as offering better value, it appears food and drink marketers may do better to think small', by H. Edwards, p. 22.
- 30/05/12 'Kellogg chief departs amid global rebrand', by S. Shearman, p. 5.

The Guardian

- 16/01/07 'The wretched price of failing to educate girls', by E. Brotherton, p. 30, reprint from 16/01/1864.
- 11/09/07 'Do postcodes define how you live?', by I. Sample, www.theguardian.com/science/2007/sep/11/postcode.
- 23/07/09 'Study finds big variations in salt contents in global food products', by R. Smithers, p. 8.
- 19/01/10 'Food scientists develop appetite-curbing gel', www.guardian.co.uk/education/2010/jan/19/gel-curb-appetite-scientists?INTCMP=SRCH.
- 09/02/10 'Teenage girls eat less healthy food than any other group, survey reveals', by R. Smithers, p. 9.
- 09/03/10 'Is it healthier to be slim but unfit or fat and fit?', by P. Daoust, p. 14.

- 03/09/10 'The domestic education of girls', reprint of 'From A Correspondent', 03/09/1901, www.theguardian.com/theguardian/2010/sep/06/the-domestic-education-of-girls.
- 15/11/10 'Advertising: time for advertisements to go up a gear', by J. Silver, p. 5.
- 30/12/10 'Speed of NHS reform means Andrew Lansley has faced a bumpy ride', www.guardian.co.uk/politics/2010/dec/30/andrew-lansley-nhs-reform?INTCMP=SRCH (accessed 02/06/12).
- 18/02/11 'Britain's fried chicken boom', by T. Meltzer, p. 6.
- 23/03/11 'Boost for convenience stores as shoppers top up on the move' (report of a study by Britvic), by R. Smithers, p. 29.
- 23/05/11 'Cut red meat and don't eat ham, say cancer researchers', by D. Campbell, p. 5.
- 25/05/11 'Supermarket sandwich maker takes bigger slice of lunch money', by S. Bowers, p. 28.
- 04/06/11 '*The Social Animal* by David Brooks – review', by A. Beckett, p. 7.
- 24/06/11 (online) Money blog: 'Are discount supermarkets any good?', www.guardian.co.uk/money/blog/2011/jun/24/discount-supermarkets-lidl-aldi#start-of-comments (accessed 11/07/11).
- 02/07/11 'Personal effects' column, Money section, p. 2.
- 09/07/11 'Effective things can come from silly places', by B. Goldacre, p. 46.
- 01/12/11 'Starbucks to brew up 5,000 jobs', by J. Treanor, p. 20.
- 20/12/11 'Matthew Freud picks up £1m-a-year contract with Department of Health', www.guardian.co.uk/media/2011/dec/20/matthew-freud-contract-department-health?INTCMP=SRCH.
- 22/12/11 'Revealed: how supermarkets plan to build thousands more stores (mostly out of town)', by R. Neate, p. 3.
- 31/12/11 'Patients with unhealthy lifestyles must be warned, say experts', by D. Campbell, p. 2.
- 15/01/12 'Ad men use brain scanners to probe our emotional response', by R. Neate, p. 29.
- 05/03/12 'Facebook: if you don't like it, don't like it', by A. Senior, p. 32.
- 07/03/12 'Krispy Kreme cashes in as Britain falls in love with the doughnut', by J. Moulds, p. 32.
- 14/03/12 'Greggs drops 2% after bakeries group says like for like sales fell in first ten weeks', by N. Fletcher, www.guardian.co.uk/business/marketforces-live/2012/mar/14/greggs-profits-up-sales-dip?INTCMP=SRCH.
- 01/06/12 'Sweet, surrender: New York mayor plans to ban the sale of super-size fizzy drinks', by E. Pilkington and K. Rogers, p. 3.
- 02/03/13 'Bring on the nanopayments: are we giving up too much economic power to the big digital companies, asks Lawrence Scott', p. 7 (Review of *Who Owns the Future?* by Jaron Lanier).
- 22/01/14 'Subway to create 13,000 jobs as it doubles outlets in UK and Ireland' (Press Association).
- 10/02/14 'Minimum alcohol pricing would save 860 lives a year, study finds', by S. Bosely.
- 28/06/14(a) 'Tesco chairman promises to turn around ailing supermarket giant', by Z. Wood, p. 41.
- 28/06/14(b) 'Lidl to spend £220m in new challenge to big four rivals', by S. Butler, p. 41.

The Independent

- 04/04/12 'Hot dog stuffed crust pizza helps Domino's unveil tasty results during cold snap', by J. Thompson, www.independent.co.uk/news/business/news/hot-dog-stuffedcrust-pizza-helps-dominos-unveil-tasty-results-during-cold-snap-8560085.html.

The Observer

- 25/04/10 'Recession-beating strategies pay off as store reveals record profits again', by J. Finch, p. 42.
- 21/11/10 'Facebook is stealing a march on Google in the battle for ad revenue', by J. Naughton, p. 21.
- 09/01/11 'UK's taste for austerity helps the pieces fall into place for Domino's Pizza', by A. Clark, p. 36.
- 24/04/11 'Obesity policy under attitude from two government advisers', by D. Boffey, p. 10.

Index

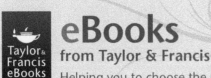
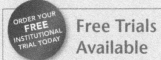
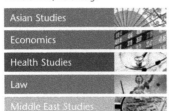

For Product Safety Concerns and Information please contact our EU
representative GPSR@taylorandfrancis.com
Taylor & Francis Verlag GmbH, Kaufingerstraße 24, 80331 München, Germany

www.ingramcontent.com/pod-product-compliance
Ingram Content Group UK Ltd.
Pitfield, Milton Keynes, MK11 3LW, UK
UKHW021032180425
457613UK00021B/1147